1995
YEAR BOOK OF
ENDOCRINOLOGY®

Statement of Purpose

The YEAR BOOK Service

The YEAR BOOK series was devised in 1901 by practicing health professionals who observed that the literature of medicine and related disciplines had become so voluminous that no one individual could read and place in perspective every potential advance in a major specialty. In the final decade of the 20th century, this recognition is more acutely true than it was in 1901.

More than merely a series of books, YEAR BOOK volumes are the tangible results of a unique service designed to accomplish the following:

- to *survey* a wide range of journals of proven value
- to *select* from those journals papers representing significant advances and statements of important clinical principles
- to provide *abstracts* of those articles that are readable, convenient summaries of their key points
- to provide *commentary* about those articles to place them in perspective

These publications grow out of a unique process that calls on the talents of outstanding authorities in clinical and fundamental disciplines, trained literature specialists, and professional writers, all supported by the resources of Mosby, the world's preeminent publisher for the health professions.

The Literature Base

Mosby subscribes to nearly 1,000 journals published worldwide, covering the full range of the health professions. On an annual basis, the publisher examines usage patterns and polls its expert authorities to add new journals to the literature base and to delete journals that are no longer useful as potential YEAR BOOK sources.

The Literature Survey

The publisher's team of literature specialists, all of whom are trained and experienced health professionals, examines every original, peer-reviewed article in each journal issue. More than 250,000 articles per year are scanned systematically, including title, text, illustrations, tables, and references. Each scan is compared, article by article, to the search strategies that the publisher has developed in consultation with the 270 outside experts who form the pool of YEAR BOOK editors. A given article may be reviewed by any number of editors, from one to a dozen or more, regardless of the discipline for which the paper was originally published. In turn, each editor who receives the article reviews it to determine whether or not the article should be included in the YEAR BOOK. This decision is based on the article's inherent quality, its probable usefulness to readers of that YEAR BOOK, and the editor's goal to represent a balanced picture of a given field in each volume of the YEAR BOOK. In addition, the editor indicates when to include figures and tables from the article to help the YEAR BOOK reader better understand the information.

Of the quarter million articles scanned each year, only 5% are selected for detailed analysis within the YEAR BOOK series, thereby assuring readers of the high value of every selection.

The Abstract

The publisher's abstracting staff is headed by a physician-writer and includes individuals with training in the life sciences, medicine, and other areas, plus extensive experience in writing for the health professions and related industries. Each selected article is assigned to a specific writer on this abstracting staff. The abstracter, guided in many cases by notations supplied by the expert editor, writes a structured, condensed summary designed so that the reader can rapidly acquire the essential information contained in the article.

The Commentary

The YEAR BOOK editorial boards, sometimes assisted by guest commentators, write comments that place each article in perspective for the reader. This provides the reader with the equivalent of a personal consultation with a leading international authority—an opportunity to better understand the value of the article and to benefit from the authority's thought processes in assessing the article.

Additional Editorial Features

The editorial boards of each YEAR BOOK organize the abstracts and comments to provide a logical and satisfying sequence of information. To enhance the organization, editors also provide introductions to sections or individual chapters, comments linking a number of abstracts, citations to additional literature, and other features.

The published YEAR BOOK contains enhanced bibliographic citations for each selected article, including extended listings of multiple authors and identification of author affiliations. Each YEAR BOOK contains a Table of Contents specific to that year's volume. From year to year, the Table of Contents for a given YEAR BOOK will vary depending on developments within the field.

Every YEAR BOOK contains a list of the journals from which papers have been selected. This list represents a subset of the nearly 1,000 journals surveyed by the publisher and occasionally reflects a particularly pertinent article from a journal that is not surveyed on a routine basis.

Finally, each volume contains a comprehensive subject index and an index to authors of each selected paper.

The 1995 Year Book Series

Year Book of Allergy and Clinical Immunology: Drs. Rosenwasser, Borish, Gelfand, Leung, Nelson, and Szefler

Year Book of Anesthesiology and Pain Management: Drs. Tinker, Abram, Chestnut, Rothenberg, Roizen, and Wood

Year Book of Cardiology®: Drs. Schlant, Collins, Engle, Gersh, Kaplan, and Waldo

Year Book of Chiropractic: Dr. Lawrence

Year Book of Critical Care Medicine®: Drs. Parrillo, Balk, Calvin, Franklin, and Shapiro

Year Book of Dentistry®: Drs. Meskin, Berry, Currier, Kennedy, Leinfelder, Roser, and Zakariasen

Year Book of Dermatologic Surgery®: Drs. Swanson, Glogau, and Salasche

Year Book of Dermatology®: Drs. Sober and Fitzpatrick

Year Book of Diagnostic Radiology®: Drs. Federle, Clark, Gross, Madewell, Maynard, Latchaw, and Young

Year Book of Digestive Diseases®: Drs. Greenberger and Moody

Year Book of Drug Therapy®: Drs. Lasagna and Weintraub

Year Book of Emergency Medicine®: Drs. Davidson, Dronen, King, Niemann, Roberts, and Wagner

Year Book of Endocrinology®: Drs. Bagdade, Braverman, Horton, Kannan, Landsberg, Molitch, Morley, Nathan, Odell, Poehlman, Rogol, and Ryan

Year Book of Family Practice®: Drs. Berg, Bowman, Davidson, Dexter, Dietrich, and Scherger

Year Book of Geriatrics and Gerontology®: Drs. Beck, Burton, Goldstein, Reuben, Small, and Whitehouse

Year Book of Hand Surgery®: Drs. Amadio and Hentz

Year Book of Hematology®: Drs. Spivak, Bell, Ness, Quesenberry, Wiernik, and Blume

Year Book of Infectious Diseases®: Drs. Keusch, Barza, Bennish, Gelfand, Klempner, Skolnik, and Snydman

Year Book of Infertility and Reproductive Endocrinology®: Drs. Mishell, Lobo, and Sokol

Year Book of Medicine®: Drs. Bone, Cline, Epstein, Greenberger, Malawista, Mandell, O'Rourke, and Utiger

Year Book of Neonatal and Perinatal Medicine®: Drs. Fanaroff and Klaus

Year Book of Nephrology®: Drs. Coe, Curtis, Favus, Henderson, Kashgarian, and Luke

Year Book of Neurology and Neurosurgery®: Drs. Bradley and Wilkins

Year Book of Neuroradiology: Drs. Osborn, Eskridge, Grossman, Hudgens, and Ross

Year Book of Nuclear Medicine®: Drs. Gottschalk, Blaufox, McAfee, Wacker, and Zubal

Year Book of Obstetrics and Gynecology®: Drs. Mishell, Kirschbaum, and Morrow

Year Book of Occupational and Environmental Medicine®: Drs. Emmett, Frank, Gochfeld, and Hessl

Year Book of Oncology®: Drs. Simone, Bosl, Glatstein, Ozols, and Steele

Year Book of Ophthalmology®: Drs. Cohen, Adams, Augsburger, Benson, Eagle, Flanagan, Grossman, Laibson, Nelson, Rapuano, Reinecke, Sergott, Tasman, Tipperman, and Wilson

Year Book of Orthopedics®: Drs. Sledge, Cofield, Dobyns, Griffin, Poss, Springfield, Swiontkowski, Weisel, and Wilson

Year Book of Otolaryngology–Head and Neck Surgery®: Drs. Paparella and Holt

Year Book of Pain: Drs. Gebhart, Haddox, Jacox, Marcus, Rudy, Shapiro, and Janjan

Year Book of Pathology and Laboratory Medicine®: Drs. Mills, Bruns, Gaffey, and Stoler

Year Book of Pediatrics®: Dr. Stockman

Year Book of Plastic, Reconstructive, and Aesthetic Surgery: Drs. Miller, Cohen, McKinney, Robson, Ruberg, and Whitaker

Year Book of Podiatric Medicine and Surgery®: Dr. Kominsky

Year Book of Psychiatry and Applied Mental Health®: Drs. Talbott, Breier, Frances, Meltzer, Schowalter, Tasman, and Yudofsky

Year Book of Pulmonary Disease®: Drs. Bone and Petty

Year Book of Rheumatology®: Drs. Sergent, LeRoy, Meenan, Panush, and Reichlin

Year Book of Sports Medicine®: Drs. Shephard, Drinkwater, Eichner, Torg, Col. Anderson, and Mr. George

Year Book of Surgery®: Drs. Copeland, Bland, Deitch, Eberlein, Howard, Luce, Seeger, Souba, and Sugarbaker

Year Book of Thoracic and Cardiovascular Surgery®: Drs. Ginsberg, Lofland, and Wechsler

Year Book of Transplantation®: Drs. Sollinger, Eckhoff, Hullett, Knechtle, Longo, Mentzer, and Pirsch

Year Book of Ultrasound®: Drs. Merritt, Babcock, Carroll, Fagin, Finberg, and Fleischer

Year Book of Urology®: Drs. deKernion and Howards

Year Book of Vascular Surgery®: Dr. Porter

Contributing Editors

Katherine Cianflone, Ph.D.
McGill Unit for the Prevention of Cardiovascular Disease, Royal Victoria Hospital, McGill University, Montreal, Quebec, Canada

Pierre Julien, Ph.D.
Centre de Recherche sur les Maladies Lipidiques, Laval University Medical Research Centre, Ste-Foy, Quebec, Canada

Allan D. Sniderman, M.D.
McGill Unit for the Prevention of Cardiovascular Disease, Royal Victoria Hospital, McGill University, Montreal, Quebec, Canada

1995

The Year Book of
ENDOCRINOLOGY®

Editor-in Chief
John D. Bagdade, M.D.

Associate Editors
Lewis E. Braverman, M.D.
Edward S. Horton, M.D.
C.R. Kannan, M.D.
Lewis Landsberg, M.D.
Mark E. Molitch, M.D.
John E. Morley, M.D.
David M. Nathan, M.D.
William D. Odell, M.D., Ph.D., M.A.C.P.
Eric T. Poehlman, Ph.D.
Alan D. Rogol, M.D., Ph.D.
Will G. Ryan, M.D.

Contributing Editors
Katherine Cianflone, Ph.D.
Pierre Julien, Ph.D.
Allan D. Sniderman, M.D.

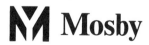 **Mosby**

St. Louis Baltimore Boston Carlsbad Chicago Naples New York Philadelphia Portland
London Madrid Mexico City Singapore Sydney Tokyo Toronto Wiesbaden

Vice President and Publisher, Continuity Publishing: Kenneth H. Killion
Director, Editorial Development: Gretchen C. Murphy
Manager, Continuity–EDP: Maria Nevinger
Developmental Editor: Catherine Flanagan
Acquisitions Editor: Shelley Scott
Illustrations and Permissions Coordinator: Maureen A. Livengood
Senior Project Manager, Production: Max F. Perez
Project Supervisor, Editing: Rebecca Nordbrock
Freelance Staff Supervisor: Barbara M. Kelly
Manager, Literature Services: Edith M. Podrazik, R.N.
Senior Information Specialist: Terri Santo, R.N.
Senior Medical Writer: David A. Cramer, M.D.
Vice President, Professional Sales and Marketing: George M. Parker
Senior Marketing Manager: Eileen Lynch
Marketing Coordinator: Lynn Stevenson

1995 EDITION
Copyright © August 1995 by Mosby-Year Book, Inc.

Printed in the United States of America
Composition by Reed Technology and Information Services, Inc.
Printing/binding by Maple-Vail

Mosby-Year Book, Inc.
11830 Westline Industrial Drive
St. Louis, MO 63146

Editorial Office:
Mosby-Year Book, Inc.
200 North LaSalle Street
Chicago, IL 60601

International Standard Serial Number: 0084-3741
International Standard Book Number: 0-8151-0443-X

Table of Contents

Mosby Document Express

Copies of the full text of the original source documents of articles abstracted or referenced in this publication are available by calling Mosby Document Express, toll-free, at **1 (800) 55-MOSBY.**

With Mosby Document Express, you have convenient, 24-hour-a-day access to literally every article on which this publication is based. In fact, through Mosby Document Express, virtually any medical or scientific article can be located and delivered by FAX, overnight delivery service, international airmail, electronic transmission of bitmapped images (via Internet), or regular mail. The average cost of a complete, delivered copy of an article, including up to $4 in copyright clearance charges and first-class mail delivery, is $12.

For inquiries and pricing information, please call the toll-free number shown above. To expedite your order for material appearing in this publication, please be prepared with the code shown next to the bibliographic citation for each abstract.

Journals Represented

Mosby subscribes to and surveys nearly 1,000 U.S. and foreign medical and allied health journals. From these journals, the Editors select the articles to be abstracted. Journals represented in this YEAR BOOK are listed below.

Acta Endocrinologica
Acta Neurochirurgica
Acta Obstetricia et Gynecologica Scandinavica
Acta Psychiatrica Scandinavica
Age and Ageing
American Journal of Cardiology
American Journal of Clinical Nutrition
American Journal of Gastroenterology
American Journal of Hypertension
American Journal of Medicine
American Journal of Neuroradiology
American Journal of Obstetrics and Gynecology
American Journal of Physiology
American Journal of Psychiatry
Annals of Internal Medicine
Annals of Rheumatic Diseases
Annals of Surgery
Annals of Thoracic Surgery
Archives of Disease in Childhood
Archives of Pathology and Laboratory Medicine
Archives of Surgery
Atherosclerosis
Bone
Bone and Mineral
British Heart Journal
British Journal of Surgery
Calcified Tissue International
Canadian Journal of Anaesthesia
Cancer
Circulation
Clinical Chemistry
Clinical Endocrinology
Clinical Investigator
Contraception
Diabetes
Diabetes Care
Diabetologia
Endocrinology
European Journal of Clinical Pharmacology
European Journal of Endocrinology
European Journal of Surgery
Fertility and Sterility
Gerontology
Gut
Human Reproduction
Journal of Applied Physiology: Respiratory, Environmental and Exercise
    Physiology
Journal of Bone and Mineral Research
Journal of Clinical Endocrinology and Metabolism
Journal of Clinical Investigation

Journal of Emergency Medicine
Journal of Endocrinology
Journal of Gerontology
Journal of Laboratory and Clinical Medicine
Journal of Pediatrics
Journal of Steroid Biochemistry and Molecular Biology
Journal of Surgical Onocology
Journal of Urology
Journal of the American Geriatrics Society
Journal of the American Medical Association
Lancet
Life Sciences
Maturitas
Mayo Clinic Proceedings
Metabolism
Modern Pathology
Nature
New England Journal of Medicine
Nuclear Medicine Communications
Obstetrics and Gynecology
Pediatric Research
Proceedings of the National Academy of Sciences
Prostate
Radiology
Southern Medical Journal
Stroke
Surgery
Transplantation Proceedings
Urologia Internationalis
Urology
World Journal of Surgery

STANDARD ABBREVIATIONS

The following terms are abbreviated in this edition: adrenocorticotropin hormone (ACTH); acquired immunodeficiency syndrome (AIDS); cardiopulmonary resuscitation (CPR); central nervous system (CNS); cerebrospinal fluid (CSF); computed tomography (CT); corticotropin-releasing hormone (CRH); deoxyribonucleic acid (DNA); electrocardiography (ECG); follicle-stimulating hormone (FSH); gonadotropin-releasing hormone (GnRH); growth hormone (GH); health maintenance organization (HMO); high-density lipoprotein (HDL); human immunodeficiency virus (HIV); insulin-dependent diabetes mellitus (IDDM); insulin-like growth factor I (IGF-I); intensive care unit (ICU); intermediate-density lipoprotein (IDL); intramuscular (IM); intravenous (IV); low-density lipoprotein (LDL); luteinizing hormone (LH); magnetic resonance (MR) imaging (MRI); multiple endocrine neoplasia (MEN); non–insulin-dependent diabetes mellitus (NIDDM); parathyroid hormone (PTH); prolactin (PRL); releasing hormone (RH); ribonucleic acid (RNA); thyrotropin-releasing hormone (TRH); thyroid-stimulating hormone or thyrotropin (TSH); thyroxine (T_4); triiodothyronine (T_3); and very-low-density lipoprotein (VLDL).

Introduction

Going. . . going. . . gone.

In my introduction to the 1991 YEAR BOOK OF ENDOCRINOLOGY, I lamented that endocrinology as a clinical subspecialty was an "endangered species" that was under siege. Nothing has happened in the past 4 years to change that characterization. For all except perhaps the molecular endocrinologist, the siege has continued for practicing and academic endocrinologists alike—relentless, painful, and mindless—driven as is most economic and governmental policy by short-term bottom-line thinking. We don't have the World Wildlife Federation or the Sierra Club on our side. Only 2 societies (the Endocrine Society and the American Association of Clinical Endocrinologists) are on our side, with agendas that should be complementary but have not been perceived as such; both are caught in the untenable position of reacting to the daunting problems of a rapidly changing health care environment rather than contributing to a comprehensive solution from the onset. It seems too late for that.

We're scrambling willy-nilly on these shifting sands, like so many special interest groups protecting their treasure from pillage or well-intentioned Robin Hoods. However, the preserve of endocrinologists is not resource-rich like the Sherwood Forest of yore, lads and lasses. Not only do we lack collective treasure, but we have precious few trees. And in what seems to be our last stand of timber, we spotted owls sit on exposed branches. Like the loggers in Oregon, there are many health care planners who love spotted owls—fried!

Long before health care reform became a household word and Harry and Louise were created on Madison Avenue to bash Hillary and her task force, James Wyngaarden lectured the Association of American Physicians ("the old Turks"). His visionary remarks, which he gave the environmentally correct title "The Clinical Investigator as an Endangered Species," were published (1). His concerns were prescient: M.D.s in the late 1970s were losing the race for grant funds to Ph.D.s because "of a failure of the M.D. investigator pool to grow at the same rate as the Ph.D. pool." To the head of the National Institutes of Health (NIH), the writing was on the wall even then. To those of us who trained in that era, our long-term prognosis was already guarded. By analogy, the same scenario can be extended to practicing endocrinologists today. Like physician-scientists being overrun by basic scientists, their activity has been increasingly limited by the ever-expanding army of general internists and family practitioners and an emerging system of delivery that has rapidly evolved in anticipation of a Clinton plan that never came to pass!

Did Wyngaarden really expect that things would get so bad that an M.D. scientist would have only a 1% to 2% chance of receiving an NIH RO1 award in 1994? Ironically, it is the VA system that now is the exclusive practitioner of conservation—of physician scientists and patient-oriented research—through their Merit Review system of support for physician-initiated medical research. In his insightful exploration of the crisis that has assuredly developed (2), E.H. Ahrens, Jr., Professor Emeritus at the Rockefeller University, identifies a number of what he characterizes as "institutional obstacles" that must be overcome to restore the species. Not only are they formidable and complex; they are, in my humble opinion, for the most part no longer capable of being corrected. The changes that have occurred since Wyngaarden's warning are so far advanced and pervasive, the intrastructure so eroded, that it is questionable whether even unlimited resources (which are hardly in the cards) applied now could reverse the situation.

Where would you start, if you could, when academic medicine has lost its mission? When the faculties of medical schools in the United States have such demands put upon them that their effectiveness as teachers, researchers, and caregivers is so compromised? When generating income to meet departmental needs is the overriding priority? When this happens, teaching, as the Macy Foundation Report (3) noted, is the first to suffer. The result is that our enrollment-swollen educational factories turn out standardized assembly-line products—men and women, now in equal numbers who may be well informed, but as Ahrens points out ". . . are not necessarily curious, imaginative, literate, or articulate." Can we expect any different when our medical schools and teaching hospitals are expected to not only meet the medical needs of the surrounding community, but to address the problems of poverty, race, drugs, AIDS, and crime?

With this burden of responsibility, how is it possible not only to train young doctors to nurture the sick, but to stimulate those with potential academic inclinations to pursue the acquisition of new knowledge about human biology and disease? Other industrialized nations have wrestled with some of these same basic issues in health care delivery and medical education. They seem to have come up with solutions that not only work better than ours but that also ensure the survival of physician scientists who never had spotted owl status. During my tenure as editor of the YEAR BOOK OF ENDOCRINOLOGY, "imported" contributions from colleagues abroad have occupied an increasing proportion of page space each year. Our "trade" deficit worsens.

John D. Bagdade, M.D.

References

1. Wyngaarden J: The clinical investigator as an endangered species. *Trans Assoc Am Physicians* 92:1, 1979.
2. Ahrens EH Jr: *The Crisis in Clinical Research: Overcoming Institutional Obstacles.* New York, Oxford University Press, 1992.
3. Macy Foundation Report: *Clinical Education and the Doctor of Tomorrow.* New York, Academy of Medicine, 1989.

Peripheral Triglyceride Clearance, the Adipsin-ASP Pathway, and Type IV Hyperlipoproteinemia

ALLAN D. SNIDERMAN, M.D., PIERRE JULIEN, PH.D.* AND KATHERINE CIANFLONE, PH.D.

McGill Unit for the Prevention of Cardiovascular Disease, Royal Victoria Hospital, McGill University, Montreal, Quebec, Canada; and *Centre de Recherche sur les Maladies Lipidiques, Laval University Medical Research Centre, Ste-Foy, Quebec, Canada

Introduction

The object of this article is to illustrate how measurement of plasma B100 levels, when it is combined with measurement of lipoprotein lipids and interpreted in the framework of the adipsin–acylation-stimulating protein (ASP) pathway, may provide new insights into the pathophysiology of peripheral triglyceride clearance and, consequently, into the pathogenesis and clinical management of type IV hyperlipoproteinemia. To do so, the major features of the adipsin–ASP pathway will be briefly reviewed; the dyslipoproteinemia that results from its dysfunction will be differentiated from that produced by heterozygotic lipoprotein lipase deficiency and from that caused by carbohydrate-induced hypertriglyceridemia; finally, the clinical significance of these distinctions will be outlined.

More than 25 years ago, it was shown that some patients with type IV hyperlipoproteinemia have an elevated level of apoB, whereas others do not (1–3). It is now clear that those with an elevated level of plasma apoB have an increased LDL particle number. When the level of plasma apoB is normal, however, the LDL particle number is normal (4). It is also now clear that in those with an increased apoB, the LDL particle number is high because of overproduction of B100 lipoproteins by the liver (5, 6). Moreover, there is considerable evidence that hypertriglyceridemic patients with an increased LDL particle number are at increased risk of vascular disease compared with hypertriglyceridemic patients with a normal LDL particle number. This was the finding in several cross-sectional studies (7–12), and this conclusion has been strongly buttressed by the findings of the Quebec Heart Study, a prospective study examining the relation of plasma lipids, lipoprotein lipids, and apoproteins to the risk of vascular disease (13). Of all the parameters examined in this study, the plasma apoB level was the single most important determinant of risk. In addition, within the hypertriglyceridemic groups, the risk of disease was 3 times higher than control for those with an elevated apoB, but it was not elevated above control for those with a normal apoB (13).

It must be accepted, therefore, that type IV hyperlipoproteinemia, as classically defined, represents a collection of different metabolic entities with different risks of vascular disease. Unfortunately, however, there has been little further progress in sorting them out. This paper is an attempt to do so. We recognize, of course, that the hypotheses and models to be presented will not turn out to be correct in every detail. But we hope that they represent a reasonable beginning and that their presentation will stir debate and experimentation.

The Adipsin–ASP Pathway

Acylation-stimulating protein is the most potent stimulant of triglyceride synthesis in human adipocytes yet described (14), and the pathway of which it is the effector is constituted as follows (15): Human adipocytes contain message for, and secrete, the 3 proteins of the alternate complement pathway. These are the third component of complement (C3), factor B, and factor D (or adipsin) (16). These 3 proteins interact extracellularly to produce a 77 amino terminal fragment of C3 known as C3a (Fig 1). Carboxypeptidases present in excess in plasma rapidly cleave the terminal arginine from C3a to produce the 76 amino acid peptide known as C3a desarg, or ASP, which then acts back upon the adipocyte, causing triglyceride synthesis to increase.

How then does ASP act upon the adipocyte to achieve this effect? In brief, it does so by increasing specific membrane transport of glucose (17) and by activating the last enzyme involved in triglyceride synthesis, diacylglycerol acyltransferase (18). The former is achieved by the same mechanism by which insulin increases glucose transport—namely, by increasing translocation of glucose transporters from the intracellular microsomal fraction to the cell membrane. However, the ASP-induced increase in membrane transport of glucose is independent of, but additive to, insulin.

The function of the adipsin–ASP pathway is to ensure that the rate of triglyceride synthesis within adipocytes is sufficiently rapid that fatty acid concentrations in the microcirculation will not increase unduly. Were

Generation of C$_{3a\ desarg}$

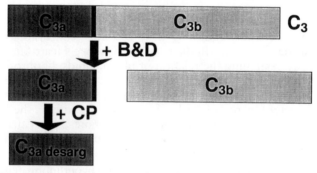

Fig 1.—The 3 proteins that interact to produce acylation-stimulating protein (ASP) are illustrated. Factor B binds to C3 (the third component of complement) and adipsin (factor D) then cleaves a 77 amino acid fragment of C3, C3a. The terminal arginine of C3a is then removed to produce C3a desarg, the form in which ASP is purified from plasma. C3a desarg is bioactive. C3a may also stimulate triglyceride synthesis, but this has not been settled with certainty. (Courtesy of Drs. Sniderman, Julien, and Cianflone.)

The Adipsin – ASP Pathway

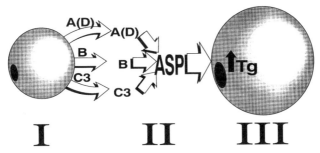

Fig 2.—Illustration of the principle of microenvironmental regulation. The adipocyte is in the subendothelial space, and a chylomicron (not illustrated) is attached to the endothelial cell within the capillary. The adipocyte synthesizes and secretes adipsin, factor B, and C3. Acylation-stimulating protein (ASP) is generated (see Figure 1) by virtue of their interaction. Chylomicrons are able to markedly accelerate the rate at which ASP is generated from these 3 precursor proteins. The model posits, therefore, that as fatty acids are being liberated from chylomicrons as a result of the action of lipoprotein lipase, ASP is also being generated. Triglyceride synthesis in adipocytes increases concurrent with the need to do so. The adipsin–ASP pathway, therefore, links events within the capillary space to the necessary metabolic response in the subendothelial space. (Courtesy of Drs. Sniderman, Julien, and Cianflone.)

this to occur, fatty acid release from triglyceride-rich lipoproteins would diminish abruptly, which would be accompanied by the series of adverse consequences that will be detailed later. Our hypothesis is that normal clearance of triglycerides in the periphery requires integration of events at the endothelial cell surface and within the adipocyte. That is, as enormous numbers of fatty acids are being rapidly liberated in the capillary space, generation of ASP allows the adipocyte to increase its triglyceride synthetic capacity, with the result that excess buildup of fatty acids in the capillary space is avoided. In this regard, it should be appreciated that the generation of ASP in a culture that contains adipocytes with an admixture of endothelial cells is not increased by the addition of fatty acids, insulin, or glucose. Rather, generation of ASP is markedly enhanced by the addition of chylomicrons (19). Thus, the factor that triggers activation of the pathway is the major triglyceride-transporting particle itself.

Integrating these observations results in the model shown in Figure 2. The essence of the adipsin–ASP pathway—and its most interesting feature—is that it permits microenvironmental metabolic regulation. By virtue of this pathway, the response of the adipocyte within the subendothelial space is linked to events within the capillary space; it is this metabolic integration that allows rapid hydrolysis of triglyceride-rich lipoproteins to continue and, consequently, rapid triglyceride clearance to occur. In support of this hypothesis are the observations that in normal subjects, plasma ASP levels rise after an oral fat load, and the degree to which they do correlates positively with the rate of triglyceride clearance from plasma (20).

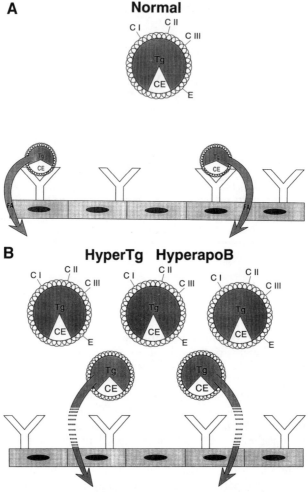

Fig 3.—**A**, normally, triglyceride-rich lipoproteins attach to the endothelial surface via interactions with lipoprotein lipase. Because adipocytes can take up and esterify the fatty acids that are released, most of the triglyceride is removed from these lipoproteins before they are released from the endothelial surface. **B**, an illustration of the situation in the capillary space when the acylation-stimulating protein receptor is defective in adipocytes in patients with hyperapoB. The rate at which triglyceride synthesis can increase is limited, and therefore fatty acid concentrations in the microcirculation rise abnormally. This increase inhibits the action of lipoprotein lipase and causes the still triglyceride-rich lipoprotein particles to be detached from the endothelial surface, from whence they pass to the liver. The increased delivery of fatty acids to the liver results in the overproduction of VLDL particles, which is also illustrated. (Courtesy of Drs. Sniderman, Julien, and Cianflone.)

Reduced Function of the Adipsin–ASP Pathway as a Cause of Hypertriglyceridemic HyperapoB

MICROENVIRONMENTAL PATHOGENESIS OF HYPERAPOB

The consequences of a fault in the receptor in the adipocyte cell membrane with which ASP interacts will now be outlined. In this instance, the maximal rate of adipocyte triglyceride synthesis would be reduced and, therefore, the maximal rate of uptake of fatty acids from the subendothelial space would be reduced. Reducing the rate of uptake of fatty acids would lead to an increase in the concentration of fatty acids within the capillary space. This increase in fatty acid concentration in the capillary space would lead to the following events. First, lipoprotein lipase (LPL)-induced triglyceride hydrolysis would be inhibited (21) and triglyceride hydrolysis would be halted. In vitro studies have shown LPL would be detached from the endothelial (22) surface and apoC II split away from it (23). Moreover, the still triglyceride-rich remnants would be prematurely detached from the endothelial surface and would reenter the circulation, from which they and the LPL could then be removed by the liver (24) (Fig 3). Delivery of fatty acids to the liver would increase, resulting in increased uptake of free fatty acids. Hepatic uptake of the triglyceride-enriched remnant particles would also occur, further increasing an unwanted delivery of lipid to this organ (25).

Then, the next round of consequences begins. The increased delivery of fatty acids to the liver results in the secretion of increased numbers of VLDL particles, whose triglyceride content is not markedly increased (26). Increased production of VLDL particles leads to increased production of LDL particles (5) and, because the capacity of the normal pathways to remove LDL from the circulation is so limited, the LDL particle number will rise as well (4–6). Finally, increased cholesterol ester-triglyceride exchanges lead to the production of increased numbers of small, dense LDL (27–29). Thus, the characteristic dyslipoproteinemia resulting from dysfunction of the adipsin–ASP pathway is hyperapoB, or familial combined hyperlipidemia. The impact on VLDL, IDL, and LDL particle number and composition is shown in Figure 4A, and these findings are contrasted with the normal, shown in Figure 4B. Note that in hyperapoB, the VLDL and IDL particle numbers are increased, as is the LDL particle number, but LDL still constitutes the vast majority of the B100 particles in plasma (3, 30). Note also that VLDL composition in terms of triglyceride-to-apoB ratio is normal or close to normal, whereas the LDL cholesterol-to–apoB ratio is often substantially reduced (30).

EVIDENCE OF DYSFUNCTION OF THE ADIPSIN–ASP PATHWAY IN PATIENTS WITH HYPERAPOB

By definition, patients with hyperapoB have an elevated LDL particle number because of overproduction of B100 lipoproteins by the liver. Impaired clearance of triglyceride-rich lipoproteins has also been demonstrated in patients with hyperapoB (31, 32). Of interest, an abnormal in-

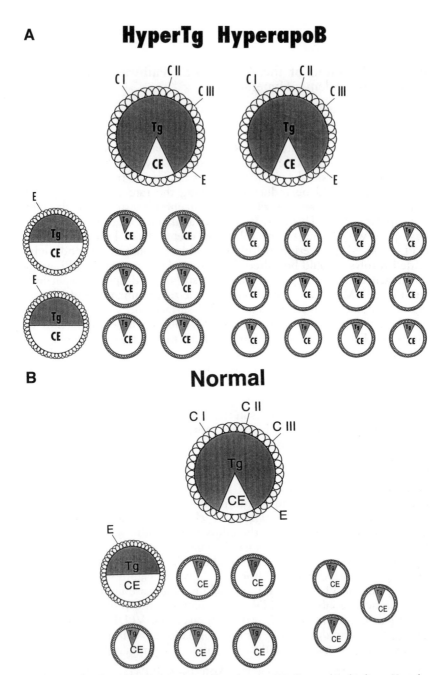

Fig 4.—A, the plasma B100 lipoprotein profile in hyperapoB is illustrated in this figure. Note that VLDL particle number is increased as well as IDL and LDL particle number. Nevertheless, more than 93% of the B100 particles are IDL and LDL. Not shown are 2 other common features of this dyslipoproteinemia: increased numbers of chylomicron remnants postprandially and a reduced HDL cholesterol level. Not only is LDL particle number increased, but many are smaller and denser than normal. **B**, the normal plasma B100 lipoprotein profile. Note there are fewer VLDL and IDL particles as well as fewer LDL particles than in normals. Note also the heterogeneity in composition of the LDL particles. This is a normal feature. However, the typical profile of hyperapoB features not only more LDL particles than normal, but many of these are smaller and denser than in normals. (Contrast the LDL particle size and composition in **A** and **B**.) (Courtesy of Drs. Sniderman, Julien, and Cianflone.)

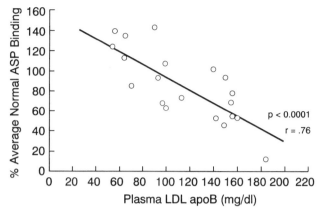

Fig 5.—The acylation-stimulating protein (ASP) stimulation of triglyceride synthesis as a percent of normal is plotted against plasma LDL apoB level. The relationship is inverse and highly significant, supporting the hypothesis that reduced peripheral triglyceride synthetic capacity is associated with increased hepatic B100 production rates. (Adapted with permission from Cianflone K, et al: *J Clin Invest* 85:722-730, 1990. Courtesy of Drs. Sniderman, Julien, and Cianflone.)

crease in plasma free fatty acids after an oral fat load has been documented in patients with hyperapoB (33), and an increased number of larger, presumably lipid-enriched, remnants has also been shown to be present postprandially (34). The increase in plasma fatty acids occurs about midway through the fat load and is often associated with a sharp decrease in HDL cholesterol, specifically HDL_2 cholesterol levels (31), a change that is probably caused by enhancement of cholesteryl ester transfer protein–mediated cholesterol ester–triglyceride exchanges in the postprandial lipolytic period (27–29). Increases in fasting free fatty acid levels have also been reported (32), and the theory that these may be responsible, at least in part, for the insulin resistance so often seen in these patients has been put forward (32).

All of these, of course, are precisely the consequences one would predict if there were impairment of the adipsin–ASP pathway leading to impaired peripheral triglyceride clearance from and premature detachment of triglyceride-rich lipoproteins. Indeed, direct evidence of such dysfunction has been obtained from studies of cultured skin fibroblasts in such patients (35–37). Specifically, it has been shown that the degree to which ASP causes triglyceride synthesis to rise in such cells is a direct function of its specific cell binding (37). Moreover, reduced responsiveness to ASP in skin fibroblasts cultured from patients with hyperapoB has been documented (35–37), the evidence in total being consistent with a reduced number of effective membrane receptors for ASP. Of interest, no defect in ASP-induced triglyceride synthesis or specific cell binding has been observed in cells from patients with familial hypercholesterolemia or in patients with hypertriglyceridemia with normal plasma apoB levels (37).

The hypothesis predicts that the degree to which fatty acids and triglyceride-rich remnants are inappropriately diverted to the liver should be directly proportional to the degree to which ASP-specific binding is reduced. As well, it predicts that the degree to which apoB levels are increased in such patients is directly related to the extent to which fatty acids and triglyceride-rich lipoproteins are inappropriately diverted to the liver. Evidence for both of these propositions is seen in Figure 5, which plots ASP-specific binding in cultured fibroblasts (as a percent of normal) against plasma LDL apoB. The relationship is inverse and highly significant, a finding that is consistent with the relation just proposed between the effectiveness of the adipsin–ASP pathway and the secretory rate of hepatic B100 lipoprotein particles.

Type IV Hyperlipoproteinemia Resulting From Heterozygotic LPL Deficiency

THE PLASMA B100 LIPOPROTEIN PROFILE IN HETEROZYGOTIC LPL DEFICIENCY

This section deals with the dyslipoproteinemia that is associated with partial LPL deficiency when that deficiency is caused by a heterozygotic defect in the gene product. An impressive number of these patients have now been studied, which allows the findings to be stated with some confidence (38). Note, however, the distinction between LPL deficiency caused by specific genetic error and LPL deficiency per se. Here, we focus on plasma B100 lipoprotein numbers and composition in patients selected because of an error in the LPL gene product. This approach differs diametrically from the studies in which LPL activity has been measured in patients known to have familial combined hyperlipidemia (39, 40). In these studies, a substantial reduction in LPL activity has been documented in an important minority of the patients. However, 2 recent studies in such patients (41, 42) have failed to detect any of the multiple known errors in the gene product; therefore, the reason the LPL is reduced is not known. Whatever the reason, the patients with familial combined hyperlipidemia who also have a reduced LPL have, by definition, an increased level of plasma apoB and their lipoprotein profile differs considerably from that which is characteristic of heterozygotic LPL deficiency per se.

In these latter patients, in whom the primary problem is undoubtedly an abnormal and dysfunctional gene product, the features of the dyslipoproteinemia are as follows (38):

- Plasma triglyceride is increased, as is VLDL apoB.

- The VLDL triglyceride–to–apoB ratio is not increased, indicating that the particles are close to normal in composition.

- The LDL cholesterol–to–apoB ratio is reduced, as is commonly the case in patients with hypertriglyceridemia.

Heterozygotic LPL Deficiency

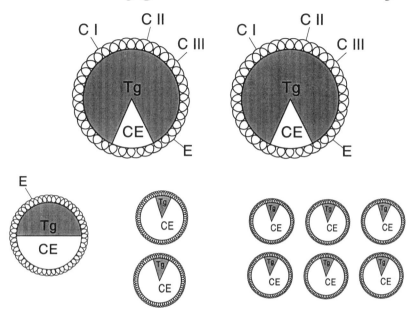

Fig 6.—The plasma B100 lipoprotein profile for a patient with heterozygotic lipoprotein lipase (*LPL*) deficiency is illustrated. Note that VLDL particle number is increased but the VLDL particles are normal in composition. Note that IDL and LDL particle numbers are normal because the B100 hepatic secretory rate is normal. More of the LDL particles are smaller and denser than normal because of the increased cholesterol ester-triglyceride core lipid exchanges, which are a consequence of the hypertriglyceridemia. (Courtesy of Drs. Sniderman, Julien, and Cianflone.)

• Most importantly, however, LDL apoB levels are not significantly elevated, clearly distinguishing these patients from those with familial combined hyperlipidemia and decreased LPL (39, 40).

These quantitative and qualitative features would result in the B100 plasma lipoprotein profile shown in Figure 6.

A Suggested Pathogenesis of the Type IV Dyslipoproteinemia Caused by Partial LPL Genetic Deficiency

The lipoprotein profile just noted is consistent with the model illustrated in Figure 7. Assume for a moment that the initial step in VLDL clearance involves binding to 1 or more LPL molecules. Reduce the number of bioeffective LPL molecules by half, and the number of VLDL particles that are bound will also be reduced. This will reduce the rate of clearance of these particles; thus, even if their production rate is normal, the number of VLDL particles in plasma will rise. However, because VLDL particles contribute so little to the total plasma apoB (30), that parameter will not be substantially affected.

Heterozygotic LPL Deficiency

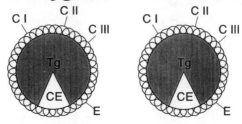

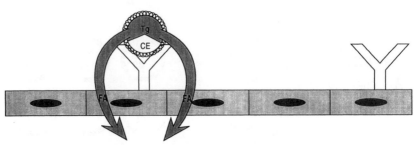

Fig 7.—A suggested model for the pathogenesis of the hypertriglyceridemia caused by heterozygotic lipoprotein lipase (*LPL*) deficiency is illustrated. Fewer VLDL particles than normal bind to the endothelial cells because of the reduction in bioactive LPL at the endothelial surface. Once bound, however, lipolysis proceeds normally because the adipsin–acylation-stimulating protein pathway is intact. Consequently, there is no excess diversion of fatty acids and triglyceride-rich remnants to the liver, and hepatic B100 production remains normal. However, the VLDL clearance rate from plasma is reduced and therefore the VLDL particle number will rise. (Courtesy of Drs. Sniderman, Julien, and Cianflone.)

What happens to the triglyceride-rich lipoproteins that are bound? Hydrolysis of triglyceride begins, and the fatty acids that are generated are rapidly cleared locally because the ASP pathway is intact. There is, therefore, no diversion of fatty acids from peripheral stores to the liver as in hyperapoB caused by dysfunction of the adipsin–ASP pathway. Consequently, the rate of production and composition of hepatic B100 particles is normal, which explains why the plasma apoB100 level is not elevated and why the VLDL triglyceride–to–apoB ratio is normal or close to normal as well. In summary, we hypothesize that the type IV hyperlipoproteinemia in such patients results from an increase in plasma of VLDL particles of normal composition caused by a reduced rate in the first step of peripheral triglyceride clearance—namely, binding of triglyceride-rich lipoproteins to LPL on the endothelial surface. As in all instances of hypertriglyceridemia, increased core lipid exchange can lead to smaller, denser LDL particles.

Carbohydrate-Induced Type IV Hyperlipoproteinemia

This is the third and final tableau—type IV hyperlipoproteinemia caused by carbohydrate-induced hepatic fatty acid synthesis that leads directly to increased triglyceride synthesis and secretion but normal hepatic apoB100 secretion from the liver (43). This was the first clearly characterized hypertriglyceridemic phenotype (44-46), which has the following features:

- Increased VLDL triglycerides with a normal VLDL apoB. The normal VLDL apoB indicates that VLDL particle number is normal, whereas the increased VLDL triglyceride–to–apoB ratio indicates that the VLDL particles contain more triglycerides than normal and are thus larger than normal.

- Total apoB is normal, and LDL apoB is on the lower side of normal.

- As in the other hypertriglyceridemic states, the LDL cholesterol-to-apoB ratio is often low, pointing to the presence of small, dense LDL.

The hallmark of the disorder is that even though hepatic triglyceride synthesis is increased, the rate at which VLDL particles are secreted is normal (43). Importantly, the secretion of triglyceride-enriched VLDL particles in response to an increased hepatic carbohydrate load has been documented in both in vitro and in vivo studies (43, 46, 47). Moreover, studies by Packard et al. (48) have suggested that the larger triglyceride-rich VLDL particles characteristic of carbohydrate-induced hypertriglyceridemia are more likely than smaller VLDL particles to be removed from the circulation without being converted to LDL particles. This accounts for the tendency of both total and LDL apoB to be on the lower side of normal. These features are illustrated in Figure 8.

Of interest, these are also the features of the dyslipoproteinemia of familial hypertriglyceridemia (49). In this instance, abnormal bile acid metabolism—specifically, decreased bile acid reabsorption and, consequently, increased bile acid synthesis—seem to be playing a pathogenic role (50, 51). Just as in carbohydrate-induced hypertriglyceridemia, hepatic fatty acid synthesis increases but apoB100 secretion does not, perhaps because, as in the carbohydrate model, cholesterol ester synthesis does not either (47). This contrasts with the response to an increased delivery of fatty acids to the liver when cholesterol ester synthesis increases in parallel with triglyceride synthesis and apoB secretion increases pari passu (26). The intracellular mechanisms responsible for these different patterns of response remain to be determined and are obviously of great interest.

Potential Pathophysiologic and Clinical Significance of These Distinctions

Why then should these distinctions be made? We would suggest there are at least 2 reasons. First, studies to determine the pathophysiology of

CHO-Induced HyperTg

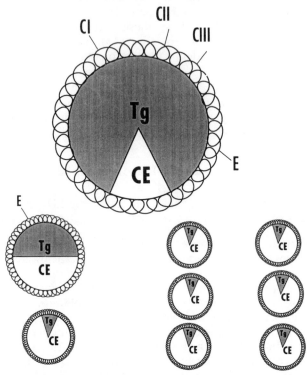

Fig 8.—The characteristics of carbohydrate-induced hypertriglyceridemia are illustrated. The VLDL particle number is normal, but the VLDL particles are triglyceride-enriched. Because fewer than normal of these particles are converted to LDL, the LDL particle number tends to be on the lower side of normal. As in the other example of hypertriglyceridemia, many of the LDL particles tend to be smaller and denser than normal. (Courtesy of Drs. Sniderman, Julien, and Cianflone.)

the various dyslipoproteinemias are unlikely to yield clear answers or novel insights if disparate entities are lumped together unknowingly. For example, much remains to be done to test the hypothesis that dysfunction of the adipsin–ASP pathway produces hyperapoB or familial combined hyperlipidemia. However, that hypothesis cannot be tested if patients are chosen with no attention to apoB levels. Equally, how can anything be learned of the pathogenesis of familial hypertriglyceridemia if, in some studies, it is characterized by normal levels of apoB (49), whereas in others (52) it is not? Is it any surprise that in some studies, familial hypertriglyceridemia is associated with an increased risk of coronary disease (53), whereas in others it is not (54)?

The second argument is quite practical: How can therapeutic strategies be appropriately chosen if patients are incompletely characterized? It is not the LDL cholesterol that interacts with the arterial wall, it is the

LDL particle. Any argument that states that the risk of vascular disease relates only to LDL cholesterol and not to the LDL particle ignores all the evidence of the past decade, which details the diverse adverse consequences of the interaction of LDL particles with the arterial endothelial and the subendothelial space.

Moreover, there now can be no doubt that small, dense LDLs are, particle for particle, of greater atherogenic potential than LDL particles of normal size and composition. The evidence for this statement is of 2 kinds—epidemiologic and basic—and each buttresses the other, the two together constituting a major advance in our understanding of the pathogenesis of vascular disease. In brief, small, dense LDLs have been shown in a series of studies to be more common in premature vascular disease (55–57) than LDL particles that are normal in size and composition. Furthermore, angiographic progression in one prospective study has correlated best with this fraction (58), whereas the extent to which regression occurs has been shown in 2 studies to relate most strongly to the decrease in this specific fraction (59, 60). Moreover, as noted earlier, in hypertriglyceridemia, several cross-sectional studies have shown increased risk with increased apoB (7–12), with evidence from 1 prospective study (13) supporting this conclusion.

That increased numbers of small, dense LDLs should be such a powerful determinant of coronary risk should not be surprising given that they enter the vascular wall more easily than normal size ones do (61). In addition, they oxidize more easily (62–65), they stimulate thromboxane synthesis more readily (66), and they stick to the glycosaminoglycans more avidly than do normal LDL particles (67). Furthermore, they are also more potent inhibitors of normal vasodilator endothelial responses in the human coronary vascular bed than are normal LDL particles (68).

To repeat, it is not the cholesterol per se that is atherogenic, it is the LDL particle, because it is the LDL particle that interacts with the arterial wall. Because of this, the LDL particle, not the LDL cholesterol, should be our primary target of therapy. Reduction of the LDL particle number slows the rate at which coronary lesions progress angiographically and diminishes the rate at which new lesions appear (69). To this can now be added the unequivocal improvement in survival in patients with coronary disease treated with a 3-hydroxy-3-methylglutaryl coenzyme A (HMG CoA) reductase inhibitor, which was demonstrated in the Scandinavian Simvastatin Survival Study (4S) trial (70). That this benefit relates to lowering of the LDL particle number rather than simply altering LDL cholesterol follows from the results of the FATS trial (71). In this study, in which all patients had an elevated apoB but only half had a frankly increased LDL cholesterol, LDL was reduced markedly by either of 2 pharmacologic therapies. It is of considerable interest that the normocholesterolemic patients with an elevated apoB did even better both in terms of angiographic and clinical outcomes than did those with an elevated LDL cholesterol and apoB, the better outcome apparently relating to the more successful normalization of LDL particle number in the former than in the latter group (72).

For all these reasons, we do not believe it remains reasonable for the physician in clinical practice to remain ignorant of LDL particle number and composition, certainly not in hypertriglyceridemic and so-called nor-molipidemic patients. Without measuring apoB, what acceptable ratio-nale is there for treating patients with hypertriglyceridemic hyperapoB with an HMG CoA reductase inhibitor rather than a fibric acid agent? The former will markedly reduce LDL particle number, the latter will diminish it modestly, if at all (73). The whole debate becomes even more pointed now that the measurement of plasma apoB has been standard-ized (74), whereas that of lipoprotein lipids has not yet been achieved. Indeed, in our present cost-conscious world, it could easily be argued that measurement of apoB is cost-effective because it would differentiate between the minority of patients with type IV hyperlipoproteinemia, who would benefit from pharmacologic therapy, and the majority, for whom no clear evidence yet exists of clinical benefit from this approach.

Thus, 3 distinct forms of hypertriglyceridemia have been explicated and a pathophysiology for each presented. Pure pictures of each have been outlined. Obviously, however, an individual patient might have fea-tures of more than one. For example, there is nothing to prevent carbo-hydrate sensitivity and a disordered adipsin–ASP pathway from coexist-ing. Nevertheless, the principles leading to recognition remain the same. In the end, all we argue for is a physiologically based approach to diag-nosis and treatment of hypertriglyceridemia, an approach that allows the incorporation of advances in understanding of lipoprotein metabolism and would move us beyond a classification scheme introduced more than 30 years ago (75). To paraphrase Gertrude Stein: A rose is a rose is a rose, but not all type IV hyperlipoproteinemia is the same.

Additional Physiologic and Pathologic Implications of the Adip-sin–ASP Pathway

This article has focused on the potential power of the adipsin–ASP pathway for the explication of the various forms of hypertriglyceridemia. However, a number of caveats must be noted before listing briefly other areas to which it may apply. In the first instance, not all hyperapoB is caused by dysfunction of this pathway. Rather, dysfunction of the path-way is only 1 cause of overproduction of hepatic B100 lipoprotein parti-cles. Numerous other causes have been documented. Among the rare but informative ones are β-sitosterolemia (76), cholesterol ester storage disease (77), and cholestanolosis (78). Moreover, overproduction of B100 lipoproteins is a major feature of the nephrotic syndrome (79). Therefore, excess delivery of fatty acids and triglyceride-rich remnants to the liver resulting from dysfunction of the adipsin–ASP pathway is not the only cause of hyperapoB, although it is an important one.

The second caveat is more important, i.e., how limited present knowl-edge is of even the most vital and simple characteristics of this new pathway we have discussed. We emphasize this limitation but do not apologize for it. New approaches require time to develop, and nothing can substitute for this requirement. Time is also required for their confirmation. In this regard, we note that all the essential observations concerning the bioactivity of ASP have now been reproduced independently (R. Parker and R. Gregg, personal communication), as have the observations of reduced ASP responsiveness in patients with hyperapoB (36, 37).

The adipsin–ASP pathway came to light based on investigation of the pathogenesis of hyperapoB. Its clinical relevance, however, may extend much beyond dyslipoproteinemias. Of these, the 2 other potential clinical connections that come immediately to mind are pathogenesis of the obese state and pathogenesis of adult-onset diabetes mellitus. Both include alterations of fatty acid metabolism and storage. Gynoid obesity may represent an instance of amplification of the activity of the ASP pathway (79), whereas android or omental obesity may represent an example of its impaired function (80). Even if dysfunction of the pathway is only a secondary feature of an excess caloric intake—as indeed is likely usually the case—it will, depending on the form the obesity takes, dictate, to an important extent, the plasma lipoprotein profile and therefore the cardiovascular risk that accompanies the increased adipose tissue mass. Moreover, the linkages between hyperapoB and insulin resistance are so intense, they now appear to be 2 sides of the same faulty coin. We believe there is a complex but critical interplay between glucose and fatty acid metabolism that we must strive to better understand, because within this dark boundary probably lie many of the origins of the most common diseases of affluent societies.

References

1. Lees RS: Immunoassay of plasma low density lipoproteins. *Science* 169:493, 1970.
2. Schonfeld G, Lees RS, George PK, et al: Assay of total plasma apolipoprotein B concentrations in human subjects. *J Clin Invest* 53:1458, 1974.
3. Durrington PN, Bocton CH, Hartog M: Serum and lipoprotein apolipoprotein B levels in normal subjects and patients with hyperlipoproteinemia. *Clin Chim Acta* 82:151, 1978.
4. Teng B, Thompson GR, Sniderman AD, et al: Composition and distribution of low-density lipoprotein fractions in hyperapobetalipoproteinemia, normolipidemia and familial hypercholesterolemia. *Proc Natl Acad Sci U S A* 80:6662–6666, 1983.
5. Teng B, Sniderman AD, Soutar AK, et al: Metabolic basis of hyperapobetalipoproteinemia: Turnover of apolipoprotein B in low-density lipoprotein and its precursors and subfractions compared with normal and familial hypercholesterolemia. *J Clin Invest* 77:663–672, 1986.
6. Venkatesan S, Cullen P, Pacy P, et al: Stable isotopes show a direct relation between VLDL apoB overproduction and serum triglyceride levels and indicate a metabolically and biochemically coherent basis for familial combined hyperlipidemia. *Arterioscler Thromb* 13:1110–1118, 1993.
7. Brunzell JD, Schrott HG, Motulsky AG, et al: Myocardial infarction in the familial forms of hypertriglyceridemia. *Metabolism* 25:313–320, 1976.
8. Durrington PN, Hunt L, Ishola M, et al: Serum apolipoproteins AI and B and

lipoproteins in middle aged men with and without previous myocardial infarction. *Br Heart J* 56:206–212, 1986.

9. Barbir M, Wile D, Trayner I, et al: High prevalence of hypertriglyceridemia and apolipoprotein abnormalities in coronary artery disease. *Br Heart J* 60:397–403, 1988.

10. Kukita H, Hamada M, Hiwada K, et al: Clinical significance of measurements of serum apolipoprotein AI, AII and B in hypertriglyceridemic male patients with and without coronary artery disease. *Atherosclerosis* 55:143–149, 1985.

11. Sniderman AD, Wolfson C, Teng B, et al: Association of hyperapobetalipoproteinemia with endogenous hypertriglyceridemia and atherosclerosis. *Ann Intern Med* 97:833–839, 1982.

12. Kwiterovich PO Jr, Coresh J, Bachorik PS: Prevalence of hyperapobetalipoproteinemia and other lipoprotein phenotypes in men (aged < 50 years) and women (aged < 60 years) with coronary artery disease. *Am J Cardiol* 72:631–639, 1993.

13. Moorjani S, Cantin B, Dagenais GR, et al: Importance of plasma apolipoprotein B in coronary artery disease: Evidence from retrospective and prospective findings in 2440 men. *J Am Coll Cardiol* 21:167A, 1993.

14. Cianflone K, Sniderman AD, Walsh MJ, et al: Purification and characterization of acylation-stimulating protein. *J Biol Chem* 264:426–430, 1989.

15. Baldo A, Sniderman AD, St-Luce S, et al: The adipsin–acylation stimulating protein system and regulation of intracellular triglyceride synthesis. *J Clin Invest* 92:1543–1557, 1993.

16. Cianflone K, Roncari DAK, Maslowska M, et al: The adipsin–acylation stimulating protein system in human adipocytes: Regulation of triacylglycerol synthesis. *Biochemistry* 33:9489–9495, 1994.

17. Germinario R, Sniderman AD, Manuel S, et al: Coordinate regulation of triacylglycerol synthesis and glucose transport by acylation stimulating protein. *Metabolism* 40:574–580, 1993.

18. Yasruel Z, Cianflone K, Sniderman AD, et al: Effect of acylation stimulating protein on the triacylglycerol synthetic pathway of human adipose tissue. *Lipids* 26:495–499, 1991.

19. Cianflone K, Maslowska M, Sniderman AD: ASP generation in differentiating human adipocytes (abstract). *Circulation* 90:Part 2:1–351, 1994.

20. Cianflone K, Vu H, Walsh M, et al: Metabolic response of acylation stimulating protein to an oral fat load. *J Lipid Res* 30:1727–1733, 1989.

21. Posner I, DeSanctis J: Kinetics of product inhibition and mechanisms of lipoprotein lipase activation by apolipoprotein C-II. *Biochemistry* 26:3711–3717, 1987.

22. Saxena U, Witte LD, Goldberg IJ: Release of endothelial cell lipoproteins by free fatty acids. *J Biol Chem* 264:4349–4355, 1989.

23. Saxena U, Goldberg IJ: Interaction of lipoprotein lipase with glycosaminoglycans and apolipoprotein C-II: Effects of free-fatty-acids. *Biochim Biophys Acta* 1043:161–168, 1990.

24. Peterson J, Bihain BE, Bengtsson-Olivecrona G, et al: Fatty acid control of lipoprotein lipase: A link between energy metabolism and lipid transport. *Proc Natl Acad Sci U S A* 87:909–913, 1990.

25. Evans AJ, Sawyez CG, Wolfe BM, et al: Lipolysis is a prerequisite for lipid accumulation in HepG2 cells induced by large hypertriglyceridemic very low density lipoproteins. *J Biol Chem* 267:10743–10751, 1992.

26. Cianflone K, Yasruel Z, Rodriguez MA, et al: Regulation of apoB secretion from HepG2 cells: Evidence for a critical role for cholesterol ester synthesis in the response to a fatty acid challenge. *J Lipid Res* 31:2045–2055, 1990.

27. Tall AR, Sammett D, Vita GM, et al: Lipoprotein lipase enhances the cholesteryl ester transfer protein-mediated transfer of cholesteryl esters from high density lipoproteins to very low density lipoproteins. *J Biol Chem* 259:9587–9594, 1984.

28. Sammett D, Tall AR: Mechanisms of enhancement of cholesteryl ester transfer protein activity by lipolysis. *J Biol Chem* 260:6687-6697, 1985.
29. Barter PJ, Chang LBF, Newnham HH, et al: The interaction of cholesteryl ester transfer protein and unesterified fatty acids promotes a reduction in the particle size of high-density lipoproteins. *Biochem Biophys Acta* 1045:81-89, 1990.
30. Sniderman AD, Vu H, Cianflone K: The effect of moderate hypertriglyceridemia on the relation of plasma total and LDL apoB levels. *Atherosclerosis* 89:109-116, 1991.
31. Genest J. Sniderman AD, Cianflone K, et al: Hyperapobetalipoproteinemia: Plasma lipoprotein responses to oral fat load. *Arteriosclerosis* 6:297-304, 1986.
32. Castro Cabezas M, de Bruin TW, de Valk HW, et al: Impaired fatty acid metabolism in familial combined hyperlipidemia: A mechanism associating hepatic apolipoprotein B overproduction and insulin resistance. *J Clin Invest* 92:160-168, 1993.
33. Sniderman AD, Kwiterovich PO Jr: *Hyperapobetalipoproteinemia and LDL and HDL$_2$ Heterogeneity: NIH Meeting Proceedings.* Washington, DC: US Dept of Health and Human Services. Proceedings of Workshop on Lipoprotein Heterogeneity, September 1987. NIH publication 87-2646.
34. Cabezas MC, deBruin TW, Kock LA, et al: Simvastatin improves chylomicron remnant removal in familial combined hyperlipidemia without changing chylomicron conversion. *Metabolism* 42:497-503, 1993.
35. Cianflone K, Maslowska M, Sniderman AD: Impaired response of fibroblasts in patients with hyperapobetalipoproteinemia to acylation stimulating protein. *J Clin Invest* 85:722-730, 1990.
36. Kwiterovich PO Jr, Motevalli M, Miller M: Acylation-stimulatory activity in hyperapobetalipoproteinemic fibroblasts: Enhanced cholesterol esterification with an additional serum basic protein, BPII. *Proc Natl Acad Sci U S A* 87:8980-8984, 1990.
37. Kwiterovich PO Jr, Motevalli M, Miller M: The effect of three serum basic proteins on the mass of lipids in normal and hyperapoB fibroblasts. *Arterioscler Thromb* 14:1-7, 1994.
38. Julien P, Gagné C, Murthy MRV, et al: Mutations of the lipoprotein lipase gene as a cause of dyslipidemias in the Québec population. *Can J Cardiol* 10(suppl B):54-60, 1994.
39. Babirak SP, Iverius P, Fujimoto WY, et al: Detection and characterization of the heterozygotic state for lipoprotein lipase deficiency. *Atherosclerosis* 9:326-334, 1989.
40. Babirak SP, Brown BG, Brunzell JD: Familial combined hyperlipidemia and abnormal lipoprotein lipase. *Arterioscler Thromb* 12:1176-1183, 1992.
41. Nevin DN, Brunzell JD, Deeb SS: The LPL gene in individuals with familial combined hyperlipidemia and decreased LPL activity. *Arterioscler Thromb* 14:869-873, 1994.
42. Gagné E, Genest J Jr, Zhang H, et al: Analysis of DNA changes in the LPL gene in patients with familial combined hyperlipidemia. *Arterioscler Thromb* 14:1250-1257, 1994.
43. Melish J, Le NA Ginsberg H, et al: Dissociation of apolipoprotein B and triglyceride production in very-low-density lipoproteins. *Am J Physiol* 239:354E-362E, 1980.
44. Ahrens EG, Hirsch J, Bette K, et al: Carbohydrate-induced and fat-induced lipemia. *Trans Assoc Am Physicians* 74:134-139, 1960.
45. Farguar JP, Frank A, Gross RC, et al: Glucose, insulin and triglyceride response to high and low carbohydrate diets in man. *J Clin Invest* 45:1648-1656, 1966.
46. Ruderman NB, Jones AL, Krauss RM, et al: A biochemical and morphological study of very low density lipoproteins in carbohydrate-induced hypertriglyceridemia. *J Clin Invest* 50:1355-1368, 1971.
47. Cianflone K, Dahan S, Monge JC, et al: Pathogenesis of carbohydrate-induced hypertriglyceridemia using HepG2 cells as a model system. *Arterioscler Thromb* 12:271-277, 1992.

48. Packard CJ, Munro A, Lorimer AR, et al: Metabolism of apolipoprotein B in large triglyceride-rich very low density lipoproteins of normals and hypertriglyceridemic subjects. *J Clin Invest* 74:2178–2192, 1984.
49. Brunzell JD, Albers JJ, Chait A, et al: Plasma lipoproteins in familial combined hyperlipidemia and monogenic familial hypertriglyceridemia. *J Lipid Res* 24:147–155, 1983.
50. Angelin B, Hershon KS, Brunzell JD: Bile acid metabolism in hereditary forms of hypertriglyceridemia: Evidence for an increased synthesis rate in monogenic familial hypertriglyceridemia. *Proc Natl Acad Sci U S A* 84:5434–5438, 1987.
51. Duane WC: Abnormal bile acid absorption in familial hypertriglyceridemia. *J Lipid Res* 36:96–107, 1995.
52. Stalenhoef AFH, Demacker PNM, Lutterman JA, et al: Plasma lipoproteins, apolipoproteins, and triglyceride metabolism in familial hypertriglyceridemia. *Arteriosclerosis* 6:387–394, 1986.
53. Goldstein JL, et al: Hyperlipidemia in coronary heart disease: II. Genetic analysis of lipid levels in 176 families and delineation of a new inherited disorder, combined hyperlipidemia. *J Clin Invest* 52:1544–1568, 1973.
54. Brunzell JD, Schrott HG, Motulsky AG, et al: Myocardial infarction in the familial forms of hypertriglyceridemia. *Metabolism* 25:313–320, 1976.
55. Crouse JR, Parks JS, Schey HM, et al: Studies of low density lipoprotein molecular weight in human beings with coronary artery disease. *J Lipid Res* 26:566–574, 1985.
56. Campos H, Genest JJ Jr, Blijlevens E, et al: Low density lipoprotein particle size and coronary artery disease. *Arterioscler Thromb* 12:187–195, 1992.
57. Coresh J, Kwiterovich PO Jr, Smith HH, et al: Association of plasma triglyceride concentration and LDL particle diameter, density, and chemical composition with premature coronary artery disease in men and women. *J Lipid Res* 34:1687–1697, 1993.
58. Krauss RM: Relationship of intermediate and low-density lipoprotein subspecies to risk of coronary artery disease. *Lancet* 113:578–582, 1987.
59. Watts GF, Mandalia S, Brunt JNH, et al: Independent associations between plasma lipoprotein subfraction levels and the course of coronary artery disease in the St Thomas' Atherosclerosis Regression Study (STARS). *Metabolism* 42:1461–1467, 1993.
60. Krauss RM, Miller BD, Fair JM, et al: Reduced progression of coronary artery disease with risk factor intervention in patients with LDL subclass pattern B (abstract). *Circulation* 86:1–63, 1992.
61. Nordestguard BG, Zilversmit DB: Comparison of arterial intimal clearances of LDL from diabetic and non-diabetic cholesterol-fed rabbits: Differences in intimal clearance explained by size differences. *Arteriosclerosis* 9:176–183, 1989.
62. de Graaf J, Hak-Lemmers HL, Hectors MP, et al: Enhanced susceptibility to in vitro oxidation of the dense low density lipoprotein subfraction in healthy subjects. *Arterioscler Thromb* 11:298–306, 1991.
63. Dejager S, Bruckert E, Chapman JM: Dense low density lipoprotein subspecies with diminished oxidative resistance predominate in combined hyperlipidemia. *J Lipid Res* 34:295–308, 1993.
64. Tribble DL, Holl LG, Wood PD, et al: Variations in oxidative susceptibility among six low density lipoprotein subfractions of differing density and particle size. *Atherosclerosis* 93:189–199, 1992.
65. Chait A, Brazg RL, Tribble DL, et al: Susceptibility of small, dense low-density lipoproteins to oxidative modification in subjects with the atherogenic lipoprotein phenotype, pattern B. *Am J Med* 94:350–356, 1993.
66. Weisser B, Locher R, de Graef J, et al: Low density lipoprotein subfractions increase thromboxane formation in endothelial cells. *BBRC* 192:1245–1250, 1993.
67. Hurt-Camejo E, Camejo G, Rosengren B, et al: Differential uptake of proteoglycan-selected subfraction of low density lipoprotein by human macrophages. *J Lipid Res* 31:1387–1398, 1990.

68. Dyce MC, Anderson TJ, Orav J, et al: The relationship between endothelial vasodilator function and LDL particle size, density and number in human coronary atherosclerosis. *Circulation* (In press).

69. Brown BG, Zhao XQ, Sacco DE, et al: Lipid lowering and plaque regression: New insights into prevention of plaque disruption and clinical events in coronary disease. *Circulation* 87:1781–1791, 1993.

70. Scandinavian Simvastatin Survival Study: Randomized trial of cholesterol lowering in 4444 patients with coronary heart disease: The Scandinavian Survival Study (4S). *Lancet* 344:1383–1389, 1994.

71. Brown BG, Albers JJ, Fisher LD, et al: Regression of coronary artery disease as a result of intensive lipid-lowering therapy in men with high levels of apolipoprotein B. *N Engl J Med* 323:1289–1298, 1990.

72. Stewart BF, Brown BG, Zhao XQ, et al: The benefits of lipid-lowering therapy in men with elevated apolipoprotein B are not confined to those with very high LDLc. *J Am Coll Cardiol* 23:899–906, 1994.

73. Vega GL, Grundy SM: Primary hypertriglyceridemia with borderline high cholesterol and elevated apolipoprotein B concentrations: Comparison of gemfibrozil vs lovastatin therapy. *JAMA* 264:2759–2763, 1990.

74. Marcovina SM, Albers JJ, Kennedy H, et al: Hannon International Federation of Clinical Chemistry standardization project for measurements of apolipoprotein A-1 and B. IV: Comparability of apolipoprotein B values by use of international reference material. *Clin Chem* 40:586–592, 1994.

75. Fredrickson DS, Levy RI, Lees RS: Fat transport in lipoproteins: An integrated approach to mechanisms and disorders. *N Engl J Med* 276:34–42; 94–103; 148–156; 215–225; and 273–281, 1967.

76. Bhattacharya AK, Conner WE: β-Sitosterolemia and xanthomatosis: A newly described lipid storage disease in two sisters. *J Clin Invest* 53:1033–1043, 1974.

77. Ginsberg HN, Le N-A, Short MP, et al: Suppression of apolipoprotein B production during treatment of cholesteryl ester storage disease with lovastatin: Implications for regulation of apolipoprotein B synthesis. *J Clin Invest* 80:1692–1697, 1987.

78. Lussier-Cacan S, Cantin M, Roy CC, et al: Tendon xanthomas associated with cholestanolosis and hyperapobetalipoproteinemia. *Clin Invest Med* 9:94–99, 1986.

79. Sniderman AD, Cianflone K, Eckel RH: Levels of acylation stimulation protein in obese women before and after moderate weight loss. *Int J Obes* 15:333–336, 1991.

80. Maslowska MH, Sniderman AD, MacLean LD, et al: Regional differences in triacylglycerol synthesis in adipose tissue. *J Lipid Res* 34:219–228, 1993.

1 Neuroendocrinology

Introduction

A major thrust in the laboratory this past year or so has been the definition of mutations that are involved in the pathogenesis of pituitary tumors, spurred by the success of defining the *gsp* mutation in 30% to 40% of patients with acromegaly. Mutations are being sought at all levels, starting with the regulation of secretion of the various releasing and inhibitory factors, through the receptors and various transduction mechanisms for these factors, and finally transcription factors. The roles of proto-oncogenes and tumor suppressors are also being explored. It is likely that multiple defects will be found. I have chosen a few representative articles to illustrate the types of approaches that are being taken (Abstracts 112-95-1–9, 112-95-1–10, and 112-95-1–11) and discuss a few more in my commentary to them.

The use of GH as therapy in adults is still under considerable investigation. The diagnosis of GH deficiency in adults must therefore be scrutinized (Abstract 112-95-1–1) as well as the type of therapy—GH vs. IGF-I (Abstract 112-95-1–3)—and the risks of therapy (Abstract 112-95-1–2).

Some large prolactinomas clearly enlarge during pregnancy. But now we learn that a GH-secreting tumor may also do so (Abstract 112-95-1–4). Therapy is still being worked out. A new, long-acting dopamine agonist, cabergoline (Abstract 112-95-1–8), has been found to be remarkably effective, but its prospects in the United States are uncertain at present. More information about the use of octreotide continues to come forth as well (Abstracts 112-95-1–5, 112-95-1–6, and 112-95-1–7). An article by Arafah and colleagues (Abstract 112-95-1–17) detailing the recovery of pituitary function after surgery will be of interest, as will an article indicating a very high risk of gliomas after pituitary irradiation (Abstract 112-95-1–16).

Although MRI continues to give us the best imaging of tumors, problems with specificity continue (Abstracts 112-95-1–13 and 112-95-1–14). I have also included a few miscellaneous items of interest, including hypophysitis associated with craniopharyngiomas (Abstract 112-95-1–15) and the endocrine changes associated with erythropoietin therapy in patients with renal failure (Abstract 112-95-1–17). The chapter finishes with an article describing the search for a mutation causing familial inherited diabetes insipidus (Abstract 112-95-1–19) and the intriguing hypothesis that explains why a mutation in a single allele could cause loss of hormone production.

Mark E. Molitch, M.D.

Growth Hormone

Diagnosis of Growth-Hormone Deficiency in Adults

Hoffman DM, O'Sullivan AJ, Baxter RC, Ho KKY (St Vincent's Hosp, Sydney, NSW, Australia; Royal Prince Alfred Hosp, Sydney, NSW, Australia)
Lancet 343:1064–1068, 1994   112-95-1-1

Background.—The optimal method for diagnosing adult (GH) deficiency has not been defined. Current cutoff values for GH deficiency are either arbitrary or based on pediatric studies; they have no statistical basis because a normal range has never been established. The diagnostic merits of stimulated GH response, 24-hour GH concentration (IGHC), IGF-I, and IGF binding protein 3 (IGFBP-3) in adults with suspected GH deficiency were investigated.

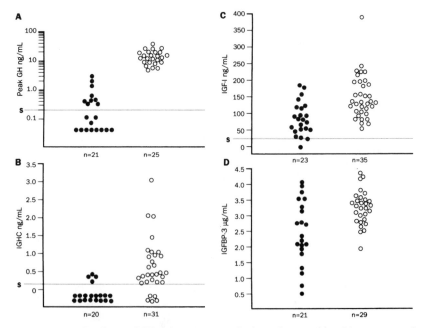

Fig 1-1.—Results of tests of GH deficiency in normal subjects (*open circle*) and hypopituitary subjects (*filled circle*). **A**, peak GH response to insulin tolerance test. **B**, mean 24-hour GH (*IGHC*). **C**, IGF-I concentration. **D**, IGF binding protein 3 (*IGFBP-3*) concentration. Note logarithmic scale for insulin tolerance test. *Abbreviations: S*, assay sensitivity for GH (.2 ng/mL) and IGF-I (25 ng/mL); *n*, number of patients tested. (Courtesy of Hoffman DM, O'Sullivan AJ, Baxter RC, et al: *Lancet* 343:1064-1068, 1994.)

Methods.—Insulin tolerance test, mean IGHC derived from 20-minute sampling, IGF-I concentration, and serum IGFBP-3 concentrations were measured in 23 patients with extensive organic pituitary disease considered GH deficient and in 35 normal subjects matched for sex, age, and body mass index.

Results.—Peak GH response to insulin tolerance test clearly differentiated subjects who had hypopituitarism from normal subjects, with the highest value in the hypopituitary group being 3 mg/mL compared with a range of 5 to 45 mg/mL in normal subjects. Hypopituitary subjects had significantly lower stimulated peak GH, mean IGHC, IGF-I, and IGFBP-3 (Fig 1–1). To overcome the age-related decline in spontaneous GH release, the diagnostic merit of IGHC and IGF-I was analyzed by stratifying subjects by age. Using the upper limit of IGHC established in hypopituitary patients would have wrongly classified 5 of 15 young and 4 of 16 elderly normal subjects as having hypopituitarism. Use of undetectable IGHC as an indicator of organic GH deficiency would have correctly identified 16 of 20 patients and 26 of 31 normal subjects. Thus, the overall predictive value of an undetectable IGHC was 70%, and for elderly subjects, it was 84%. Using the upper limit of young and elderly hypopituitary IGF-I values as a diagnostic cutoff would have correctly classified 10 of 35 normal subjects; the lower IGF-I limits in normal subjects would have identified correctly 9 of 23 hypopituitary subjects. Combining IGF-I and IGFBP-3 measurements did not improve diagnostic accuracy achieved with either measurement alone.

Conclusion.—Adult GH deficiency is most reliably identified by stimulatory testing; IGF-I and IGFBP-3 are poor diagnostic tests for adult GH deficiency.

▶ As Yogi Berra once said, "It's déjà vu all over again." Of course, here we are dealing with adults rather than children. There are a number of additional confounding variables as well, such as age, obesity, and gonadal status. I have alluded to this question regarding gonadal status before (1991 YEAR BOOK OF ENDOCRINOLOGY, p 9; 1993 YEAR BOOK OF ENDOCRINOLOGY, p 4).

In this paper, the patients appear to have had appropriate gonadal hormone replacement. In addition, Dysken et al. (*Biol Psychiatry* 33:610, 1993) remind us of the tremendous intrasubject variability on repeated GH stimulation tests. Therefore, a single negative test must be repeated. Some years ago, Rose et al. (*N Engl J Med* 319:201, 1988) concluded from studies in children carried out at the National Institutes of Health that stimulation tests were better than measurement of spontaneous secretion in diagnosing GH deficiency. The stimulation tests get around the problem that in completely normal individuals, most of the time GH levels are extraordinarily low. Iranmanesh et al. (*J Clin Endocrinol Metab* 78:526, 1994) have shown, using a chemiluminescence assay with a sensitivity down to .005 ng/mL, that in normal men GH levels frequently go down to as low as .18 to .30 ng/mL and that the mean 24-hour GH was in the .4 to .7 ng/mL range in young and middle-aged men, .07 to .3 ng/mL in older men, and .08 to .15 in obese men. It is no wonder that there is considerable overlap between normal adults and hypopituitary adults when looking solely at spontaneous secretion. The resistance of some endocrinologists to performing insulin-hypoglycemia stimulation tests continues to amaze me. These tests are relatively easy to perform, highly reliable, and safe, provided that a physician is nearby to stop the test when significant symptoms develop. I do not perform them in patients older than age 60 years, in those with known cardiovascular disease, or in those with seizure disorders.

Why measure GH levels so precisely in adults? Well, to replace them with GH, of course. The benefits of doing so have been discussed previously (1990 YEAR BOOK OF ENDOCRINOLOGY, p 10; 1992 YEAR BOOK OF ENDOCRINOLOGY, p 7; YEAR BOOK OF ENDOCRINOLOGY, p 8). Rosén et al. (*Acta Endocrinol* 129:195, 1993) remind us of the increased mortality from cardiovascular disease present in GH-deficient patients (1991 YEAR BOOK OF ENDOCRINOLOGY, p 31) and now report that these GH-deficient patients had higher triglyceride and lower HDL cholesterol levels and increased hypertension, all potential cardiovascular risk factors.

Two studies have now evaluated cardiac function in GH-deficient adults before and after replacement. Beshyah et al. (*Eur J Endocrinol* 130:451, 1994) showed that a mildly decreased exercise time increased, and isovolumic relaxation time, a measure of left ventricular diastolic function, decreased significantly with 6 months of GH treatment compared with placebo. Cittadini et al. (*Am J Physiol* 267:E219, 1994) found that resting and exercise-stimulated systolic function (ejection fraction, cardiac index) were markedly impaired, and treatment with GH for 6 months caused significant improvement in these parameters. Thus, there may be added benefits of GH therapy with respect to cardiovascular function.

How about possible adverse effects of GH therapy?—M.E. Molitch, M.D.

Risk of Leukemia After Treatment With Pituitary Growth Hormone
Fradkin JE, Mills JL, Schonberger LB, Wysowski DK, Thomson R, Durako SJ, Robison LL (Natl Inst of Diabetes and Digestive and Kidney Diseases, Bethesda, Md; Natl Inst of Child Health and Human Development, Bethesda, Md; Ctrs for Disease Control and Prevention, Atlanta, Ga; et al)
JAMA 270:2829–2832, 1993   112-95-1–2

Background.—An earlier estimate of a twofold greater incidence of leukemia in GH recipients was based on incomplete databases from Europe and North America. This report presents the incidences of leukemia and lymphoma derived from a study evaluating the risk for Creutzfeldt-Jakob disease and other adverse effects of GH among U.S. National Hormone and Pituitary Program participants.

Methods.—Eighty-four percent of 6,284 GH recipients or their proxies were contacted and interviewed; medical records or death certificates were reviewed for the deceased. Reported diagnoses of leukemia or lymphoma were confirmed by reviewing medical records. Person-years of risk for each subject were established from the date of first GH treatment to the date of interview, death, or diagnosis of leukemia or lymphoma.

Results.—In 59,736 patient-years of follow-up, there were 3 cases of leukemia, which was not significantly higher than the 1.66 cases expected in an age-, race-, and sex-matched United States general population. However, extension of follow-up revealed 3 additional cases, yielding a minimum leukemia rate of 6, which is significantly higher than the expected 2.26. Leukemia was not associated with idiopathic GH deficiency but significantly correlated with craniopharyngioma. Five patients who had leukemia required GH after antecedent cranial tumor; 4 had undergone radiotherapy. Lymphoma was not excessive in this cohort.

Conclusion.—The overall incidence of leukemia is 2.25 times higher among patients treated with pituitary GH compared with the general population. This increase is attributable to patients with antecedent tumors, primarily craniopharyngioma. Whether GH administration, underlying risk factors, or an interaction of the 2 components caused the heightened leukemia rate must be determined. Growth hormone–related malignancy should continue to be evaluated in patients receiving recombinant GH.

▶ In this paper, the specter of an increased risk of leukemia occurring with GH treatment is raised. Actually, it has been raised before, but the data are becoming more unsettling as we progress into an era in which large numbers of adults as well as children may be treated. Although the risk was increased about twofold in this study, 5 of these 6 children had antecedent tumors (4 craniopharyngiomas and 1 astrocytoma) and 4 had had previous cranial radiotherapy. The authors cite studies showing a higher risk of second tumors and leukemia for all patients with brain tumors. Perhaps my more pathologic colleagues (I guess the correct term is pathologists) could help me: Are craniopharyngiomas true neoplasms?

Anyway, in this paper the association with craniopharyngiomas was striking—more than 20-fold higher than would be expected. Two other similar populations have been reported from other countries recently. Job et al. (*Horm Res* 38:355, 1992) reported on 5,418 patients treated with GH in France between 1959 and 1990, finding no increased frequency of leukemia, lymphoma, or other malignancies. On the other hand, Watanabe et al. (*J Pediatr Endocrinol* 6:99, 1993) found 12 cases of leukemia among 16,428 children treated with GH in Japan, resulting in an increased risk of leukemia of 7.8:1. Interestingly, an abstract by Redmond et al. (*Pediatr Res* 31:83, 1992) reports leukemia developing in 6 patients with documented GH deficiency who had never received GH treatment; 4 of these had received cranial irradiation, including 1 who had a craniopharyngioma. The full article has not yet been published as of the time that this comment was being written and a MEDLINE search carried out (1/6/95).

The relationship of GH to neoplasms has been discussed for years. One additional issue is whether GH therapy can cause an increase in the relapse rate of the brain tumors for which the surgery/irradiation was initially given. Ogilvy-Stuart et al. (*BMJ* 304:1601, 1992) reported that of 207 children treated for brain tumor, 47 of whom received GH, and of 161 children with acute lymphoblastic leukemia, 15 of whom were treated with GH, there was no increase in tumor recurrence associated with GH therapy. However, Bourguignon et al. (*Lancet* 341:1505, 1993) reported that GH therapy of 19 patients caused a twofold increased growth rate of melanocytic nevi. These authors noted no neoplasms or malignant transformation of these nevi and stated that there are no reports of increased frequency of skin tumors in GH-treated or acromegalic patients, but we should all be careful about watching such nevi in our patients. The increased risk of malignancies in patients with acromegaly has been mentioned previously, and the role of GH-dependent growth factors acting in an autocrine and paracrine fashion has been discussed (1992 YEAR BOOK OF ENDOCRINOLOGY, p 16).

I think the bottom line is not clear on this subject. Certainly, patients with acromegaly appear to be at increased risk, particularly for gastrointestinal malignancies. Patients treated with GH will have to undergo close scrutiny to determine whether there is truly any increased risk.—M.E. Molitch, M.D.

Effect of Growth Hormone and Insulin-Like Growth Factor-I on Immunoglobulin Production by and Growth of Human B Cells
Kimata H, Yoshida A (Kyoto Univ, Japan)
J Clin Endocrinol Metab 78:635–641, 1994   112-95-1–3

Background.—Growth hormone enhances the proliferation of T cells, erythrocytes, and retinal microvascular endothelial cells in vitro and mesangial cell growth in vivo. It also increases human B-cell immunoglobulin (Ig) production and proliferation in vitro in serum-free medium. Insulin-like growth factor-I also enhances proliferation of myeloid cells, B cells, and thyroid cells in vitro and spleen and thymus growth in vivo. In many patients, GH-induced enhancement is mediated by endogenously produced IGF-I.

Methods and Findings.—The effect of human GH and IGF-I on Ig production by and proliferation of human B cells in serum- and hormone-free medium was investigated. The production of Ig by and thymidine uptake of the human lymphoblastoid B-cell lines CBL and GM-1056 were enhanced by GH and IGF-I, but not IGF-II or insulin. The GH-induced enhancement was not mediated by IGF-I; enhancement was blocked by anti-GH antibody but not by anti-IGF-I antibody or anti-IGF-I receptor antibody. By contrast, anti-IGF-I antibody and anti-IGF-I receptor antibody but not anti-GH antibody blocked IGF-I-induced enhancement. In addition, GH and IGF-I increased Ig production by and proliferation of the cell lines CESS, GM-1500, SKW, and GM-3332. Growth hormone and IGF-I increased production of IgG_1, IgG_2, IgG_3, IgG_4, IgA_1 IgA_2, and IgM by and thymidine uptake of tonsillar B cells stimulated with *Staphylococcus aureus* Cowan strain I. The

GH-induced increase was blocked by anti-GH antibody. The IGF-I-induced enhancement was blocked by anti-IGF-I antibody or anti-IGF-I receptor antibody but not vice versa.

Conclusion.—Both GH and IGF-I enhance Ig production by and proliferation of B-cell lines and B cells. By contrast, IGF-II and insulin do not. Growth hormone and IGF-I did not mediate one another.

▶ These experiments continue the investigations in the GH/IGF-I–immune axis. In previous studies, GH and IGF-I were reported to be produced by B lymphocytes, IGF-I was said to be chemotactic to T lymphocytes, and GH was reported to stimulate natural killer cell activity (see 1991 YEAR BOOK OF ENDOCRINOLOGY, p 9; 1992 YEAR BOOK OF ENDOCRINOLOGY, p 5). On the other hand, neutrophil chemotaxis is decreased in patients with acromegaly (Fornair et al. *Eur J Endocrinol* 130:463, 1994). The clinical relevance of all this and whether GH supplements will help postoperative or immunosuppressed patients still remain uncertain.

The effects of GH vis-à-vis IGF-I are still being worked out (see 1990 YEAR BOOK OF ENDOCRINOLOGY, p 51; 1992 YEAR BOOK OF ENDOCRINOLOGY, p 7; 1993 YEAR BOOK OF ENDOCRINOLOGY, p 6). In contrast to the report of Rosén et al. (*Acta Endocrinol* 129:195, 1993), Cuneo et al. (*Metabolism* 24:1519,1993) found that patients with GH deficiency have not only elevated triglycerides and lowered HDL cholesterol levels but also elevated LDL cholesterol levels; GH treatment decreased the elevated LDL cholesterol levels but caused no increase in HDL cholesterol levels. However, these lipid changes were not correlated with changes in IGF-I levels.

When GH and IGF-I therapy were compared directly in GH-deficient patients, Hussain et al. (*J Clin Invest* 94:1126, 1994) found that both therapies promoted lipolysis and lipid oxidation, but IGF-I does this via suppression of endogenous insulin secretion whereas GH does this by directly enhancing the activity of hormone-sensitive lipase. Interestingly, when IGF-I was given to normal individuals by this group (Hussain et al: *J Clin Invest* 92:2249, 1993), insulin secretion was reduced, glucose tolerance was unaltered, protein oxidation was reduced, and resting energy expenditure and lipid oxidation were increased. Gee, when looking at this grouping of effects, it makes me wonder whether IGF-I would be a good treatment for patients with NIDDM or impaired glucose tolerance.—M.E. Molitch, M.D.

Visual Loss in Pregnant Women With Pituitary Adenomas
Kupersmith MJ, Rosenberg C, Kleinberg D (New York Univ, New York)
Ann Intern Med 121:473–477, 1994   112-95-1–4

Objective.—Women with pituitary adenomas may have loss of vision develop during pregnancy either because the adenoma enlarges or because the pituitary gland itself naturally increases in size during pregnancy, putting pressure on the optic system. The results of high-resolution CT and MRI to study the relationship between tumor size and vision loss during pregnancy were reported.

Methods.—Sixty-six pregnant patients (aged 21–38 years) with previously untreated pituitary adenomas underwent neuroimaging analysis. Prospective visual and ocular motor data were collected, and PRL levels were measured. One patient, who had her pregnancies terminated, was excluded from the study.

Results.—In 111 pregnancies, visual field defects were detected in 11 of 12 eyes of 6 patients, although visual acuity was 20/30 or better in all eyes but 1. Color vision acuity decreased in 1 eye. Eight patients had adenomas 1.2 cm or larger; 6 of these had vision loss. Four were successfully treated with bromocriptine and 2 with transsphenoidal adenomectomy. The 57 patients who had adenomas with a vertical height of 1.0 cm or less had no vision loss.

Conclusion.—Patients with adenomas larger than 1.2 cm have a high risk of vision loss developing during pregnancy and need to be followed carefully with visual field examinations during pregnancy.

▶ You may wonder why I have included this article in the growth hormone section and not in the prolactin section. Molitch must be confused again! To me, the most interesting facet of this article, which otherwise really doesn't say much new, was the fact that 1 patient whose tumor enlarged had acromegaly with a tumor that produced only GH and not PRL. I don't think that this has been reported previously, and the authors did not highlight this aspect. As for the rest of the patients, the rather high frequency of field defects in the patients with macroadenomas may, in part, reflect some selection bias in that these were patients selected from neuro-ophthalmology and not endocrinology records. If I have a patient with a 1.3-cm prolactinoma that extends inferiorly into the sphenoid sinus and has no suprasellar extension, I do not routinely get visual fields, even when pregnancy is anticipated. On the other hand, I probably would obtain them each trimester in such a patient.

In other studies, Nyquist et al. (*Neurosurgery* 35:179, 1994) found that 73% of acromegalic patients with tumors that contained both GH and PRL were women, whereas only 43% of tumors that stained for GH occurred in women. Of greater clinical importance was the fact that 78% of the GH-only tumors were "cured" (GH < 5 ng/mL) by surgery, whereas only 21% of the combined GH-PRL tumors were "cured" using this criterion. This was not because of significantly higher GH or IGF-I levels in the GH-PRL patients preoperatively nor because of larger size or greater invasiveness of these tumors. It is not clear from their analysis how many GH-PRL patients had normalization of PRL levels despite persistently elevated GH levels after surgery, but the mean preoperative to postoperative change for GH was only 79.8 to 67.2 ng/mL, but for PRL, it was 40.2 to 8.4 ng/mL. One issue that was not looked at was the electron microscopic appearance of the GH-PRL tumors to determine their cells of origin. The GH-PRL tumors may be acidophil stem cell adenomas, mammosomatotroph adenomas, or combined somatotroph-lactotroph adenomas and may be sparsely or densely granulated. Careful delineation of tumor type in this fashion may show that some are more amenable to surgical cure than are others. The trick will be to sort these tumor types out clinically before surgery.

Previous studies have been conflicting as to whether the increased GH pulse frequency seen in patients with acromegaly returns to normal or not (1991 YEAR BOOK OF ENDOCRINOLOGY, p 11), but the data have been problematic as a result of the relatively poor sensitivities of the assays. This question has been readdressed by Ho et al. (*J Clin Endocrinol Metab* 88:1403, 1994) using a more sensitive assay, who found the pulse frequency went down to a level intermediate between that found preoperatively and that found in normal controls matched for age, sex, and body weight. These studies are still inconclusive, I think, with respect to settling the issues surrounding the pathogenesis of acromegaly.

Is excessive sweating in acromegalic patients the result of GH or IGF-I? Main et al. (*J Clin Endocrinol Metab* 77:821, 1993) have shown that patients with GH insensitivity syndrome (Laron-type dwarfism) have greatly decreased sweating, implying that this phenomenon is mediated by IGF-I rather than by GH.—M.E. Molitch, M.D.

Effects of Octreotide on Insulin-Like Growth Factor I and Metabolic Indices in Growth Hormone–Treated Growth Hormone–Deficient Patients

Laursen T, Jørgensen JOL, Orskov H, Møller J, Harris AG, Christiansen JS (Aarhus Kommunehospital, Denmark; Cedars-Sinai Med Ctr, Los Angeles)
Acta Endocrinol 129:399–408, 1993   112-95-1–5

Objective.—In addition to inhibiting GH secretion, octreotide inhibits hepatic or peripheral IGF-I generation in animals. These observations were studied in patients with GH deficiency. Whether octreotide used for the treatment of acromegaly causes a greater change in IGF-I action than could be explained by simply decreasing GH levels was tested.

Methods.—Ten patients with GH deficiency were studied during 2 occasions with at least a 4-week interval. In 5 patients, regular GH therapy was discontinued 3 days before each study. For both occasions, the patients received subcutaneous (sc) injection of GH (3 IU/m²) at 6 PM. In a single-blinded manner, the patients were randomly assigned to receive continuous 38-hour sc infusion of 200 μg/24 hour of octreotide or saline. Blood was sampled frequently.

Results.—The pharmacokinetics of exogenous human GH were identical during continuous sc infusion of either octreotide and placebo on the 2 occasions. Growth hormone administration significantly increased serum IGF-I levels, but the increase was similar during infusion of octreotide (from 85.3 to 174.25 mU/L) and placebo (from 97.0 to 158.8 mU/L for placebo). Likewise, GH administration caused identical increases in IGF binding protein 3 (IGFBP-3) during octreotide and placebo infusion. Octreotide infusion significantly lowered mean serum insulin levels and inversely increased IGFBP-1 levels. Blood glucose levels increased significantly during octreotide infusion, whereas levels of lipid intermediates were identical during octreotide and placebo infusion.

Conclusion.—Short-term continuous sc infusion of octreotide does not directly affect the generation of IGF-I or the pharmacokinetics of exogenous GH in GH-deficient human beings.

▶ The hypothesis that octreotide independently lowers IGF-I levels was generated by the following findings: (1) Those patients with acromegaly seemed to have a disproportionate reduction in IGF-I compared to GH levels than those who were successfully treated with octreotide (see 1992 YEAR BOOK OF ENDOCRINOLOGY, p 17; 1993 YEAR BOOK OF ENDOCRINOLOGY, p 7); (2) rat studies showed that octreotide appeared to decrease IGF-I generation in response to injected GH (1992 YEAR BOOK OF ENDOCRINOLOGY, p 19); and (3) in acromegalic patients, octreotide caused an increase in IGFBP-1 levels. In this study of GH-deficient humans treated with GH, octreotide caused no change in IGF-I generation but did cause a borderline increase in IGFBP-1 levels. I think there is something here. As I said in the 1992 YEAR BOOK, such studies should also be carried out with bromocriptine.

Without question, octreotide improves the morbidity of acromegaly as well as GH and IGF-I levels. As pointed out previously (1992 YEAR BOOK OF ENDO-CRINOLOGY, p 15), sleep apnea is common in patients with acromegaly. Grunstein et al. (*Ann Intern Med* 121:478, 1994) have shown a 50% decrease in respiratory disturbances and a 40% decrease of total apnea time with octreotide along with an improved state of alertness. In a smaller study, Leibowitz et al. (*J Intern Med* 236:231, 1994) reported similar findings along with a decrease in daytime sleepiness and fatigue. Oxygen saturation was improved by octreotide in both studies. Previous studies (see 1992 YEAR BOOK OF ENDOCRINOLOGY, p 18; 1994 YEAR BOOK OF ENDOCRINOLOGY, p 15) have demonstrated benefits of octreotide on various abnormal echocardiographic parameters, and a new case report (Legrand et al: *Eur Heart J* 15:1286, 1994) documents dramatic clinical and echocardiographic improvement with octreotide and subsequent transsphenoidal surgery in a patient with severe dilated cardiomyopathy. What was unique about this case was the before- and after-treatment myocardial biopsies that were done, which showed regression of cell myofibrilolysis with reduced myocytolysis.—M.E. Molitch, M.D.

Morphological Effects of Octreotide on Growth Hormone–Producing Pituitary Adenomas

Ezzat S, Horvath E, Harris AG, Kovacs K (Univ of Toronto; Univ of California, Los Angeles)
J Clin Endocrinol Metab 79:113–118, 1994   112-95-1–6

Objective.—Octreotide is a potent GH-inhibiting agent that effectively lowers circulating blood GH levels in patients with acromegaly. The morphologic changes induced by octreotide on GH adenomas were systemically examined.

Methods.—Eighty-six adenomas from patients with acromegaly who participated in a multicenter, randomized study were studied. Tissue samples from 43 patients who were treated with octreotide for 4 months before transsphenoidal pituitary surgery and 43 patients who underwent surgery without pretreatment with octreotide were studied by histology, immunohistochemistry, and transmission electron microscopy, light microscopy, and ultrastructural morphometry.

Findings.—The preoperative administration of octreotide did not result in consistent morphologic changes in the different subtypes of GH-secreting pituitary adenomas, compared with control adenomas. In fact, other than the higher prevalence of perivascular and interstitial fibrosis in the octreotide group (72%), not 1 cellular alteration could be consistently associated with octreotide treatment. In some octreotide-treated tumors, the morphologic response did not differ from that of untreated adenomas. Necrotic changes were not evident. Acidophilia and GH immunoreactivity were more pronounced in octreotide-treated adenomas, and an increase in hormone granularity was obvious in only 4 of 15 densely granulated tumors and in 2 of 9 sparsely granulated tumors. Decreased cell size was evident in only 4 of 15 densely granulated and 2 of 10 sparsely granulated adenomas, but decreased cell size was not linked with increased granularity. Morphometric studies showed a slight downward trend in the cell and cytoplasm size in all treated tumors and a slight upward trend in secretory granule size in treated sparsely granulated adenomas. Only 2 of 9 sparsely granulated adenomas in the octreotide-treated group displayed significant reduction in cell and cytoplasmic size. There were no significant changes in the sizes of nuclei, secretory granules, or lysosomes between the 2 groups.

Conclusion.—There are no morphologic changes in GH pituitary adenomas that can be consistently associated with octreotide treatment. Octreotide treatment does not eliminate the tumor as successfully as it ameliorates the clinical and biochemical features of acromegaly.

▶ This is really a very nice study. The authors did not know whether the patients had received octreotide when they examined the adenomas, avoiding all possibilities of bias. The differences in morphologic responses to octreotide and bromocriptine (1983 YEAR BOOK OF ENDOCRINOLOGY, p 36) are striking—essentially no morphologic changes were observed after octreotide. However, there is one resemblance to bromocriptine, i.e., the increase in perivascular and interstitial fibrosis (see 1987 YEAR BOOK OF ENDOCRINOLOGY, p 43). This relative lack of morphologic change is in accordance with the clinical findings of only modest tumor size reduction occurring with octreotide treatment. We await the final surgical outcome paper from this study. Based on the morphologic changes, fibrosis may impair rather than help surgical cure.

To which of the 5 types of somatostatin receptors does octreotide bind? You mean you didn't know that there are 5 somatostatin receptors? They belong to a class of receptors that has 7 hydrophobic transmembrane domains with amino acid homologies ranging from 42% to 60% and differing abilities to couple G-proteins and inhibit adenylate cyclase, according to Greenman and Melmed (*J Clin Endocrinol Metab* 78:393, 1994, and 79:724, 1994). Octreotide binds with highest affinity to receptors 2 and 5; receptor 2 was expressed in 9 of 10 GH-secreting adenomas, 5 of 9 nonfunctioning adenomas, and 0 of 5 prolactinomas, and receptor 5 was expressed in 10 of 11 GH-secreting adenomas. They also found that receptor 5 is expressed predominantly in mammosomatotroph adenomas. Eventually, perhaps, knowledge of the somatostatin-binding domains of the specific receptors will allow the development of even more specific analogues for the treatment of acromegaly and perhaps other tumors.

Somatostatin analogue scintigraphy is now available as a diagnostic agent to localize neuroendocrine tumors. In an interesting paper in which it was used in patients with ACTH-secreting tumors causing Cushing's disease, it successfully localized most ACTH-secreting ectopic tumors but not those in the pituitary (EUTOPIC) (De Herder et al: *Am J Med* 96:305, 1994). Interestingly, this technique also localized a CRH-producing tumor and an otherwise occult ACTH-secreting bronchial carcinoid (Weiss et al: *Ann Intern Med* 121:198, 1994). The clinical use of octreotide in the treatment of Cushing's disease has been discussed previously (see 1991 YEAR BOOK OF ENDOCRINOLOGY, p 18; 1994 YEAR BOOK OF ENDOCRINOLOGY, p 24). In a recent report, Fornari et al. found that octreotide inhibited CRH-stimulated ACTH release from pituitary adenomas in vitro but not in vivo from the same adenomas (*Eur J Endocrinol* 130:125, 1984).—M.E. Molitch, M.D.

A Comparison of Octreotide, Bromocriptine, or a Combination of Both Drugs in Acromegaly
Fløgstad AK, Halse J, Grass P, Abisch E, Djøseland O, Kutz K, Bodd E, Jervell J (Natl Hosp, Oslo, Norway; Sandoz Pharma Ltd, Basel, Switzerland)
J Clin Endocrinol Metab 79:461–465, 1994   112-95-1-7

Objective.—The pharmacokinetics, pharmacodynamics, and tolerability of bromocriptine and octreotide, administered both individually and in combination, were studied in 12 patients with acromegaly.

Methods.—The patients received bromocriptine from days 1 through 28. After an initial titration period, bromocriptine, 5 mg orally twice daily, was administered starting on day 8. Octreotide was given at a dose of 200 μg subcutaneously twice daily from days 15 through 42. Plasma bromocriptine and octreotide profiles were obtained on days 0, 14, 28, and 42. The pharmacodynamics of the drugs were assessed by measurements of 12-hour profiles of GH secretion and IGF-I.

Results.—During bromocriptine treatment, both the area under the GH day curves (AUC) and the mean IGF-I levels decreased to 64% of initial values. During octreotide treatment, the AUC for GH decreased to 23% and mean IGF-I levels decreased to 32% of initial values, and these decreases were greater than those during bromocriptine treatment. With combined treatment, the AUC for GH was reduced to 16% and IGF-I to 25% of initial values. This combination was more effective and caused a more sustained suppression of GH than did either drug alone. Coadministration of bromocriptine did not change the pharmacokinetics of octreotide. However, the bioavailability of bromocriptine increased by approximately 40% when administered together with octreotide, compared with bromocriptine alone. Bromocriptine disposition parameters were not altered during combined treatment. There were no serious adverse effects of treatment, and combined treatment with bromocriptine and octreotide did not lead to more serious side effects than treatment with either drug alone.

Implications.—For patients with acromegaly, combined treatment with octreotide and bromocriptine increases the bioavailability of bromocriptine and reduces both GH and IGF-I levels more effectively than treatment with either drug alone. The combination treatment presents the possibility of fewer drug administrations because of the sustained GH suppression and, consequently, lower doses of octreotide and lower treatment costs.

▶ This study is more interesting than the title alone suggests. Although the blood levels for octreotide are completely superimposable with and without bromocriptine, profiles differ. With octreotide, there is a delay of the bromocriptine peak by more than 2 hours, creating a broader and longer peak with a greater AUC. When the GH AUC is inspected more closely, the AUC for the first 6 hours after octreotide administration is the same and very low with and without bromocriptine, but 6–12 hours after octreotide, the level is lower when bromocriptine is added. Thus, the inhibitory action of octreotide trails off after 6–8 hours as its concentration declines, and this is where bromocriptine's inhibitory effect seems to be felt. A similar effect has been shown previously (Wagenaar et al: *Acta Endocrinol* 125:637, 1991). We have all learned that octreotide has to be given at least every 8 hours and sometimes even more frequently. It would be interesting to have these authors repeat this study with the octreotide given every 8 hours to see whether this additive effect of bromocriptine persists. It may well be that a lower dose of octreotide is as effective when bromocriptine is added. Several previous studies have documented that some patients respond better to the combination than to either drug alone (1987 YEAR BOOK OF ENDOCRINOLOGY, p 40; 1988 YEAR BOOK OF ENDOCRINOLOGY, p 37).

What is happening with the long-acting somatostatin analogue preparations discussed last year (1994 YEAR BOOK OF ENDOCRINOLOGY, p 14)? In 1 study, Marek et al. (*Eur J Endocrinol* 131:20, 1994) showed that in 13 patients treated with lanreotide, 30 mg twice per month for 9 months, GH levels decreased from 32 ng/mL to 19.1 ng/mL, and IGF-I levels decreased from 1,193 to 621 µg/L (normal up to 270 to 450, depending on age). Clinical improvement was noted in all patients. In only 3 patients did GH levels fall below 5 ng/mL and in only 2 were IGF-I levels normalized. In a second study in which patients were crossed over from octreotide to lanreotide, 30 mg every 14 days with a 1-week washout, Morange et al. (*J Clin Endocrinol Metab* 79:145, 1994) found a normalization of GH and IGF-I levels after 3 months in 6 of 19 patients. Ten who did not normalize were then treated with lanreotide every 10 days, and GH and IGF-I levels normalized in 7. These studies were done on the Continent.

Across the Channel, lanreotide seems to be called by a different name: somatuline. If I understand these papers correctly, somatuline and lanreotide are both preparations of a somatostatin analogue with the structure D-Nal-Cys-Tyr-D-Trp-Lys-Val-Cys-Thr-NH$_2$ that is dispersed in polylactide glycolide acid-biocompatible biodegradable polymer and made by Ipsen Biotech from Paris; both have the code name BIM 23014. Johnson et al. (*Eur J Endocrinol* 130:229, 1994) found that 30 mg of somatuline given every 2 weeks for 6 months to 8 patients resulted in normal GH levels in 7 patients and normal IGF-I levels in 4. Thus, this appears to be a worthwhile treatment, although the dose may need to be adjusted for various patients. In the meantime, Sandoz appears to be readying a long-acting octreotide preparation. All of the above are welcome news for the many patients with acromegaly who receive subcutaneous injections of octreotide 3 times per day.—M.C. Molitch, M.D.

Prolactin

A Comparison of Cabergoline and Bromocriptine in the Treatment of Hyperprolactinemic Amenorrhea
Scanlon MF, for the Cabergoline Comparative Study Group (Univ of Wales, Cardiff)
N Engl J Med 331:904–909, 1994   112-95-1–8

Background.—Cabergoline, a long-acting dopamine agonist, suppresses PRL secretion and restores gonadal function in women with hyperprolactinemic amenorrhea. The efficacy and tolerability of bromocriptine and cabergoline were compared in a randomized, multicenter trial.

Methods.—Four hundred fifty-nine women with hyperprolactinemic amenorrhea were given cabergoline, .5 to 1 mg twice a week, or bromocriptine, 2.5 to 5 mg twice per day. The drugs were administered for 8 weeks in a double-blind fashion and for 16 weeks in an open fashion. Dose adjustments were made according to response. The patients were followed up for 6 months.

Findings.—Stable normoprolactinemia was achieved in 83% of the women given cabergoline and in 59% treated with bromocriptine. Ovulatory cycles or pregnancy occurred in 72% of those given cabergoline and 52% of those given bromocriptine. Amenorrhea persisted in 7% of the women treated with cabergoline and in 16% treated with bromocriptine. Adverse effects occurred in 68% and 78%, respectively. Three percent in the cabergoline group stopped therapy because of drug intolerance, compared with 12% in the bromocriptine group. The women treated with cabergoline had significantly less frequent, less severe, and shorter-lived gastrointestinal symptoms.

Conclusion.—Cabergoline is a very effective, well-tolerated treatment in most women with hyperprolactinemic amenorrhea. It is both more effective and tolerable than bromocriptine, making it an important advance in the treatment of hyperprolactinemia.

▶ This very large European study group has clearly shown that cabergoline is more effective and better tolerated than bromocriptine. I've been involved in preliminary studies in the United States and would agree with this assessment. We've been able to give cabergoline on a once-a-week basis with really great success. Fortunately, patients unable to tolerate bromocriptine, pergolide, or quinagolide (CV 205-502) because of gastrointestinal side effects experience no side effects from cabergoline. At the moment, further development of cabergoline in the United States appears to be stymied by political problems in the company producing it (Adria Laboratories) and equivocation about further development in the United States by its Italian parent company. Now, things have become even more complicated because of Adria's sale to the Swedish firm, Pharmacia. The new alliance has not yet made a decision about where they want to go with this medication. It can be obtained on a compassionate-use basis at the moment for patients who have macroadenomas who have failed surgery or who are inoperable and who have failed bromocriptine and pergolide.

Although Glaser et al. (*J Reprod Med* 39:449, 1994) reported successful treatment of 9 patients with prolactinomas using quinagolide (CV 205-502) who previously could not tolerate bromocriptine because of adverse side effects (nausea, dizziness, sleep disturbance, hallucinations), my own experience was less impressive. It does work about as well as bromocriptine, but I have not been impressed that its side effects are substantially less. Those patients who are truly intolerant of bromocriptine are usually also intolerant of quinagolide and pergolide. However, it is always worth trying a different drug; some clearly have fewer side effects with different drugs and some clearly respond better hormonally (see also the 1992 YEAR BOOK OF ENDOCRINOLOGY, p 20; 1993 YEAR BOOK OF ENDOCRINOLOGY, p 11). There is yet another drug starting in the pipeline. Roxindol, a nonergot D_2 dopamine agonist that also has 5-hydroxy-tryptamine type 1A receptor agonist activity and serotonin reuptake inhibitory effects (*Clin Investigator* 72:451, 1994), is made by Merck (Germany). This drug may cause fewer side effects, but it also may not work as well.

A couple years ago, Hattori et al. reported that anti-PRL autoantibodies may be present in the sera of some individuals, possibly affecting their PRL measurements (*J Clin Endocrinol Metab* 75:1226, 1992). In 2 new papers they now clarify the clinical importance of this finding (Hattori et al: *Eur J Endocrinol* 130:434, 438, 1994): (1) the measured PRL was generally lower than the actual total PRL in standard double antibody radioimmunoassays; (2)

PRL levels measured by an immunoradiometric assay (IRMA) assay are generally normal; (3) autoantibodies are present in increased frequency in patients with idiopathic hyperprolactinemia (16% vs. 4.8% with drug-induced hyperprolactinemia, 2.7% with prolactinoma, and 1.3% of 228 normal controls); (4) the proportion of PRL that is IgG bound was 69.5% to 95.9%; (5) PRL levels tend to be higher than those in the usual patient with idiopathic hyperprolactinemia (8 of 12 had levels above 100 ng/mL and 5 had levels above 200 ng/mL); and (6) most had normal menses and no galactorrhea. Thus, in patients with "incidental" (they would have to be if there were no indication to draw a PRL) idiopathic hyperprolactinemia, it may be worth measuring PRL by IRMA or using polyethylene glycol to look for antibodies.—M.E. Molitch, M.D.

▶ Cabergoline is a much longer acting dopamine agonist than is bromocriptine, and in this large clinical study, there were fewer side effects. It will be interesting to see whether patients are compliant when taking medications twice weekly than twice daily.—W.D. Odell, M.D., Ph.D.

Normal Structural Dopamine Type 2 Receptor Gene in Prolactin-Secreting and Other Pituitary Tumors

Friedman E, Adams EF, Höög A, Gejman PV, Carson E, Larsson C, De Marco L, Werner S, Fahlbusch R, Nordenskjöld M (Karolinska Hosp, Stockholm; Kopfklinikum, Erlangen, Germany; Natl Inst of Mental Health, Bethesda, Md; et al)

J Clin Endocrinol Metab 78:568–574, 1994   112-95-1–9

Background.—Dopamine, acting through its type 2 receptor (DRD2), tonically inhibits pituitary PRL secretion and lactotroph proliferation. In addition, dopamine agonist therapy for pituitary prolactinomas reduces PRL secretion and tumor size. Given these considerations, it is hypothesized that functional dopamine uncoupling may release lactotrophs from the inhibitory effects of dopamine and contribute to the development of PRL-secreting pituitary tumors. Such uncoupling may occur by inactivating mutation(s) of the DRD2, and 1 common indicator for an existing inactivating mutation is allelic loss. The recent cloning of the DRD2 and its localization to the long arm of chromosome 11, a region that displays allelic losses in some prolactinomas, allows screening for mutations in this gene in pituitary tumors.

Methods.—Seventy-nine pituitary tumors, mostly prolactinomas and mixed GH/PRL-secreting, were examined for mutations in the coding exons of the DRD2 gene. After polymerase chain reaction amplification, the samples were analyzed for migration abnormalities by denaturing gradient gel electrophoresis, complemented by direct DNA sequencing.

Results.—There were no mutations detected in the DRD2 gene, and all abnormal migration patterns detected by denaturing gradient gel electrophoresis resulted from polymorphisms within the DRD2 gene. Furthermore, allelic losses in the MEN type 1 region in 11q13 were not found in all 5 informative prolactinomas.

Conclusion.—Mutations in the DRD2 gene could not be demonstrated in PRL or GH/PRL-secreting pituitary tumors, and allelic loss of the long arm of chromosome 11 was uncommon in prolactinomas. The role of other proteins in inhibitory signal transduction pathway in pituitary development should probably be directed at postreceptor events.

Invasive Human Pituitary Tumors Express a Point-Mutated α-Protein Kinase-C

Alvaro V, Lévy L, Dubray C, Roche A, Peillon F, Quérat B, Joubert D (Centre CNRS-INSERM de Pharmacologie et d'Endocrinologie, Montpellier, France; Laboratoires Sandoz, France; INSERM U223, CHU Pitié-Salpêtrière, Paris; et al)

J Clin Endocrinol Metab 77:1125–1129, 1993   112-95-1-10

Purpose.—The eukaryotic kinase, protein kinase-C (PKC), serves an important function in transmembrane signaling and influences vital cellular processes such as proliferation. Adenomatous pituitary glands show increased PKC activity and expression, protein expression being highest in invasive pituitary tumors. However, although the increase in expression is about ninefold, the increase in activity is about threefold, suggesting a dysfunction of PKC in invasive pituitary tumors. Investigation demonstrated the overexpression of the PKC α-isoform (αPKC) in human pituitary tumors as well as the presence of a point mutation in invasive pituitary tumors.

Observations.—Expression of αPKC was increased in both the membrane and soluble fraction of 5 human pituitary tumors. On complete sequencing of PKC complementary DNA, 4 invasive tumors had a point mutation that was not present in any of the noninvasive tumors analyzed. Located at position 294, in the V3 region, the observed mutation caused a substitution of a negatively charged aspartic acid by an apolar glycine.

Conclusion.—The α-isoform of PKC may be overexpressed in human pituitary tumors and that may be structurally altered in invasive pituitary tumors. The observed point mutation appears to play an important role in enzymatic function. Given the importance of PKC in regulating cell growth, PKC inhibitors could play a potentially important role as antineoplastic agents.

Ras Mutations in Human Prolactinomas and Pituitary Carcinomas

Cai WY, Alexander JM, Hedley-Whyte ET, Scheithauer BW, Jameson JL, Zervas NT, Klibanski A (Harvard Med School, Boston; Mayo Clinic and Found, Rochester, Minn)
J Clin Endocrinol Metab 78:89–93, 1994   112-95-1–11

Background.—The clonal nature of human pituitary tumors has been demonstrated, indicating that 1 or more somatic mutations may play a key role in the pathogenesis of these tumors. *Ras* proto-oncogenes have been shown to play a role in tumorigenesis, and mutated forms of *ras* proteins have been identified in thyroid adenomas and carcinomas. Although no *ras* mutations have been identified in somatotroph or glycoprotein-secreting pituitary tumors, a mutation in the H-*ras* gene (Gly-Val) at codon 12 in a highly invasive prolactinoma was shown. It is possible that *ras* mutations underlie the development of PRL-secreting pituitary tumors and/or may be a marker for tumor invasiveness and malignant transformation.

Methods.—Fifty-nine prolactinomas, 13 invasive prolactinomas, and 6 pituitary carcinomas were analyzed for activating point mutation in the 3 *ras* genes (N-*ras*, K-*ras*, and H-*ras*) using oligonucleotide-specific hybridization. Synthetic oligonucleotides specific for each *ras* mutation were used as controls.

Results.—None of the 55 oligonucleotide probes detected *ras* mutations in any of the prolactinomas, invasive prolactinomas, or pituitary carcinomas.

Conclusion.—*Ras* mutations are rare in prolactinomas and pituitary carcinomas. The previous finding of a *ras* mutation in a single highly invasive prolactinoma is not representative of a common mechanism in lactotroph tumor formation. In contrast, 20% to 50% of thyroid tumors contain activating *ras* mutations, indicating that *ras* mutations may play a role in a subset of endocrine neoplasms but not in pituitary tumorigenesis.

▶ With evidence now showing that most pituitary adenomas are monoclonal (1992 YEAR BOOK OF ENDOCRINOLOGY, p 10), current approaches now center on efforts to identify mutations that may be involved in their pathogenesis. Thus far, only the *gsp* mutation has been identified in about 40% of cases of acromegaly (1989 YEAR BOOK OF ENDOCRINOLOGY, p 5). These 3 papers nicely illustrate the types of ongoing investigations used to explore this question and give a flavor to the thinking that is involved.

Friedman et al. (Abstract 112-95-1–9) are focusing on a possible defect in a receptor for hypophysiotropic factors (i.e., trying to determine whether mutations exist in the gene for the dopamine D_2 receptor in prolactinomas that decrease responses to normal levels of dopamine). Unfortunately, they did not find one. Those of us who do clinical research and who have been in this business for awhile could have predicted this one, however. A number of studies done more than a decade ago using graded-dose dopamine infusions showed no "resistance" to dopamine in patients with prolactinomas. Because most mutations will likely cause defective function of a given protein product, it is appropriate to look for receptor mutations in inhibitory hypophysiotropic receptors such as dopamine or somatostatin but probably not worthwhile to look for such mutations in stimulatory hypophysiotropic receptors. Mutations in the guanine nucleotide regulatory proteins that couple these stimulatory receptors to intracellular transduction mechanisms have been found, however, such as the activating *gsp* mutation referred to above. There may well be racial/genetic differences in the mutation frequencies in various populations. For example, in Japan, *gsp* mutations were found only in 2% of GH-secreting tumors (Hosoi et al: *Acta Endocrinol* 129:301,1993), whereas this figure is in the 30% to 40% range for Caucasian populations.

Alvaro et al. (Abstract 112-95-1–10) have looked at one of the next steps in signal transduction after the guanine regulatory proteins, i.e. the gene for protein kinase–C, which is a calcium- and phospholipid-dependent protein kinase involved in hormone secretion and cell proliferation, and found an almost 9-fold increase in protein kinase–C gene expression but only a 2.6-fold increase in kinase activity in invasive pituitary tumors. How this would result in neoplastic transformation is another question.

Cai et al. (Abstract 112-95-1–11) used yet another approach, that of looking for proto-oncogenes. These investigators were unable to detect a significant increase in *ras* mutations in prolactinomas, regardless of the invasiveness or whether they were true carcinomas. Mutations in *ras* genes have been found in other neoplasms, including thyroid cancer, serving to convert the *ras* gene into an active oncogene. Pei et al. (*J Clin Endocrinol Metab* 78:842, 1994) found no mutations of the *ras* genes in any pituitary carcinomas or invasive adenomas but did find point mutations of the H-*ras* gene in some metastatic tumor sites.

Yet another gene of interest in pituitary adenomas is that of the transcription factor Pit-1 (1993 YEAR BOOK OF ENDOCRINOLOGY, p 2). Asa et al. (*J Clin Endocrinol Metab* 77:127, 1993), Friend et al. (*J Clin Endocrinol Metab* 77:1281, 1993), Lloyd et al. (*Lab Invest* 69:570, 1993), and Pellegrini et al. (*J Clin Endocrinol Metab* 79:189, 1994) found no abnormalities of Pit-1 in their analyses in pituitary tumors, although there appears to be some controversy about whether Pit-1 expressed in tumors that do not produce PRL, GH, or TSH-β.—M.E. Molitch, M.D.

ACTH

Recombinant Interleukin-6 Activates the Hypothalamic-Pituitary-Adrenal Axis in Humans
Mastorakos G, Chrousos GP, Weber JS (Natl Inst of Child Health and Human Development, Bethesda, Md; Natl Cancer Inst, Bethesda, Md)
J Clin Endocrinol Metab 77:1690–1694, 1993   112-95-1–12

Background.—Inflammatory cytokines can activate the hypothalamic-pituitary-adrenal (HPA) axis. Tumor necrosis factor-α and interleukin (IL)-1, studied in animals and human beings, produce significant toxicity, primarily severe hypotension. By contrast, IL-6 has shown modest toxicity in animal experiments.

Methods.—The ability of recombinant IL-6 to stimulate the human HPA axis was investigated in 5 patients with cancer and a good performance status. The patients were 4 women and 1 man, aged 36–63 years. Injections of IL-6, 30 μg/kg, were administered subcutaneously every morning for 7 consecutive days.

Findings.—Substantial, prolonged increases of plasma ACTH and cortisol occurred on the first day. Blunted ACTH responses were recorded on day 7. However, the overall cortisol response on day 7 was of similar magnitude, suggesting a new equilibrium in the feedback regulation of the HPA axis with chronic IL-6 administration. The toxic effects associated with IL-6 were modest.

Conclusion.—The subcutaneous administration of IL-6, 30 μg/kg daily, had a profound, prolonged stimulatory effect on the human HPA axis. Because its adverse effects are modest, IL-6 may be useful in the clinical testing of the HPA axis as an alternative to the insulin tolerance test.

▶ Most previous experiments showing activation of CRH, ACTH, and cortisol secretion by lymphokines have been performed in animals (1987 YEAR BOOK OF ENDOCRINOLOGY, pp 15 and 49; 1990 YEAR BOOK OF ENDOCRINOLOGY, p 20), but the experiments here were done in human beings. Interestingly, Jones et al. (*J Clin Endocrinol Metab* 78:180, 1994) showed that about 50% of pituitary adenomas of all types make IL-6, where it may serve to stimulate cell growth and proliferation. Complicated. The area of neuroendocrine-immune interaction was reviewed concisely in 1993 by Si Reichlin (*N Engl J Med* 329:1246, 1993).

In reviewing papers for this section, I stumbled across one particularly worthy of comment that compared ACTH and cortisol responses to CRH vs. metyrapone in children with hypopituitarism (*Pediatric Res* 36:215, 1994). What I was taught and have subsequently told now to hundreds of students and house officers is that a full metyrapone test should not be carried out in patients who are severely ACTH-deficient because you could knock out their last remaining bit of cortisol reserve and kill them. In this paper, the kids had even been taken off their glucocorticoid replacement for a minimum of 3 weeks before testing. I just find this a very dangerous situation. Am I wrong? Do others agree? By the way, metyrapone is available again from Ciba-Geigy for use in diagnostic testing. It is now considered to be an experimental medication, however, and IRB approval may be required before you can use it. It can be obtained by writing to them.

Petrosal sinus sampling has been discussed previously (1985 YEAR BOOK OF ENDOCRINOLOGY, p 272; 1989 YEAR BOOK OF ENDOCRINOLOGY, p 16; 1991

YEAR BOOK OF ENDOCRINOLOGY, p 19; 1992 YEAR BOOK OF ENDOCRINOLOGY, p 22; 1993 YEAR BOOK OF ENDOCRINOLOGY, p 21). The new wrinkle this year is extending the sampling catheter into the cavernous sinus itself. Teramoto et al. (*J Clin Endocrinol Metab* 76:637, 1993) showed that the central to peripheral gradient for ACTH increased from a range of 1 to 52 for petrosal sinus sampling to 12 to 111 for cavernous sinus sampling for the same patients. They found that the increased basal gradients were so high that the further stimulation with CRH was unnecessary. Apparently, a new soft, very fine catheter is used and, I suspect, the angiographer has to be pretty slick.—M.E. Molitch, M.D.

General

Pituitary Magnetic Resonance Imaging in Normal Human Volunteers: Occult Adenomas in the General Population

Hall WA, Luciano MG, Doppman JL, Patronas NJ, Oldfield EH (Natl Inst of Neurological Disorders and Stroke, Bethesda, Md; The Clinical Ctr, NIH, Bethesda, Md)
Ann Intern Med 120:817–820, 1994   112-95-1–13

Objective.—The prevalence of focal pituitary lesions consistent with adenoma was determined in 100 healthy individuals 18 to 60 years of age. Magnetic resonance images of the pituitary fossa were acquired in the coronal and sagittal planes before and after the IV administration of gadolinium-diethylenetriaminepentaacetic acid.

Observations.—All 3 reviewers agreed that a normal pituitary was present in 59 of the 100 subjects. At least 1 reviewer found a site of abnormal signal intensity in the pituitary in 21 subjects before contrast administration. Seven others had focal areas of reduced signal. After contrast injection, 41 sites of abnormal signal intensity were found in 34 subjects, 10 of whom had changes interpreted as representing pituitary adenoma in the view of at least 2 of the reviewers. These 10 patients all had normal endocrine studies.

Patient Review.—Of 50 patients with Cushing's disease who had an adenoma identified operatively, 56% had focal areas of low signal intensity on MRI after contrast administration. In 4 instances, however, the site of the adenoma was incorrectly read on the MR study.

Conclusion.—Approximately 10% of normal adults have MR changes in the pituitary that are consistent with pituitary adenoma. Most of these adenomas remain asymptomatic and need not be treated.

▶ It's not so much the finding of abnormalities in 10% of "normal" individuals that bothers me, as this has been found multiple times before by CT and autopsy studies, but the relative inaccuracy of this procedure in making a diagnosis. Here, 3 experienced neuroradiologists at the NIH cannot agree on most of the cases! Of the 42 MRI scans suggesting adenoma after gadolinium as judged by at least 1 radiologist, only 10 of these were judged to be abnormal by 2 radiologists, and only 2 were considered to be abnormal by all 3 radiologists. The Cushing's data are even worse. In another study in which the radiologists were not blinded to the information that all patients had a surgically confirmed ACTH-secreting adenoma, 12 of 16 MRI scans (with gadolinium) were found to be true positives, 3 had MRI findings on the opposite side of the actual lesions, and 1 patient had a false negative MRI (Colombo et al: *AJNR* 15:1591, 1994).

In a study of normal volunteers similar to that done at the NIH, but without the inter-radiologist comparisons, Chong et al. *AJNR* 15:675, 1994) found that the MRI scans of 20 of 52 volunteers contained focal hypointense areas 2–5 mm in diameter compatible with pituitary adenomas.

Where does this leave us? It leaves us with lots of false positives and false negatives, which means that we have to be very sure of our biochemical diagnoses. Fortunately, things sort themselves out. If the diagnosis of acromegaly is clearly established, a negative MRI might suggest doing a GHRH measurement, but, by-and-large, those patients will end up undergoing pituitary surgery regardless of the MRI finding. If the diagnosis of Cushing's disease vs. ectopic ACTH is pretty well established, then with equivocal MRI findings and/or biochemical findings, the patient will need petrosal sinus sampling. Fortunately, few prolactinomas will need surgery and so dopamine agonists suffice regardless of equivocal MRI findings. Equivocal clinically nonfunctioning or gonadotroph adenomas don't really need surgical resection either (but they do need follow-up). Most TSH-secreting tumors are large, and if you have a negative MRI, it is important to separate this from selective pituitary resistance to thyroid hormone. Voilà!—M.E. Molitch, M.D.

Sequential MR Enhancement Pattern in Normal Pituitary Gland and in Pituitary Adenoma
Yuh WTC, Fisher DJ, Nguyen HD, Tali ET, Gao F, Simonson TM, Schlechte JA (Univ of Iowa, Iowa City)
AJNR 15:101–108, 1994   112-95-1-14

Objective.—The pattern of enhancement of the pituitary gland was measured and evaluated prospectively using dynamic-contrast MRI in 30 healthy individuals and 10 patients with sellar pituitary macroadenomas.

Methods.—Dynamic MRI was performed using an image-acquisition process with increased temporal resolution (5–10 seconds) during a bolus injection of gadolinium. An automated method of time-intensity curve analysis was used that allowed relative enhancement time to be calculated quantitatively at fractional temporal resolutions.

Findings.—In normal individuals, qualitative visual analysis revealed a consistent sequential pattern of pituitary enhancement in which the posterior lobe enhanced first, followed by the stalk, and then the anterior lobe. The posterior lobe enhanced earlier than the anterior lobe by an average of 35 seconds. Quantitative analysis showed that the posterior lobe enhanced significantly earlier (mean, 9.8 seconds) than the anterior lobe; the straight sinus, a venous system, enhanced consistently before the anterior and posterior lobes. In patients wth pituitary adenoma, tumor enhancement occurred consistently 9.3 seconds after straight-sinus enhancement, and occurred slightly, although not significantly, before the posterior lobes and significantly before the anterior lobes.

Conclusion.—The sequential enhancement pattern of the normal pituitary gland is consistent with its vascular anatomy. Because the straight sinus rapidly and consistently enhances after contrast administration, it may serve as a reliable reference structure, particularly when pituitary adenomas disrupt pituitary lobar anatomy. Contrary to previous reports, pituitary adenomas enhance earlier than the anterior lobe, suggesting that pituitary adenomas may have a direct arterial (neovasculature) blood supply that is similar to that of the posterior pituitary lobe.

▶ It may be that sequential dynamic studies such as these will provide more definitive information than the more static studies discussed in the previous abstract. The early filling of adenomas is interesting, and the authors postulate a neovascular arterial supply to the adenomas and provide supporting arguments in their discussion based on other angiographic and histopathologic studies. That there is a partial arterial supply to the normal pituitary is clear (1988 YEAR BOOK of ENDOCRINOLOGY, p 53). That it is important is also clear, in light of the common finding of metastases in the pituitary. Whether this arterial supply is of pathogenetic significance, allowing tumors to escape from hypothalamic control, as has been put forward (1990 YEAR BOOK of ENDOCRINOLOGY, p 13), is uncertain. Can tumors be embolized via this route? In other studies, Kucharczyk et al. (*Am J Radiol* 163:671, 1994) found that dynamic MRI with early images was considerably better at diagnosing microadenomas than conventional imaging.

Kobayashi et al. (*Neuroradiology* 36:298, 1994) have tried to evaluate a number of histologic factors with adenoma appearance on MRI. They analyzed the age of the patient, size of the tumor, cell density, and proportion of hormone-positive cells vs. signal intensity by multiple regression analysis and found that the greatest influence on signal intensity was the proportion of hormone-positive cells.

The next new technique is intraoperative ultrasound. Dr. Doppman and colleagues from the NIH are now using intraoperative ultrasound to try to localize pituitary tumors (*Radiology* 192:111, 1994). They were able to visualize 7 of 13 microadenomas but stated that more experience is needed. What we need is external pituitary ultrasound that endocrinologists could do and bill for!—M.E. Molitch, M.D.

The Anterior Pituitary Lobe in Patients With Cystic Craniopharyngiomas: Three Cases of Associated Lymphocytic Hypophysitis

Puchner MJA, Lüdecke DK, Saeger W (Univ Hosp Hamburg-Eppendorf, Germany; Marienkrankenhaus, Hamburg, Germany)
Acta Neurochir (Wien) 126:38–43, 1994   112-95-1-15

Introduction.—Minor inflammatory reactions within the pituitary gland were reported in 7% of a large autopsy series. Extensive infiltration that leads to a histologic appearance typical of lymphocytic hypophysitis has not been previously described in patients with craniopharyngioma. To investigate further, specimens of the anterior pituitary lobe were investigated histologically in 28 patients with craniopharyngioma operated on transsphenoidally.

Findings.—In 3 patients, the anterior pituitary gland was invaded by numerous inflammatory cells, mainly lymphocytes. The histologic appearance was typical of lymphocytic hypophysitis, for an incidence of 11% among patients with craniopharyngiomas located intrasellarly. The inflammation was most pronounced in the transition zone between the pituitary parenchyma and the cystic wall of the craniopharyngioma, giving the impression that the inflammation spread in continuity with the tumor to the pituitary gland (Fig 1–2).

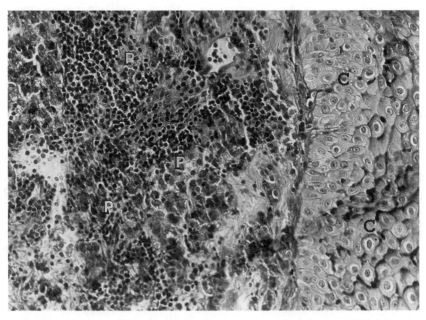

Fig 1–2.—Near the transition zone between the spinocellular craniopharyngioma (C) and the anterior pituitary lobe (P), the concentration of lymphocytes is pronounced, giving the impression of a local induction of inflammation. Periodic acid-Schiff reaction: original magnification, ×340. (Courtesy of Puchner MJA, Lüdecke DK, Saeger W: *Acta Neurochir (Wien)* 126:38–43, 1994.)

The symptoms at diagnosis and preoperative endocrinologic findings did not differ significantly between the 3 patients with associated lymphocytic hypophysitis and the 25 patients without associated lymphocytic hypophysitis. However, after surgery all 3 patients with associated lymphocytic hypophysitis had complete pituitary insufficiency compared with only 36% of those without associated lymphocytic hypophysitis.

Discussion.—Lymphocytic hypophysitis is rare, partly because of failure to systematically examine the anterior pituitary lobe in patients with craniopharyngioma. To date, 60 cases have been reported, mostly in women during late pregnancy or shortly after delivery. The pathophysiologic mechanism appears to be an autoimmune disorder. In contrast, it is hypothesized that inflammation in the 3 study patients was "locally induced" by the cystic fluid of the craniopharyngioma. The additional damage to the anterior pituitary gland by the inflammation may explain the poor postoperative endocrine status in these patients.

▶ The authors postulate that the hypophysitis they are seeing is caused by some chemical irritation from leaking cyst fluid, similar to the meningitis that sometimes can be seen. This is in contrast to the more usual form of lymphocytic hypophysitis, which is thought to be an autoimmune phenomenon. In both forms, however, the hypophysitis appears to be destructive, and these 3 patients had no return of pituitary function after resection of the craniopharyngioma, whereas one third of the patients without hypophysitis had return of function.

There have been a number of other case reports that represent additional variations on this theme. Mau et al. (*South Med J* 87:267, 1984) reported a woman who was seen with partial hypopituitarism post partum with positive antipituitary antibodies who had a completely normal MRI scan. Naik et al. (*J Neurosurg* 80:925, 1994) described another woman who was seen 8 years after delivery with symptoms of hypopituitarism and was found to have a pituitary mass that on biopsy turned out to be hypophysitis. She had had an episode of headache, vomiting, and transient diplopia 7 months after delivery, but these symptoms resolved and she had been well with normal menses until the time of presentation. Could she have had a tumor with apoplexy 7 months after delivery with the subsequent hypophysitis being a reaction to the apoplexy? It has never been reported.

In yet another case, 25-year-old woman had hypopituitarism and diabetes insipidus develop unrelated to a pregnancy and caused by hypophysitis (Paja et al: *Postgrad Med J* 70:220, 1994). This patient may represent yet another example of infundibuloneurohypophysitis discussed here last year (1994 Year Book of Endocrinology, p 40). Incidentally, the pathologist on this last paper is listed as S. Ramón y Cajal. Could this individual be related to the famous neuropathologist of a generation past?

In another case, the mass decreased in size and the hypopituitarism resolved while 60 mg of prednisone was being taken (Beressi et al: *Neurosurgery* 35:505, 1994). Cause and effect? As stated previously, some of these patients get better by themselves without such therapy so cause and effect is hard to prove (1992 YEAR BOOK OF ENDOCRINOLOGY, p 33). Finally, 2 more men have been reported (Lee et al: *Neurosurgery* 34:159, 1994); in at least 1 of these, the infundibulum was involved, as demonstrated by MRI, similar to the above patients with diabetes insipidus, but this patient did not have diabetes insipidus.—M.E. Molitch, M.D.

Glioma Arising After Radiation Therapy for Pituitary Adenoma: A Report of Four Patients and Estimation of Risk
Tsang RW, Laperriere NJ, Simpson WJ, Brierley J, Panzarella T, Smyth HS
(Princess Margaret Hosp, Toronto; Wellesley Hosp, Toronto)
Cancer 72:2227–2233, 1993   1 12-95-1–16

Background.—Cranial radiation therapy has often been linked to the development of brain tumors. The risk of second brain tumors in children treated by irradiation has been studied, but there is little information of this type for patients treated as adults.

Methods.—The risk of secondary brain tumors in 305 adults treated with megavoltage radiation therapy for pituitary adenoma was investigated. This population was considered ideal for study because the treatment volume often involves only small areas of brain tissue and because long-term survival is good. Most patients received postoperative radiation therapy. The radiation dose was usually between 43 and 50 Gy. Records were reviewed for the subsequent development of brain tumors, the risk of which was estimated by calculating the observed/expected ratio.

Findings.—Four patients had gliomas of the brain (table). All these lesions occurred within the previous radiation fields 8–15 years after treatment. All 4 tumors were fatal; treatment was limited by the location of the gliomas and the previous administration of moderately high levels of radiation. The relative risk of brain tumor for the study cohort was 16 times higher than that of the general population. The 10-year cumulative actuarial risk of secondary glioma after radiation therapy was 1.7%, and the 15-year risk was 2.7%. Excess relative risk per Gy of radiation administered was 0.37.

Discussion.—Patients who undergo radiation therapy for pituitary adenoma are at a clinically significant increased risk of subsequent brain malignancy. This increased risk is thought to arise from irradiation, because pituitary adenoma per se does not appear to be associated with glioma. This risk should be taken into account before advising patients with pituitary adenomas to undergo irradiation.

▶ This article is very disturbing. Certainly there have been anecdotal reports of brain tumors developing after irradiation, but the relative risk of 16:1 over the general population shown here is impressive. The authors quote other studies showing that the relative risk for gliomas is 2.6:1 for low-dose irradia-

Data on 4 Patients Who Had Brain Gliomas After Pituitary Irradiation

	Case			
	1	2	3	4
Diagnosis	Nonfunc adenoma	GH adenoma	Nonfunc adenoma	Prolactinoma
Age when radiated (yr)	26	34	42	38
Year	1972	1974	1975	1979
XRT dose (Gy)	45	42.5	50	50
No. of fields (size [cm])	6 (5)	2 (8)	2 (6)	2 (8)
Second tumor (biopsy)	Pontine glioma (not done)	Left temporal glioblastoma (+)	Pontine glioblastoma (+)	Left frontoparietal m astrocytoma (+)
Latency (yr)	10	10	15	8
Treatment	Palliative XRT (to 10 Gy)	Surg debulking and XRT (30 Gy)	None	Surg debulking and I^{125} implant
Occurrence of death (mo)	< 1	19	2	23

Abbreviations: *Nonfunc,* nonfunctional; *XRT,* radiation; *m,* malignant; *Surg,* surgical; +, positive; *I,* iodine.
(Courtesy of Tsang RW, Laperriere NJ, Simpson WJ, et al: *Cancer* 72:2227–2233, 1993.)

tion for tinea capitis and 22:1 for children with acute lymphoblastic leukemia. We are familiar with the high rate of hypopituitarism after irradiation, and last year (1994 YEAR BOOK OF ENDOCRINOLOGY, p 36) this complication was pointed out regarding radiotherapy for all brain tumors. In addition, there may also be an increased risk of stroke (1993 YEAR BOOK OF ENDOCRINOLOGY, p 36). Radiotherapy does work, however, in controlling growth of tumors. Hughes et al. (*Int J Radiat Oncol Biol Phys* 27: 1035, 1993) state that of 108 patients treated with radiotherapy alone, overall tumor control was achieved in 83 (77%), with a mean follow-up of 12.75 years. I think that what they mean by "tumor control" is lack of radiologic (CT) evidence of progression and/or no worsening of clinical signs and symptoms. They have no untreated controls, of course.

I have certainly seen a few patients who have refused all therapy and whose tumors have not changed in size over many years, probably because of fibrosis. In addition to all the above ill effects of irradiation, I also think that irradiation tends to fry people's brains so that they think less clearly. As I think about it, I don't think I have sent a single patient for radiotherapy in the past 5–6 years. I admit I am biased, but the more articles I see like the one cited, the less excited I am about sending a patient for radiotherapy. Certainly, with MRI and CT available, there is no role for routine postoperative radiotherapy if no tumor is visible on scan.—M.E. Molitch, M.D.

Immediate Recovery of Pituitary Function After Transsphenoidal Resection of Pituitary Macroadenomas
Arafah BM, Kailani SH, Nekl KE, Gold RS, Selman WR (Case Western Reserve Univ, Cleveland, Ohio)
J Clin Endocrinol Metab 79:348–354, 1994   112-95-1-17

Introduction.—Patients with pituitary macroadenomas that do not secrete PRL commonly have mild hyperprolactinemia along with hypopituitarism, suggesting that hypopituitarism may result from compression of portal vessels. It this is so, hypothalamic control over pituitary function should return immediately after adenomectomy.

Methods.—This hypothesis was tested by evaluation of pituitary function before and after transsphenoidal adenomectomy in 26 ACTH-deficient patients. Twenty-three subjects with normal adrenal and thyroid function served as controls. The ACTH-deficient patients received glucocorticoids, which were withdrawn 36 hours after surgery. All subjects underwent twice-daily measurement of ACTH, cortisol, and PRL.

Results.—In controls, ACTH and PRL levels increased within hours after surgery, returning to baseline over 4 days. The hypopituitary patients showed a 50% decrease in PRL levels within hours of adenomectomy, and this decrease persisted until discharge. In 65% of the hypopituitary patients, ACTH levels increased within hours; all these patients had normal adrenal function by the time they were discharged. The remaining patients required cortisol replacement for low ACTH levels.

Conclusion.—In patients with pituitary macroadenomas that do not secrete PRL, hypopituitarism appears to be reversible and to result largely from compression of the portal vessels and the resulting interruption in delivery of hypothalamic hormones. Hypopituitarism persists in some patients, however, suggesting that ischemic necrosis of the anterior pituitary can limit recovery.

▶ This is how clinical research should be done. The hypotheses are clearly stated, the experimental approach is elegant yet straightforward, and the results are clear. This paper is the culmination of a series of superb papers by Dr. Arafah and his colleagues detailing the recovery of pituitary function after pituitary surgery for large, clinically nonfunctioning tumors (1987 YEAR BOOK OF ENDOCRINOLOGY, p 57) or for apoplexy (1992 YEAR BOOK OF ENDOCRINOLOGY, p 30). It is amazing to see how rapidly ACTH levels increased—within 2–4 hours after tumor resection, even in those receiving exogenous steroids. Levels of PRL declined during this same period from slightly elevated to normal, but only in those who had subsequent recovery of pituitary function. I am still struck by the fact that a hypothalamic or stalk lesion can be large enough to cause a decrease in dopamine reaching the pituitary yet often cause only minimal if any effects on other aspects of pituitary function.

Farnoud et al. (*Virchows Arch* 424:75, 1994) provide some interesting pathologic findings to help explain why neurosurgeons often do not cure patients. They debunk the idea that the tumor compresses normal tissue with the formation of a pseudocapsule. Their staining techniques do not reveal a sharp demarcation between tumor and normal tissue but rather a transition zone in which there is an intermingling of tumor and normal cells. However, this intermingling occurs only on the adenomatous side of the transition zone and not the normal cell side. Thus, a wide surgical margin around each tumor is necessary to remove this transitional zone.

A few years ago (1992 YEAR BOOK OF ENDOCRINOLOGY, p 25), Peter Snyder and colleagues showed that gonadotroph adenomas could be distinguished from truly nonsecreting adenomas with high reliability in women by measuring the FSH, LH, and LH-β responses to TRH. Now they show similar data for men (Daneshddost et al: *J Clin Endocrinol Metab* 77:1352, 1993). As with GnRH antagonists (1991 YEAR BOOK OF ENDOCRINOLOGY, p 22), the GnRH analogue, nafarelin, had no effect on shrinking such tumors (Colombo et al: *Eur J Endocrinol* 130:339, 1994). Perhaps one reason gonadotroph tumors do not respond to GnRH agonists and antagonists is that they do not express GnRH receptors. Alexander and Klibanski (*J Clin Invest* 93:2332, 1994) found that many such tumors do not express the receptor and that this is detectable clinically by the response to pulsatile GnRH stimulation. Unfortunately, this does not explain everything, in that many of the tumors that have hormone responses to GnRH agonists and antagonists still have no change in tumor size.—M.E. Molitch, M.D.

The Effects of Corticotropin and Growth Hormone Releasing Hormones on Their Respective Secretory Axes in Chronic Hemodialysis Patients Before and After Correction of Anemia With Recombinant Human Erythropoietin

Ramirez G, Bittle PA, Sanders H, Rabb HAA, Bercu BB (James A Haley VA Hosp, Tampa, Fla; Univ of South Florida, Tampa)
J Clin Endocrinol Metab 78:63–69, 1994   1 1 2-95-1–18

Background.—Endocrine abnormalities in patients on long-term hemodialysis are partly corrected by controlling anemia with recombinant human erythropoietin (rHu-EPO). After such correction, changes occur in hypothalamic-pituitary secretion in thyroidal and gonadal axes. Abnormalities in adrenocortical and GH responses may also be altered by rHu-EPO.

Methods.—Responses to the administration of 2 hypothalamic hormones (GHRH and ovine CRH) were studied in 5 men with anemia on chronic hemodialysis before and after anemia correction with rHu-EPO. Five age-matched healthy male volunteers were also tested.

Findings.—Compared with healthy volunteers, the patients had high basal GH levels, an exaggerated GH response to exogenous GHRH, elevated IGF-I levels, and increased concentrations of IGF-I binding protein-3. The 2 groups had comparable ACTH responses to CRH. The cortisol response to endogenous ACTH release was prolonged. Cortisol binding globulin in patients was similar to that in volunteers. Basal increases in GH were no longer seen after anemia was corrected, but the exaggerated response of GH to exogenous GHRH continued. In patients, IGF-I and IGF-I binding protein-3 concentrations remained high. The ACTH response to CRH was normal before anemia correction, then increased. However, prolonged cortisol response continued.

Conclusion.—In patients on long-term hemodialysis, controlling anemia with rHu-EPO can partly correct perturbations in the GH secretory axis. However, this treatment may result in new abnormalities in the CRH-ACTH axis.

▶ In a previous paper, this group found that EPO resulted in a normalization of low free T_4 and T_3 levels, elevated PRL levels, and depressed FSH levels, with an improvement but not normalization of low testosterone levels (1993 YEAR BOOK OF ENDOCRINOLOGY, p 28). This all sounds very good, but have others had the same experience? Yes and no. Bommer et al. (*Nephrol Dial Transplant* 5:204, 1990) and Watschinger et al. (*Horm Res* 36:22, 1991) found no improvement in elevated PRL levels with EPO, but Schaefer et al. (*Int J Artif Organs* 12:445, 1989) did. Furthermore, Bernini et al. (*Nephron* 65:522, 1993) found no effect of EPO acutely on PRL secretion in normal individuals.

With respect to gonadal function, neither Bommer et al. nor Watschinger et al. found improvement in testosterone or FSH levels. Although Watschinger et al. also found low free T_4 levels, they did not find any change with EPO. Tomodo et al. (*Nephron* 66:307, 1994) found that there indeed was an improvement in free T_4 and T_3 levels, but it only occurred in those individuals responding to the EPO with a significant increase in hematocrit. I guess not all patients respond to EPO with an increase in hematocrit, but for most it makes a real difference.—M.E. Molitch, M.D.

Posterior Pituitary

Familial Neurohypophyseal Diabetes Insipidus Associated With a Signal Peptide Mutation

McLeod JF, Kovács L, Gaskill MB, Rittig S, Bradley GS, Robertson GL (Northwestern Univ, Chicago; Comenius Univ, Bratislava, Slovakia; Univ of Aarhus, Denmark)

J Clin Endocrinol Metab 77:599A–599G, 1993   112-95-1–19

Background.—Linkage studies in 3 kindreds with familial neurohypophyseal diabetes insipidus (FNDI) provide strong circumstantial evidence that exon 2 mutations of the gene that codes for the vasopressin-neurophysin-II (VP-NPII) are responsible for FNDI (Fig 1–3). However, alleles associated with these mutations are not present in affected members in 5 other FNDI kindreds. Detailed clinical and molecular genetic studies of arginine vasopressin (AVP) function were performed in 1 of these latter kindreds, and preliminary evidence was provided for the same genetic mutation in 2 others.

Patients.—Thirty-five members from 3 generations of a white American kindred in which FNDI is segregating were studied. In addition, 2 affected members from a Danish and an American kindred in which FNDI is segregating in an autosomal dominant mode were studied.

Findings.—In the white American kindred, 12 members had polyuria and deficiency of plasma AVP, which progressed in severity over time. Another member had normal urine volume and plasma AVP at age 3 years but had severe plasma AVP deficiency develop at about 6 years of age. For unknown reasons, another man had normal urine volume and

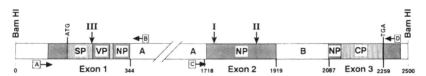

Fig 1–3.—The arginine vasopressin–neurophysin-II (AVP-NPII) gene. The *shaded segments* of each exon indicate the areas that code for specific parts of the vasopressin (VP)-NPII precursor. Exon 1, the signal peptide (*SP*), AVP (*VP*), and the variable N-terminal portion of neurophysin-II; exon 2, the conserved middle portion of neurophysin and the glycopeptide, copeptin (*CP*). The annealing positions of the oligopeptide primers used for polymerase chain reaction are indicated by the boxes labeled A–D, with the *arrows* indicating primer orientation. The *numbers under the vertical bars* indicate nucleotide positions. The *vertical arrows and roman numerals* indicate the location of mutations associated with familial neurohypophyseal diabetes insipidus in the previous (I and II) and present studies (III). (Courtesy of McLeod JF, Kovács L, Gaskill MB, et al: *J Clin Endocrinol Metab* 77:599A–599G, 1993.)

osmolality despite severe AVP deficiency and a history of severe polyuria during childhood and adolescence. From 1 affected member, full-length nucleotide sequences were determined from 12 distinct genomic clones of exon 1 and 10 clones of exon 2/3. There were no abnormalities in exon 2/3, the area in which mutations were previously identified in other kindreds with FNDI. However, 7 of 12 clones of exon 1 contained a substitution of adenosine for guanosine in the first nucleotide of the codon for amino acid 19, predicting a substitution of threonine for alanine at the propeptide cleavage site between the signal peptide and the first amino acid of vasopressin. By restriction analysis, this mutation was present in all 14 affected members but in none of the 41 unrelated controls or 19 adult members with normal urine volumes and plasma or urinary AVP. The mutation was also present in 2 infants with normal AVP secretion at ages 6 and 9 months. When these 2 infants and another child with apparently normal AVP secretion were assigned an indeterminate phenotype, the lod score for association of the FNDI phenotype attained a maximum of 5.70 at $0 = 0.0$, indicating that this mutation was very close, if not identical, to that lesion responsible for FNDI in this kindred. The same mutation was also present in 2 affected members of unrelated FNDI kindreds in Denmark and America.

Conclusion.—It is hypothesized that a mutation in exon 1 of the VP-NPII gene causes FNDI in this kindred by making an abnormally processed precursor that gradually destroys vasopressinergic neurons.

▶ One of the most interesting aspects of this disorder, apart from the identification of the specific mutation itself, is the development of a hormone deficiency from an autosomal dominant lesion. Only 1 allele is affected by the mutation, and therefore 50% of vasopressin should be secreted normally, which is certainly an adequate amount. The authors postulate:

. . . the precursor produced by the mutant allele gradually destroys the neurosecretory neurons that express it. By analogy with the cirrhosis caused by accumulation of denatured peptides in the endoplasmic reticulum of patients with some forms of α_1-antitrypsin deficiency, this incompletely processed VP-NPII precursor could accumulate within the cytoplasm or neurosecretory apparatus of magnocellular neurons, forming large and poorly soluble complexes that eventually destroy the cell.

In their paper they report children with the mutation who went from partial to severe vasopressin deficiency over a 3-year time period. Autopsies in these patients show lack of magnocellular neurosecretory vasopressinergic neurons, which the authors postulate to have resulted from their degeneration rather than from their congenital absence.

Another form of inherited central diabetes insipidus has been reported by Yagi et al. (*J Clin Endocrinol Metab* 78:884, 1994), in which there is associated anterior hypopituitarism. Magnetic resonance imaging in the 3 brothers reported showed absence of the pituitary stalk, severely hypoplastic anterior pituitaries, and an absent posterior pituitary bright spot in 2, with an ectopic bright spot adjacent to the median eminence in the third. This "ectopic" location of the posterior pituitary bright spot has been discussed previously (1991 YEAR BOOK OF ENDOCRINOLOGY, p 33). Thus, this particular familial defect would fall within the spectrum of midline cleft defects. I wonder what happens to all these kids with congenital hypopituitarism. As an adult endocrinologist, I very rarely have one passed along to me.

Physicians often have difficulty clinically differentiating patients with primary polydipsia from those with partial diabetes insipidus. Dehydration testing or hypertonic saline infusions usually will sort these out, especially when vasopressin levels are measured. However, Moses and Clayton (*Am J Physiol* 265:1247R, 1993) now demonstrate that patients with primary polydipsia actually downregulate their release of vasopressin in response to hypertonicity. Thus, their osmotic threshold for vasopressin release is higher and they release vasopressin at lower rates.

As we have discussed previously, vasopressin has a number of extrarenal actions mediated by different receptors. The V_2 receptor is on the distal tubule, and the V_1 receptor is on vascular smooth muscle and mediates vasoconstriction (1987 YEAR BOOK OF ENDOCRINOLOGY, p 60; 1993 YEAR BOOK OF ENDOCRINOLOGY, p 39). The V_1 receptors, stimulation of which activates phospholipase C and mobilization of intracellular calcium, have been broken down further into V_{1b} receptors, which are involved with mediating the stimulating effect on ACTH, and the V_{1a} receptors, which mediate all other known vasopressin actions. Serradell-Le Gal et al. (*J Clin Invest* 92:224, 1993) report a new, potent, selective, orally active, nonpeptide vasopressin antagonist, called SR 49059, which is specific for V_{1a} receptors. This drug inhibits vasopressin-induced platelet aggregation and pressor activity. Whether this drug or similar ones will have human applications remains to be seen.—M.E. Molitch, M.D.

Suggested Reading

The following articles are recommended to the reader:

Acromegaly Therapy Consensus Development Panel: Consensus statement: Benefits versus risks of medical therapy for acromegaly. *Am J Med* 97:468–473, 1994.
> ▶ It is not clear to me how this panel was organized, but their approach is reasonable. Surgery is primary. Medical therapy is secondary, the choices being dopamine agonists or octreotide. Irradiation fits in there somehow.

Aguilera G: Regulation of pituitary ACTH secretion during chronic stress. *Front Neuroendocrinol* 15:321–350, 1994.
> ▶ A thorough review of this subject from the experimental animal's perspective.

Allen DB, Brook CGD, Bridges NA, et al: Therapeutic controversies: Growth hormone (GH) treatment of non-GH deficient subjects. *J Clin Endocrinol Metab* 79:1239–1248, 1994.
> ▶ This is an interesting collection of opinions by noted pediatric endocrinologists, all experts in treating growth disorders with GH, on the uses of GH in children who are not absolutely GH deficient. Highly recommended.

Bertagna X: Proopiomelanocortin-derived peptides. *Endocrinol Metab Clin North Am* 23:467–485, 1994.

▶ This is an updating of the POMC-derived peptides and includes aspects of their measurement in clinical states, including renal failure and Cushing's syndrome resulting from pituitary tumors and ectopic secretion.

Biller BMK: Pathogenesis of pituitary Cushing's syndrome: Pituitary versus hypothalamic. *Endocrinol Metab Clin North Am* 23:547–554, 1994.

▶ In this review, Dr. Biller reviews the controversy surrounding the primary pituitary vs. hypothalamic etiology of Cushing's disease.

LeRoith D, Baserga R, Helman L, et al: Insulin-like growth factors and cancer. *Ann Intern Med* 122:54–59, 1995.

▶ In this review, the various IGFs and other growth factors and their binding proteins and receptors in cell growth are reviewed. The role of these growth factors in the development of breast cancer, osteosarcoma, and Wilms' tumor are also reviewed.

Loosen PT: Cushing's syndrome and depression. *Endocrinologist* 4:373–382, 1994.

▶ The neuropsychiatric manifestations of all causes of Cushing's syndrome are discussed here. An attempt is made at the pathophysiology of the neuropsychiatric symptoms, but this is a very difficult area.

Miller WL: Molecular genetics of familial central diabetes insipidus. *J Clin Endocrinol Metab* 77:592–595, 1993.

▶ The molecular defects causing familial diabetes insipidus are described in this brief review.

Rosenfeld RG, Rosenbloom AL, Guevara-Aguirre J: Growth hormone (GH) insensitivity due to primary GH receptor deficiency. *Endocr Rev* 15:369–390, 1994.

▶ This is the politically correct term for Laron dwarfism. Clinical features, therapeutic aspects, biochemical features, and the molecular biology are discussed.

Saccà L, Cittadini A, Fazio S: Growth hormone and the heart. *Endocr Rev* 15:555–573, 1994.

▶ The effects of GH deficiency and excess on the heart are discussed.

Vance ML: Hypopituitarism. *N Engl J Med* 330:1651–1662, 1994.

▶ This is a thorough review of this topic, including etiologic and treatment aspects. Written for the clinician.

2 Pediatric Endocrinology

Introduction

What has happened since the last installment of the chapter on pediatric endocrinology in the 1994 YEAR BOOK OF ENDOCRINOLOGY? Peace and war continue to be intertwined with Bosnia, Rwanda, the Middle East, and the Republics and dissident areas of the former Soviet Union, choosing one or the other depending on what day it is. These events notwithstanding, I have again placed particular emphasis on the issues of growth and adolescent development. One will note in both the chapter itself and in the Suggested Reading list that I have emphasized a few contributions that have made use of modern molecular biological techniques to not only unravel the precise genetic lesion, but also to give promise to earlier (even prenatal) diagnosis of particular familial disorders. This is not to say that the clinical evaluation is less important but to note that we must have even sharper clinical skills and biological reasoning to put together various signs and symptoms into a syndrome complex to permit proper molecular hypotheses to be tested in the proper biological context.

The first section on growth and GH begins with one of the difficulties in testing children for GH deficiency. Should one use sex-hormone "priming?" Data are presented to show more homogeneous responses if estrogen is used, but what do the results mean for a prepubertal child with growth failure? The GH axis is dissected in the 2 following contributions to note that body composition, probably a metabolic signal from the adipose tissue compartment, has a profound effect on spontaneous GH release. The analogues of GH-releasing peptide are active in children and adolescents and may presage oral and/or intranasal *therapy* for a majority of GH-deficient children.

A number of studies of the growth-promoting activity of GH therapy in children and adolescents with chronic renal insufficiency (CRI) were published within the past year. I have chosen several that emphasize both pre– and post–renal transplantation efficacy of GH therapy to augment the growth rate of slowly growing children with CRI. It should be no surprise that none of the investigations have followed treated children to *measured adult height*. The first report in this subsection reminds us of the inadequate tools that we had before GH to permit children with CRI to meet their genetically programmed target height; however, treatment with vitamin D analogues did represent a major advance in therapy several decades ago.

The section on puberty begins with a short report on the incidence and etiology of precocious puberty at a large clinic in central London; however, our own practices may differ based on the referral pattern of our patients. Two reports follow that are concerned with the heights of children treated with GnRH analogues (GnRH$_a$). The first shows efficacy using the gold standard—*measured* adult height. The second, in children with idiopathic short stature, predicts taller adult height based on 4 years of GnRH$_a$ therapy; however, the critical data—what happens after discontinuation of therapy—are yet to be gathered.

The final 2 reports in this section remind us that the real issues of the endocrinology of puberty involve *bioactive* gonadotropin fractions that may or may not be predicted from the usual gonadotropin immunoassays. It is heartening to note that the newer, third-generation immunoradiometric (and chemiluminescent) assays that can measure gonadotropin fluctuations in prepubertal and early pubertal children more closely track the classical, but cumbersome, biological assays. The report on the development of bone mass and bone density emphasizes the importance of sex steroid hormones (and thus gonadotropins) in the accrual of skeletal calcium.

I close this year's Pediatric Endocrinology chapter with 2 reports on hereditary diabetes insipidus (DI), not because it is an overwhelmingly prevalent problem, but because it points to the power of the molecular tools for families with well-evaluated syndromes of DI. Of course, each type mentioned could have had the pathophysiology noted, but the 2 sets of investigators took their clinically based molecular hypotheses to their logical conclusion.

The final report emphasizes the practical use of potent, *locally* active glucocorticoids to treat children with severe asthma. Remarkable efficacy was demonstrated without the concomitant serious side effects of growth retardation and adrenal insufficiency often noted during systemic glucocorticoid therapy in severely affected children with asthma.

As I close the introductory portion of the chapter, I remind the reader that I take full responsibility for the unbalanced emphasis on growth and adolescent development. These areas have a profound influence on our practice, and the newer developments have great practical value for diagnosis and therapeutics for the children and adolescents under our care.

Alan D. Rogol, M.D., Ph.D.

Growth and Growth Hormone

The Effects of Estrogen Priming and Puberty on the Growth Hormone Response to Standardized Treadmill Exercise and Arginine-Insulin in Normal Girls and Boys

Marin G, Domené HM, Barnes KM, Blackwell BJ, Cassorla FG, Cutler GB Jr

(Natl Inst of Child Health and Human Development, Bethesda, Md)
J Clin Endocrinol Metab 79:537–541, 1994   112-95-2–1

Introduction.—Although GH stimulation tests are used to diagnose GH deficiency, the criteria for diagnosis are controversial. One of the difficulties preventing the definitive establishment of diagnostic criteria is the paucity of research documenting normative data. To document normative GH data exploring the effects of puberty and estrogen administration on GH stimulation tests, 84 normal boys and girls at all 5 pubertal stages performed a standardized treadmill exercise test and underwent the arginine–insulin tolerance test. The tests were performed both before and after 2-day ethinyl estradiol administration in a subset of prepubertal patients.

Methods.—Endocrine function and growth were evaluated and pubertal stage was assessed in 41 girls and 43 boys. All had normal endocrine function and growth. The patients performed a treadmill exercise test, with the velocity and inclination adjusted for age, on 2 consecutive days. The patients fasted overnight between test days. On the second day, they rested in a bed for an hour before the test. Blood samples were obtained at baseline, immediately before exercise, and every 5 minutes after exercise for 30 minutes, and GH levels were analyzed. The arginine–insulin tolerance test (AITT) was performed on the second day, and blood was obtained every 15 minutes for 2 hours to analyze plasma GH and glucose. Eleven prepubertal children were randomly assigned to receive either oral ethinyl estradiol or placebo for 2 days before testing. Six weeks later, they were crossed over to the other protocol and retested.

Results.—The peak GH responses to either exercise or AITT were progressively higher with increasing pubertal stage but did not differ significantly between boys and girls. Using the conventional criterion of a GH peak exceeding 7 μg/L, 61% of the children at stage 1 of puberty, 44% at stage 2, 11% at stage 3, and 0% at stages 4 and 5 would have been considered GH deficient. Estrogen priming significantly increased the peak GH responses to either exercise or AITT. Peak GH response to exercise or AITT also correlated positively with bone age.

Discussion.—Both puberty and estrogen administration significantly affected the results of GH stimulation tests. These data show the inadequacy of current criteria for the diagnosis of GH insufficiency in the early pubertal years, because the conventional criterion of peak GH response was appropriate only for children at stages 4 and 5 of puberty.

▶ Should we or should we not? What do the results mean? There has long been debate on whether pharmacologic tests for GH adequacy in children should be preceded by estrogen priming. The argument is that somatotropes may be sex-hormone dependent, and only those patients whose somatotropes are not awakened by gonadal steroid hormones are truly GH deficient. But what does one do with a 6-year-old child who is failing to grow adequately, has a delayed bone age, low circulating levels of IGF-I and IGFBP-3, low response to pharmacologic stimuli to GH release, and no other definable cause of the growth failure? Even if GH release is augmented by sex steroids, as the results show for the controls in the later stages of puberty, are such children to be treated with sex steroid hormones? The results of this study indicate that in all prepubertal GH-sufficient children the lower 95% confidence limit after sex steroid priming rose from 1.7 to 7.2 μg/L, a value similar to the late pubertal patients.

The real question is what to do therapeutically for those prepubertal children who meet the auxological and "testing" criteria for GH deficiency. It would be prudent to treat them as they are, i.e., with growth hormone and no sex steroids. One will find 10% to 20% of them who, after retesting as adults, will respond to pharmacologic testing as GH sufficient. If the children are at the pubertal age and the bone age is 10 years or above for girls and 11 years or above for boys, one might administer low-dose gonadal steroid hormone and re-measure levels of IGF-I and IGFBP-3. If these rise to the normal range, a longer trial is indicated, with the change in growth rate the most important parameter to follow. The treatment of this variety of patient is controversial, but I believe that a significant number of children experiencing the preadolescent "dip" in growth rate (i.e., with significantly delayed puberty) are not GH deficient but have somatotropes that require sex steroid hormones (probably through an estrogen-dependent mechanism) to function adequately to support the pubertal growth spurt (Metzger et al: *Trends Endocrinol Metab* 5:290, 1994; Mauras et al: *Am J Pediatr Hematol Oncol* 10:9, 1988).—A.D. Rogol, M.D., Ph.D.

Body Composition and Spontaneous Growth Hormone Secretion in Normal Short Stature Children
Abdenur JE, Solans CV, Smith MM, Carman C, Pugliese MT, Lifshitz F (Maimonides Med Ctr, Brooklyn, NY)
J Clin Endocrinol Metab 78:277–282, 1994   112-95-2-2

Purpose.—Abnormal spontaneous GH secretion (SGHS) has been reported in children of normal and short stature as well as in those with other clinical conditions. Previous studies have not considered that body composition may play a role in explaining the observed discrepancies in the SGHS. The relationship between adiposity—measured and estimated—and SGHS was assessed in normal children of short stature.

Methods.—The study sample comprised 37 healthy children referred for evaluation of short stature, which was below the fifth percentile for age in all cases. There were 15 pubertal patients—10 males and 5 females—and 22 prepubertal patients—17 males and 5 females. In addition to a review of their medical histories, all patients underwent a physical examination, relevant laboratory tests, and nutritional assessment, including anthropometry and bioelectrical impedance measurement of body composition. Adiposity was measured as body fat percentage and

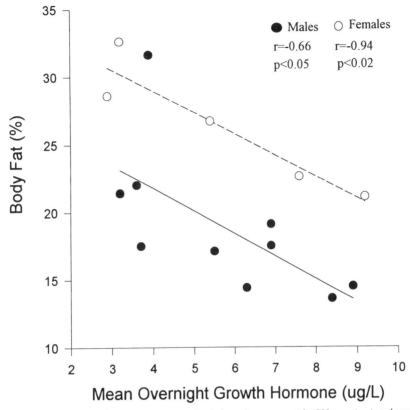

Fig 2–1.—Correlation between percentage of body fat and mean overnight GH secretion in pubertal patients. *Closed circles,* males; *open circles,* females. (Courtesy of Abdenur JE, Solans CV, Smith MM, et al: *J Clin Endocrinol Metab* 78:277–282, 1994.)

body fat mass index and estimated by weight-for-height ratio, body mass index, and body mass index z-score.

Results.—The degree of adiposity had a marked influence on SGHS. The strongest negative correlation was found with measured indices of adiposity. Females needed greater adiposity levels than males before decreases in SGHS occurred (Fig 2–1). Attenuation of mean SGHS was associated with changes in the amplitude of GH pulses in pubertal children and with the number of pulses in prepubertal children.

Conclusion.—In the assessment of children of short stature, interpretation of SGHS values must consider not only pubertal status but also body composition and sex. In a patient with mildly increased body fat, SGHS levels that appear decreased may actually be normal; in a lean patient, apparently normal SGHS values may actually be decreased. Larger studies will provide confidence intervals for use in defining the normal values of SGHS according to body composition and gender.

▶ How accurately does the pattern of SGHS reflect the "growth hormone status" of an individual child? Although some investigators have attempted to use cutoff levels for mean GH level, there is enough variability among normally growing children (and values well below these standards) that it is very difficult to determine whether slowly growing children with diminished (by these standards) GH release are in fact GH deficient or might respond to GH therapy with not only an augmented growth rate but also an increased adult height.

There are many players in the GH axis, e.g., GH, GH-binding protein, IGF-I, IGF binding proteins, and the GH and IGF receptors, to preclude any simple relationship between spontaneous GH release, growth rate, and adult height. Abdenur and co-workers add an important caveat with reference to body composition. Using a crude measure of body composition, the body mass index [weight (kg) divided by height^2 (m^2)], 2 groups of investigators have noted a highly significant negative correlation between mean *normal range* (Rose et al: *J Clin Endocrinol Metab* 73:428, 1991; Martha Jr et al: *J Clin Endocrinol Metab* 74:336, 1992). Abdenur and co-workers have taken the analysis to the next level in evaluating short children whose body fat percentage was based on a more accurate method, bioelectrical impedance, than just using the body mass index. The inverse correlations between body fat [(%) most within the normal range and mean overnight GH concentration] are striking—$r = -0.94$ in females and $r = -0.66$ in males—making the point that in children of normal short stature, the spontaneous GH secretion is *greatly influenced* by the degree of adiposity. In addition to many of the well-known factors that regulate the GH system, e.g., GH itself, IGF-I, and glucose, one must add the dominant negative influence of a metabolic signal that is proportional to the relative fat composition of the body.

Despite the low levels of GH, most obese children are tall for their calendar age but have an advanced bone age. It is quite the opposite for a small, delayed GH-deficient child despite similarly low GH levels. The more we isolate one component of the GH-IGF-I axis, often the less we really know. However, once a diagnosis of GH deficiency (or subsufficiency) is made, one must consider the individual child, that is, auxology, far more than any single laboratory value.—A.D. Rogol, M.D., Ph.D.

Growth Hormone–Releasing Activity of Growth Hormone–Releasing Peptide-1 (A Synthetic Heptapeptide) in Children and Adolescents
Laron Z, Bowers CY, Hirsch D, Almonte AS, Pelz M, Keret R, Gil-Ad I (Tel Aviv Univ, Israel; Tulane Med School, New Orleans, La; Rafa Pharmaceutical Labs, Jerusalem)
Acta Endocrinol 129:424–426, 1993   112-95-2-3

Background.—Recently, synthesized small GH-releasing peptides (GHRPs), consisting of 6 or 7 amino acids, have been found to release GH specifically in several animal species and in human beings. Studies in normal adults have shown that GHRPs release human GH (hGH) more effectively than GHRH. The small previous experience with GHRPs in children was extended by studying children and adolescents with known normal or abnormal GH secretion.

Methods.—Twenty-three patients received the heptapeptide GHRP-1 as a 1-μg/kg IV bolus. Fifteen of the patients were short but healthy children, 9 pubertal and 6 prepubertal. The other 8 were juvenile males with pituitary insufficiency: 4 had isolated GH deficiency, 2 had multiple pituitary hormone deficiencies, and 1 each had partial GH deficiency and GHRH deficiency. An intravenous GHRH (1–29) test was performed in 11 patients.

Results.—In response to GHRP-1, all the healthy children showed a progressive increase in plasma hGH. The hGH increase, which peaked at 15 to 30 minutes, was significantly greater in the pubertal children. Healthy children tested by GHRH (1–29) showed similar or slightly higher peak responses. In 6 of the hypopituitary patients, there was no response to either GHRP-1 or GHRH. The patient with partial GH deficiency showed an hGH peak of 6.5 μg/L 5 minutes after GHRP-1 and an hGH peak of 9.2 μg/L 15 minutes after GHRH. The remaining hypopituitary patient had no hGH response to hypoglycemia, clonidine, or GHRP-1, although his plasma hGH level increased to 10 μg/L in response to GHRH. Administration of GHRP-1 was followed by a significant increase in plasma free T_4 and a decrease in TSH, although both of these values remained within normal limits. Plasma cortisol increased transiently, whereas plasma PRL, LH, and FSH were unchanged.

Conclusion.—Intravenous bolus administration of GHRP-1 effectively and rapidly releases hGH in children and adolescents. The effect is similar to that obtained with intravenous GHRH, although there is evidence that the mechanisms of these 2 peptides differ—GHRP may act at least partially on the hypothalamus. As a potent GH-releasing drug that also acts when administered orally, GHRP-1 has potentially great pharmaceutical and clinical applications.

▶ What's new in the GH axis? Perhaps most promising from a therapeutic point of view for both children and adults is the clinical investigation of GHRPs. Although not all are peptides (some are organic compounds), they all have the property of GH release from the anterior pituitary, whether administered intravenously, subcutaneously, or orally. The peptide members of this family all derive from the pioneering work of Dr. Cy Bowers (Bowers et al: *Endocrinology* 114:1537, 1984). This biological action is not abrogated by somatostatin—a critical issue because, as noted in GHRH-deficient children, there remains a circadian rhythm of somatostatin (Martha Jr et al: *J Clin Endocrinol Metab* 67:449, 1988) that could significantly diminish the effective GH release evoked by this family of peptides.

This report by Laron et al. investigates the GH release of a heptapeptide derivative, GHRP-1. In most children, increased GH levels were seen as early as 5 minutes after the administration of GHRP-1. Slight, but statistically significant, increases also were noted in cortisol and PRL levels.

Further molecular "tinkering" has developed more potent peptide and non-peptide analogues (Bowers et al: *Endocrinology* 128:2027, 1991; Aloi et al: *J Clin Endocrinol Metab* 79:943, 1994; Penalva et al: *Clin Endocrinol (Oxf)* 38:87, 1993). Thus, the GH-releasing properties of this family of simple structure offers great promise for a number of patients with disordered GH release but intact pituitary glands: most GH-deficient children, some GH-deficient adults, and the population of elderly individuals whose GH release has naturally declined. The next few years should be exciting as we await the results of a large number of trials already under way and others waiting on the launching pad.—A.D. Rogol, M.D., Ph.D.

GROWTH IN CHRONIC RENAL INSUFFICIENCY

A Prospective, Double-Blind Study of Growth Failure in Children With Chronic Renal Insufficiency and the Effectiveness of Treatment With Calcitriol Versus Dihydrotachysterol
Chan JCM, McEnery PT, Chinchilli VM, Abitbol CL, Boineau FG, Friedman AL, Lum GM, Roy S III, Ruley EJ, Strife CF (Children's Med Ctr, Richmond, Va; Med College of Virginia, Richmond; Univ of Cincinnati, Ohio)
J Pediatr 124:520–528, 1994   112-95-2–4

Objective.—Calcitriol was compared with dihydrotachysterol in children with chronic renal insufficiency. Metabolites of vitamin D are administered to reverse the osteodystrophic process and resulting growth failure in children, but there are concerns that renal functional deterioration may be accelerated with this treatment.

Methods.—Participants were children between ages 18 months and 10 years who were receiving treatment for chronic renal insufficiency at 25 centers in the United States and Canada. All had a calculated glomerular filtration rate between 20 and 75 mL/min per 1.73 m² body mass and elevated serum parathyroid hormone concentrations. Growth was retarded in all patients. Eighty-two patients completed a period of control observations and at least 12 months of treatment with calcitriol (average dose, 17.1 ng/kg body weight per day) or dihydrotachysterol (average dose, 13.8 µg/kg per day). The occurrence of hypercalcemia was recorded for each patient in addition to the dates when treatment was started and stopped.

Results.—Neither treatment affected linear height z scores. During the treatment periods, the glomerular filtration rate significantly decreased in both groups. The rate of decrease was significantly steeper in the calcitriol group. Time to development of hypercalcemia, the number of episodes of hypercalcemia, and the severity of hypercalcemia were similar in the 2 treatment arms. No significant effects of serum calcium in the glomerular filtration rate were observed.

Conclusion.—Neither calcitriol nor dihydrotachysterol treatment significantly changed z scores during a mean follow-up of almost 2 years. Both groups had significant decreases in the glomerular filtration rate during the treatment phase, showing the need for careful follow-up of renal function. Because dihydrotachysterol is less expensive than calcitriol, it can be substituted for calcitriol with equal efficacy.

▶ With all the emphasis on the studies of GH therapy to increase the growth rate of children with chronic renal insufficiency, it is becoming difficult to remember "the way it was." The authors remind us of one of our former therapeutic agents, dihydrotachysterol, a pseudo 1-position hydroxylated derivative of vitamin D that becomes biologically active after hepatic 25-hydroxylation. In this multicenter comparative trial, well-defined subjects with a moderate decline in glomerular filtration rate and abnormal calcium–phosphorus homeostasis, as defined by an increased level of C-terminal serum parathyroid hormone level, were randomly assigned to receive either calcitriol or dihydrotachysterol in addition to standard therapy for chronic renal insufficiency. There were no differences in height z scores between pre- and post-therapy assessment within groups or between groups. Both groups had a decline in renal function and the same incidence of hypercalcemia; therefore, the investigators recommend the less costly agent, dihydrotachysterol.

Because historical "control" groups often had a decline in height z score, there may very well have been a salutary effect of vitamin D analogue therapy. Recent studies with GH have shown increases in height z scores that have continued to increase over several years (see also Fine et al: *J Pediatr* 124:374, 1994, on which Abstract 112-95-2–5 was based; Hokken-Koelega et al: *Pediatr Res* 36:323, 1994). Although there have been questions of accelerated decline in renal function in those children receiving GH, there do not seem to be any significant differences in this parameter with the results shown in this study.—A. D. Rogol, M.D.,Ph.D.

Growth After Recombinant Human Growth Hormone Treatment in Children With Chronic Renal Failure: Report of a Multicenter Randomized Double-Blind Placebo-Controlled Study
Fine RN, for the Genentech Cooperative Study Group (State Univ of New York, Stony Brook)
J Pediatr 124:374–382, 1994   112-95-2–5

Objective.—Growth retardation is an important aspect of renal insufficiency in children and may be what leads to the diagnosis. A randomized, double-blind, placebo-controlled trial of recombinant human GH (rhGH) was carried out in 125 children seen at 17 pediatric nephrology centers from 1988 to 1990.

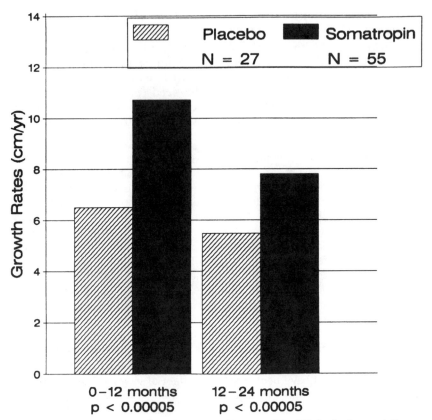

Fig 2–2.—Mean growth rates by treatment group. (Courtesy of Fine RN, for the Genentech Cooperative Study Group: *J Pediatr* 124:374–382, 1994.)

Study Design.—All participants had irreversible renal insufficiency with a creatinine clearance of 5 to 75 mL/min/1.73 m² and a height below the third percentile for chronological age. The children all were prepubertal. Bone age was less than 10 years for girls and less than 11 years for boys. Two thirds of the children received rhGH subcutaneously in a daily dose of .05 mg/kg. The remaining children received an equivalent volume of placebo. The GH dose was adjusted for change in body weight at 3-month intervals.

Results.—Mean growth rates in the first 2 years were significantly greater for rhGH-treated children (Fig 2–2). Mean standardized height improved in the actively treated patients but did not change in placebo recipients. Bone age had increased 2.3 years in the treated group after 2 years and 1.6 years in the placebo group. Predicted adult height increased significantly in treated children. There also was a significantly greater mean body weight gain in the GH-treated patients. The serum creatinine rose similarly in both groups in the first 2 years. In the second

25

year of the study, 8 GH-treated patients and no placebo patients experienced wheezing or asthma after upper respiratory tract infection. Glucose tolerance was not impaired by GH treatment.

Conclusion.—Treatment with rhGH safely promotes growth in children with chronic renal failure whose growth has been retarded.

▶ These data and analysis of them form the backbone of the successful new drug application for the use of GH in children with chronic renal insufficiency. The results that growth rate and standardized height were significantly increased in growth-retarded prepubertal children without undue advancement of bone age are promising for the children to reach their genetically based target height. Concordant with many other studies of GH therapy in other conditions, such as GH deficiency and the Turner syndrome, the growth velocity declines during the second year; however, compared to an appropriately followed control (placebo) group, there was virtually a 1.5-SD gain in height (approximately 6.5 cm) after 2 years. This difference translated into an increase in predicted adult height, although one must be very wary of making such predictions definitively, especially in children who have not yet begun puberty and who may undergo progressive deterioration in renal function and/or renal transplantation with its attendant growth-retarding medications. However, the prospects are very encouraging for additional adult height as the children attempt to reach their genetically determined target height. One's enthusiasm must be tempered, however, because the conclusions are solely based on the predicted adult height. The measured adult height is the important parameter, and the predicted and measured may differ significantly, as already discussed for children stopping GnRH analogue therapy for precocious puberty (See Abstract 112-95-2-9). —A.D. Rogol, M.D., Ph.D.

Growth Hormone Treatment in Growth-Retarded Adolescents After Renal Transplant

Hokken-Koelega ACS, Stijnen T, de Ridder MAJ, de Muinck Keizer-Schrama SMPF, Wolff ED, de Jong MCJW, Donckerwolcke RA, Groothoff JW, Blum WF, Drop SLS (Sophia Children's Hosp, Rotterdam, The Netherlands; Erasmus Univ, Rotterdam, The Netherlands; Univ Hosp of Nijmegen, The Netherlands; et al)
Lancet 343:1313–1317, 1994   112-95-2-6

Introduction.—The majority of patients who undergo renal transplantation before the age of 15 years experience marked growth retardation after transplantation. Studies of GH treatment have reported accelerated growth in these patients, but there are concerns about the effect of GH on graft function. A 2-year, double-blind, dose-response trial of GH treatment in growth-retarded pubertal patients who had received renal allografts evaluated the effects of treatment on both growth and renal graft function.

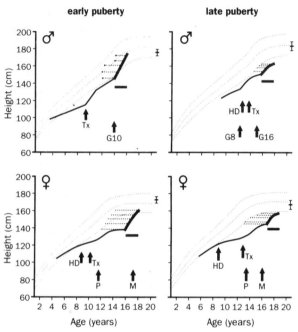

Fig 2–3.—Growth charts of 4 pubertal renal allograft recipients who received GH. *Dashed lines,* bone age; *black bar,* period of GH therapy; *HD,* start of hemodialysis; *Tx,* renal transplantation; ‡, target height ± 4 cm; *P,* girls, start of puberty (Tanner stage M2); *M,* menarche; *G,* boys, testicular volume in mL. (Courtesy of Hokken-Koelega ACS, Stijnen T, de Ridder MAJ, et al: *Lancet* 343:1313–1317, 1994.)

Methods.—Sixteen growth-retarded adolescents (10 boys and 8 girls), aged 11.3–19.5 years and with stable renal allografts received at least 12 months earlier, were receiving prednisone to achieve immunosuppression. They were stratified for pubertal stage and randomly and blindly assigned to receive either 4 or 8 IU/m²/day of biosynthetic GH for 2 years. Radiographs were taken of the left hand and wrist to assess bone age. Glomerular filtration rate (GFR) and effective renal plasma flow (ERPF) were evaluated. Blood and urine were sampled and analyzed regularly to monitor renal function and IGF. The 1-year and 2-year height changes in the treated patients were compared with the same measures in matched controls.

Results.—Height increases were significantly higher in the GH-treated patients than in the matched controls: 10 cm vs. 2.4 cm at 1 year and 15.7 cm vs. 5.8 cm at 2 years. Both pubertal and prepubertal patients had significantly increased growth; the changes were greatest in prepubertal patients (Fig 2–3). There were no dose-related differences in growth. Episodes of rejection and deteriorating renal function were related to reduced immunosuppressive doses or infection, not to GH treatment. The incidence of significant reductions in GFR occurring in the GH-treated patients was similar to that seen in the non–GH-treated patients. Plasma IGF concentrations increased significantly with GH treatment but did not correlate with bone age parameters.

Discussion.—Pubertal patients receiving either 4 or 8 IU/m²/day of GH for 2 years experienced marked, persistent height increases after renal transplantation. Because bone age was not affected, the patients may experience further growth. Although renal graft function deteriorated in some patients, there was no evidence of an association with GH treatment. As this deterioration was generally associated with reduced or noncompliant prednisone therapy, it is recommended that patients on GH therapy be maintained on an optimal daily prednisone regimen.

▶ This is the third abstract that evaluates the important aspects of growth in children with chronic renal failure. Growth hormone, but not vitamin D analogue alone, is able to increase the growth velocity in children with moderate renal insufficiency (Abstracts 112-95-2-4 and 112-95-2-5). The Dutch cooperative group has studied a large number of pretransplant subjects and found that GH therapy could increase the growth rate in such children who commonly fail to grow at an adequate (for age) rate. Often the rate of growth will increase after renal transplantation, but the increase is rarely sustained. The reasons for the failure to achieve full catch-up growth after transplantation are incompletely understood, but the antirejection drugs, especially glucocorticoids, are likely contributors.

This report shows highly statistically significant and biologically relevant growth and, importantly, a nonsignificantly higher rate of decline of GFR or acceleration of bone age maturation (see Fig 2–3 for individual examples). If the growth rates are sustained until epiphyseal closure, these children have a much greater chance to reach their genetically determined target height.

In summary, it is apparent that GH is effective in increasing the growth rate in prepubertal patients with moderate renal failure (Abstract 112-95-2-5) and in pubertal patients after renal transplantation. Predicted adult height is clearly increased, because the bone age did not accelerate as rapidly as the growth velocity; however, as pointed out numerous times, not all subjects, especially those abnormally growing ones, reach their "predicted" height. One must follow the children to measured adult height, which is now being done for children and adolescents after withdrawal of therapy for precocious puberty or those children with idiopathic short stature whose adult heights are predicted to increase.—A.D. Rogol, M.D., Ph.D.

GROWTH IN ASTHMA

Growth and Pituitary–Adrenal Function in Children With Severe Asthma Treated With Inhaled Budesonide

Volovitz B, Amir J, Malik H, Kauschansky A, Varsano I (Hasharon Hosp, Petach-Tiqva, Israel)
N Engl J Med 329:1703–1708, 1993   112-95-2-7

Background.—Inhaled corticosteroids are considered the best treatment choice for patients with severe persistent asthma. However, the effects of these agents on young children have not been studied. Their effect on growth and pituitary function are of particular concern. A study documenting both efficacy and long-term safety is necessary.

Methods.—Fifteen children, aged 2–7 years, whose asthma could not be controlled with cromolyn sodium, terbutaline sulfate, theophylline, and prednisone, entered the trial and were followed for 3–5 years. They received 100-μg doses of inhaled budesonide twice daily, with occasional increased doses or additional agents during periods of exacerbation. The children were assessed monthly for the first year, then every 3 months. Their assessments included height, weight, and height velocity to evaluate growth and serum cortisol concentration to evaluate pituitary–adrenal function. The children's parents kept daily records of symptoms for the first year. Each child had a slit-lamp eye examination.

Results.—Clinical evaluation and parental records documented significantly improved control of asthma symptoms within the first month of budesonide therapy, which was maintained throughout the treatment period. Discontinuation of therapy was attempted with all 15 children 46 times. All but 2 attempts were unsuccessful. In most unsuccessful attempts, symptoms returned within 1 month after discontinuation. Height, weight, and height velocity were age-appropriate in all children. All measures of serum cortisol concentrations were normal. No children had cataracts. One child had brief dysphonia. There were no other side effects.

Discussion.—Long-term budesonide therapy is both effective and safe when used in relatively low doses in young children. The most common adverse effects of inhaled corticosteroid therapy are related to the dosage. The use of spacer devices and the use of lower doses could account for the absence of oral candidiasis in these children. There were also no children with cataracts; it may be that the formation of cataracts is associated only with orally administered corticosteroids.

▶ Do they or don't they—that is, does the regular use of inhaled corticosteroids impair physiologic adrenal function in children? This report seems so clear; the young children receiving budesonide for the vast majority of days did not show growth failure and had a completely normal hypothalamic-pituitary-adrenal axis. These are excellent results, not only in terms of the control of the disease (airway hyperresponsiveness), but also in terms of the growth of the children; however, the study includes only 15 subjects. Previous investigations using this and other potent inhaled glucocorticoids have shown equivocal results; some studies show the expected dose-dependent toxic effects of growth failure and a partially suppressed adrenal axis (Wolthers and Pederson: *Pediatrics* 89:839, 1992; Balfour-Lynn: *Lancet* 1:476, 1988). Others have shown promising results consistent with the study abstracted here. The general precept that the least amount of steroid, for the shortest amount of time, to the smallest area will serve young children with severe asthma well. It is clear that systemic steroid therapy often leads to growth failure, making trials with inhaled, poorly systemically absorbed preparations highly desirable; however, the underlying respiratory compromise must be reversed. The long duration of the present trial, the decrease in other anti-bronchoconstricting medications, and the improvement in symptoms and in peak expiratory flow rate show marked efficacy and safety. Thus, even in young children, the relatively low dose of budesonide (200 μg per day) is safe and effective.—A.D. Rogol, M.D., Ph.D.

Puberty

Sexual Precocity: Sex Incidence and Aetiology
Bridges NA, Christopher JA, Hindmarsh PC, Brook CGD (Middlesex Hosp, London)
Arch Dis Child 70:116–118, 1994   112-95-2–8

Purpose.—Experience with the differential diagnosis of sexual precocity, defined as the appearance of secondary sexual characteristics before age 8 in girls and age 9 in boys, was reviewed. The study period was 15 years, beginning in 1975 and continuing to 1990.

Patients and Methods.—A total of 213 children, including 197 girls and 16 boys, were evaluated. All underwent standard anthropomorphic measures. Patients were assigned to diagnostic categories on the basis of clinical assessment, endocrine evaluation, radiologic imaging, and pelvic ultrasonography (Fig 2–4).

Results.—Central precocious puberty was identified in 91 girls and 4 boys (female-to-male ratio 23:1). Endocrine studies showed a dominance of LH over FSH, and stimulation with GnRH resulted in a response similar to that found during normally timed puberty. In each boy, a cause was identified: 1 brain tumor, 1 hypothalamic hamartoma, 1 severe head trauma, and 1 congenital adrenal hyperplasia resulting from 21-hydroxylase deficiency. In girls, a cause was found in only 6. In those patients, central precocious puberty was secondary to previously diagnosed intracranial disorder, including 2 instances of isolated hydrocephalus, 2 brain tumors, 1 hypothalamic hamartoma, and 1 arachnoid cyst. Sexual precocity associated with raised gonadotropins was distinguished from central precocious puberty. It was associated with either isolated breast development, where FSH concentration predominated and pelvic

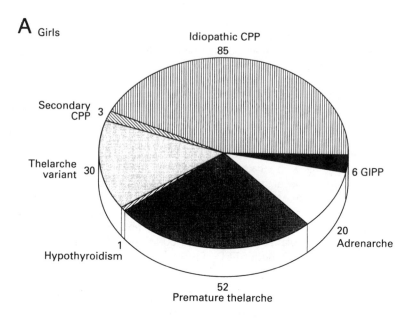

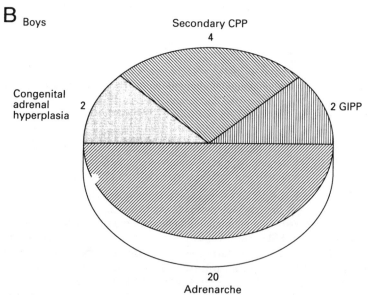

Fig 2–4.—Pie charts showing numbers of children seen with sexual precocity with each diagnosis in girls (**A**) and boys (**B**). *Abbreviation:* CPP, central precocious puberty. (Courtesy of Bridges NA, Christopher JA, Hindmarsh PC, et al: *Arch Dis Child* 70:116–118, 1994.)

ultrasonography generally revealed a single cyst in 1 ovary, or with primary hypothyroidism with predominating FSH concentrations. Thelarche variant, noted in 20 girls, was associated with raised serum LH concentrations, although not to the same extent as in central precocious puberty. Neither growth rate nor skeletal maturation was accelerated in patients with this condition. Gonadotropin-independent precocious puberty was noted in 3 girls and 2 boys. In those individuals, stimulation with GnRH showed low baseline LH and FSH concentrations and an absent response. Adrenarche, characterized by isolated pubic and axillary hair development, was common, found in 50% of boys and 15% of girls.

Conclusion.—In boys with precocious puberty, detailed investigations should be performed. In girls, investigations should revolve around clinical findings, particularly the consonance of puberty. Improvements in imaging techniques and therapeutic alternatives have led to a more dynamic classification of sexual precocity.

▶ Most of us who evaluate patients for disorders of early pubertal development have no idea what the incidence is or what the relative proportions are among sexual precocity, either central or peripheral, or those variants that are seemingly more common: premature thelarche and adrenarche. These data from a referral center in a very large city give some indication and some very important guidelines for the clinical, biochemical, and imaging evaluation of children with early sexual development.

As noted in many other studies, girls were referred more often than boys (197 vs. 16). In the vast majority of girls with central precocious puberty, a specific anatomical cause could not be identified. Smaller numbers of girls were referred for premature thelarche, thelarche variant (1992 YEAR BOOK OF ENDOCRINOLOGY, p 55) and adrenarche. In my own referral practice, the latter are far more common and suggest that these "variants of normal" are diagnosed and the patients and their parents are counseled at the local or regional level rather than referred to central London. The few gonadotropin-independent forms of sexual precocity are in line with a number of previous studies.

What can we learn from this compilation of well-evaluated patients? First and foremost is that children with early puberty or with any deviation from the regular smooth progression through puberty require an explanation. The recent improvements in noninvasive structural studies of the hypothalamus and pituitary as well as the pelvis and ovary have permitted more precise diagnoses and have shown that most hamartomas of the hypothalamus are static lesions. The biochemical differentiation of the various forms of sexual precocity is important in terms of the individual targeting of pharmacologic therapy: GnRH analogues for central precocious puberty and inhibitors of steroid hormone biosynthesis for gonadotropin-independent sexual precocity.—A.D. Rogol, M.D., Ph.D.

Adult Height in Girls With Idiopathic True Precocious Puberty

Brauner R, Adan L, Malandry F, Zantleifer D (Hopital et Faculté Necker-Enfants Malades, Paris)
J Clin Endocrinol Metab 79:415–420, 1994   112-95-2-9

Introduction.—Precocious puberty results in an increased rate of bone maturation that may lead to reduced adult height. In some girls with idiopathic true precocious puberty, however, bone age progression is accompanied by an appropriate acceleration of growth. Thus, indications for treatment with GnRH analogues are not fully established, and the ability of GnRH analogues to preserve adult height remains uncertain. Thirty-four girls with idiopathic true precocious puberty were analyzed for growth and adult height after being treated or not treated with a GnRH analogue.

Methods.—Nineteen patients received a GnRH analogue. (Decapeptyl) for at least 2 years, and 15 were followed without therapy. The criterion for therapy was a predicted final height of less than 155 cm at initial examination or at subsequent 6-month evaluations. To exclude the spontaneously regressive forms of precocious puberty, treatment was started 6 months or more after the onset of breast development. Estrogen activity was fully blocked during GnRH therapy. In most cases, therapy was stopped at a bone age greater than 12 years. Target height was calculated from midparental heights.

Results.—For those in the treatment group, GnRH analogue therapy was initiated at a mean age of 7.5 years and discontinued at a mean age of 10.6 years. During treatment, mean bone age increased from 10.5 to 12.3 years and mean height from 131 to 147.7 cm. Adult height in the treatment group was greater (mean, 159 cm) than the predicted height before therapy (mean, 152 cm). The mean target heights of the 2 groups were similar (difference, 0.9 cm). Adult heights of the treatment and nontreatment groups were also similar (difference, 3 cm) and close to target heights. Only 3 girls, 1 treated and 2 untreated, reached an adult height that was more than 5 cm below the target height. The treated girl had intrauterine growth retardation and short stature before puberty.

Conclusion.—Girls with true precocious puberty and low adult height prediction who received GnRH analogue therapy achieved a mean height gain of 6.5 cm between predicted and adult heights. The decision to treat was based on the difference between predicted and target height, level of estrogen activity, and gonadotropin peak ratio. Girls who were not treated had a predicted height of more than 155 cm on the basis of tests of bone age and sex steroid secretion. Such patients appear to have a slow evolutive form of precocious puberty and need to be followed, although target height may be achieved without therapy.

▶ One of the outcome measures for children who have had precocious puberty is their adult height, especially in relationship to their genetic potential (target height). When patients are first evaluated, an adult height is predicted based on the height at presentation and a bone age determination; however, the evolution of the prepubertal development cannot necessarily be predicted. Some may have only a slowly progressive form that permits attainment of the genetically targeted height.

Although this study is relatively small, there is at least one important new factor when considering therapy with GnRH analogues—that of predicted adult height of above or below 155 cm. It should be obvious that those predicted to be below 155 cm had the most discrepancy between height age and bone age and thus are the more severely affected. Only those with lower predicted adult height (group 1) were treated with GnRH analogue. Those with an adult predicted height of more than 155 cm were evaluated at 6-month intervals without therapy. The outcome measure was *assessed adult height* rather than predicted adult height, as is used in most studies. For group 1 patients, the net "gain" of almost 7 cm (159 cm at the end compared with 152 cm at the beginning) is both highly statistically significant and biologically meaningful. Not only did the group 2 patients reach their adult height predicted at the onset of therapy, but they also reached their target height, making it clear that the biological height potential was not affected by the onset of puberty earlier than expected. Group 2 patients also had less "intense" pubertal development at first evaluation.

What does this all mean? Perhaps the most conservative interpretation is that the girls in group 2 represent the tail of Gauss, that is, those girls have normal sexual development despite their chronological age of less than 8 years. One should recall that the lower 5% boundary for "normal" pubertal development is 8 years, and we should expect a small number of subjects to "normally" begin adolescent development before that age. Undoubtedly, timing and tempo genes are involved, and I suspect that very careful family histories of siblings and mothers and aunts would show significantly earlier pubertal onset in the group 2 individuals compared with similar relatives in a population who had average or delayed adolescent development. For the individual subject, the markers of a large difference between the predicted and target heights as well as a greater peak LH/FSH ratio after GnRH stimulation (as is proper for the later stages of puberty) predict a need for and a response to GnRH analogue therapy.—A.D. Rogol, M.D., Ph.D.

Effect of Deslorelin-Induced Pubertal Delay on the Growth of Adolescents With Short Stature and Normally Timed Puberty: Preliminary Results

Municchi G, Rose SR, Pescovitz OH, Barnes KM, Cassorla FG, Cutler GB Jr (Natl Inst of Child Health and Human Development, Bethesda, Md; Univ of New Mexico, Albuquerque; Indiana Univ, Indianapolis)
J Clin Endocrinol Metab 77:1334–1339, 1993   112-95-2-10

Objective.—In children with LH-releasing hormone (LHRH)–dependent precocious puberty, LHRH agonist treatment can effectively slow bone maturation and increase adult height. However, within the normal range, the timing of puberty does not appear to affect average final height, calling into question the effects of delaying a normally timed puberty on adult height. A randomized, double-blind trial was conducted to ascertain whether pubertal delay induced by LHRH agonist treatment can increase final height in children with short stature and a normally timed puberty.

Methods.—The study included 43 children with short stature, with height or predicted height at least 2.25 SD below the mean for age. There were 28 girls and 15 boys. All were randomly selected to receive either placebo or the LHRH agonist deslorelin, 4 μg/kg per day subcutaneously, for 4 years. This preliminary analysis includes 16 children—9 in the deslorelin group and 7 in the placebo group—who completed at least 4 years of treatment. Four patients—3 in the deslorelin group and 1 in the placebo group—also received concurrent GH treatment.

Results.—The deslorelin group showed a 7.6-cm increase in predicted adult height compared with the pretreatment baseline and a 10.3-cm increase compared with the placebo group. Even after omission of the children who received concurrent GH, the results were essentially the same: the deslorelin group had a 7.2-cm increase in predicted adult height compared with baseline and a 10.9-cm increase compared with the placebo group. There were no significant adverse effects.

Conclusion.—In children with short stature and normally timed puberty, an LHRH agonist–induced pubertal delay appears to increase predicted adult height. Longer follow-up will be needed to determine whether deslorelin treatment increases final height. Pending these results, LHRH agonist treatment of these children should be considered investigational.

▶ The use of long-acting GnRH agonist analogues has revolutionized the therapy of central precocious puberty. The evidence is overwhelming that a substantial number of the children will reach an adult height much closer to their target height (based on midparental stature) than they would have had they not been treated or had they been treated with the formerly used agent, medroxyprogesterone acetate. These GnRH analogues, of which deslorelin is but one, would really be desirable agents if they permitted short, normally developing children to have a greater adult height. However, the predictions are made while these children remain in "gonadal arrest." How rapidly the change in height age vs. the change in bone age would be once the analogue therapy was stopped is a critical bit of data. Would their theoretical gains *predicted* during the conduct of this study remain once natural puberty was reinitiated? In children with precocious puberty, this same research group has reported a loss of approximately one third of the increase predicted after the conclusion of therapy (1993 YEAR BOOK OF ENDOCRINOLOGY, p 46).

No mention is made of the psychosocial aspects of significantly delayed puberty. The children with precocious puberty discontinue the medication and attain prepubertal development at a time that is concordant with their peers. After 4 years of therapy, the children in the present study were ap-approximately 16 years of age and were still very early in puberty (their heights or height ages are not listed). How well did they fit in with their age peers? Did they have some of the same concerns as severely constitutionally delayed children? Before this therapy is considered for a much larger group of children, the present children must be followed to *measured* adult height and to when proper inventories of psychosocial well-being are evaluated. It is clear that if these children do not really end up significantly taller than they might have been, the psychosocial downside may significantly tilt the risk:-benefit ratio toward the numerator.—A.D. Rogol, M.D., Ph.D.

Serum Bioactive Luteinizing and Follicle-Stimulating Hormone Concentrations in Girls Increase During Puberty

Kasa-Vubu JZ, Padmanabhan V, Kletter GB, Brown MB, Reiter EO, Sizonenko PC, Beitins IZ (Univ of Michigan, Ann Arbor; Tufts Univ, Springfield, Mass; Univ of Geneva)
Pediatr Res 34:829–833, 1993   112-95-2-11

Introduction.—Given the key role played by FSH in folliculogenesis and ovarian growth, it is surprising that there is no apparent increase in bioactive FSH (B-FSH) during the gonadal changes of puberty. Studies of this issue to date have been cross-sectional in nature and thus prone to intersubject variability. For this reason, a longitudinal study was con-

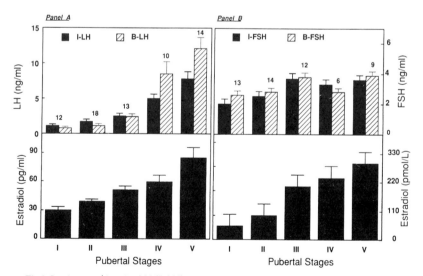

Fig 2–5.—**A,** mean bioactive LH (B-LH), immunoreactive LH (I-LH) using LER 960 standard, and estradiol levels relative to pubertal stages I through V. **B,** mean bioactive FSH (B-FSH), immunoreactive FSH (I-FSH), and estradiol levels relative to pubertal stages I through V. *Numbers above bars* in top graphs represent the number of individuals at each pubertal stage. (Courtesy of Kasa-Vubu JZ, Padmanabhan V, Kletter GB, et al: *Pediatr Res* 34:829–833, 1993.)

ducted to determine whether B-FSH increases during pubertal maturation in girls.

Methods.—Thirty healthy girls were enrolled in the study at pubertal stages I to IV. Every 6 months, the girls were followed up for pubertal staging, radiographic bone age determination, and measurement of adrenal and ovarian steroids. In addition, 14 had measurement of serum immunoreactive FSH (I-FSH) and B-FSH, and 18 had measurement of immunoreactive LH (I-LH) and bioactive LH (B-LH).

Results.—Clinical and hormonal characteristics of puberty were present in all subjects. Relative elevations in I-FSH and B-FSH were present before puberty, whereas I-LH and B-LH levels were low. Modest but significant increases in serum I-FSH and B-FSH occurred from pubertal stages I to III. The expected pubertal changes in serum I-LH and B-LH occurred as well, with B-LH showing a greater increase than I-LH (Fig 2–5).

Conclusion.—Serum B-FSH and I-FSH increase during pubertal maturation in girls. From early to midpuberty, relative elevations in B-FSH concentrations are noted; this may play an important role in ovarian growth at a time when circulating LH and estrogen levels are low. Continued and selective increases in LH occur as puberty progresses, inducing an increase in estradiol and ultimately leading to ovulation.

▶ Doesn't everybody know that gonadotropin concentrations increase at puberty? Why review such a straightforward concept? This work was very carefully done in a longitudinal cohort of normally developing girls using well-validated in vitro bioassays. The data show the quantitative alterations that occur during puberty and point to the early rise in biologically effective FSH concentrations. These data are also the benchmark for the newer gonadotropin immunoassays that use chemiluminescent marker antibodies to ensure that these assays, which are much easier to perform than the bioassays, measure the biologically relevant charge and size isomers of FSH.

The critical data are shown in Figure 2–5 and illustrate that bioactive LH and immunoactive estradiol rise after the effective concentrations of bioactive FSH, but before the external signs of puberty are prominent. Presumably, these are important to folliculogenesis and are required for the induction of aromatase P450 within the small follicle.—A. D. Rogol, M.D., Ph.D.

Development of Bone Mass and Bone Density of the Spine and Femoral Neck: A Prospective Study of 65 Children and Adolescents
Kröger H, Kotaniemi A, Kröger L, Alhava E (Kuopio Univ, Finland; Rheumatism Found Hosp, Heinola, Finland)
Bone Miner 23:171–182, 1993   112-95-2–12

Background.—Adults show great biological variation in bone mass and bone mineral density (BMD). Peak bone mass may be affected by a number of variables, including genetic factors, physical activity, and nutrition. Data on BMD in growing children could provide useful information on the mechanisms of differences in bone mass accumulation; however, there have been few longitudinal studies on the development of BMD. The magnitude and timing of the increase in BMD, bone mineral content (BMC), and bone size in the spine and proximal femur were studied in healthy children and adolescents.

Methods.—Sixty-five Finnish children and adolescents, ranging in age from 7 to 20 years, were studied twice in a 1-year interval. There were 37 females and 28 males; none had any chronic disease or growth rate abnormality. Lumbar spine and femoral neck BMD and BMC were measured by dual-energy x-ray absorptiometry. Bone volumetric density was calculated by a previously described method using the BMD values corrected for bone size.

Results.—At both anatomical sites, the greatest annual increase in BMD and bone volumetric density occurred at the time of menarche in females and between the ages of 13 and 17 years in males. Mean annual incremental rates of femoral BMC and femoral neck width were significantly higher in males; there were no sex-related differences in spinal measures. By the age of 20 years, bone mass and bone density acquisition had ceased or markedly decreased. The rate of incremental increase in bone density was not significantly related to physical activity or calcium uptake.

Conclusion.—Puberty is a key time in the development of bone mass and density. Genetic factors, especially the hormonal effects of puberty, appear to be the main components of this process. The findings support the hypothesis that the largest portion of peak bone mass is attained in late adolescence. Prevention of osteoporosis should begin during the maximum phase of growth in children.

▶ Diminished bone density is a major public health problem in middle-aged and elderly individuals. The processes leading to this condition don't occur overnight but are usually attributed to the slow, insidious process of bone loss, both structurally as well as in mass, over many years. However, bone, like most tissues, is a still frame of a moving picture of accrual and breakdown. From this premise, one is compelled to consider the attainment of peak bone mass much earlier than previously, i.e., in adolescence and early adulthood. What are the determinants of maximal bone density? When do they occur? Are there dietary and activity issues when considered in the context of the genetic background that will steer the individual to a healthy bone mass?

This study, along with a number of others (DeSchepper et al: *J Nucl Med* 32:216, 1991; Theintz et al: *J Clin Endocrinol Metab* 75:1060, 1992), reports the longitudinal trajectory of bone density in adolescent boys and girls, the precise time of greatest accrual of bone since fetal life and arguably the most important time for the prevention (or amelioration) of senile osteoporosis and its attendant health and financial morbidity. The noninvasive, very-low-radiation technique of dual x-ray absorptiometry (also known as DEXA or DXA) has been used in this study and in many others, replacing the less precise technique of dual photon absorptiometry and the much higher radiation doses of quantitative CT. The short-term precision in children in this study was .8% for the spine and 2.3% for the femoral neck. These permit the determination in a longitudinal study of half-yearly or yearly evaluations during the time of rapid change. Using measured bone size, the values for bone mineral density were corrected to yield a volumetric density, the parameter of greatest interest. This point is important during times of rapid growth.

Not surprisingly, the greatest rate of accrual of bone occurred in girls in the 2 years before menarche, a time of greatest change in the levels of sex steroid hormones, especially estradiol; however, there still was quite an increase in bone density up to age 20 years. In boys, the maximal increase occurred later, usually during the period of the growth spurt, with slower accrual of mineral up to the 20th year. Although in the small study no effects of physical activity (Slemenda et al: *J Bone Miner Res* 6:1227, 1991) and current daily calcium intake were found on the increase in BMD or BMD_{vol}, the statistical power to find such effects, given the present methodology, was quite low. In a recent study of twins, an effect of calcium supplementation on BMD was found (Johnston et al: *N Engl J Med* 327:82, 1992).

This study shows the normal physiologic rise in BMD and BMD_{vol} in adolescent boys and girls and emphasizes the importance of puberty on the development of peak bone mass. One must understand the factors that drive this increase before designing properly controlled studies that will benefit patients both as adolescents and young adults, but perhaps more importantly, as middle-aged and elderly adults.—A.D. Rogol, M.D., Ph.D.

Hereditary Diabetes Insipidus

Novel Mutations in the V2 Vasopressin Receptor Gene in Two Pedigrees With Congenital Nephrogenic Diabetes Insipidus
Yuasa H, Ito M, Oiso Y, Kurokawa M, Watanabe T, Oda Y, Ishizuka T, Tani N, Ito S, Shibata A, Saito H (Nagoya Univ, Japan; Niigata City Gen Hosp, Japan; Niigata Univ, Japan)
J Clin Endocrinol Metab 79:361–365, 1994   112-95-2-13

Background.—Congenital nephrogenic diabetes insipidus (CNDI) is an X-linked form of the disorder associated with impaired production of cyclic adenosine monophosphate (cAMP). Linkage studies have localized the gene responsible for CNDI to the Xq28 region. Because hybrid cells carrying this region of the X chromosome express V_2 vasopressin receptors, an abnormality of the gene producing defective receptors may be a cause of CNDI. The V_2 receptor is one of the family of G protein-coupled receptors that contain 7 distinctive transmembrane domains. The V_2 receptor gene itself is encoded by 3 exons.

New Mutations.—Novel mutations of the V_2 vasopressin receptor gene were identified in 2 Japanese pedigrees with X-linked CNDI. In one of them, 1 of 4 consecutive guanine sequences in the second exon was deleted, resulting in a frame shift starting at codon 154 in the second intracellular domain and a premature termination at codon 161. In the other pedigree, a missense mutation (A to G) was identified at nucleotide position 310 in the second exon. This point mutation changed a histidine at codon 80 in the second transmembrane domain to an arginine that is more positively charged than histidine in a neutral environment. Each of the mutations cosegregated with the phenotype of diabetes insipidus.

Conclusion. —The mutations of the V_2 vasopressin receptor gene that have been identified in CNDI pedigrees result in either premature termination secondary to a frame shift, or single amino acid substitutions in the extracellular, transmembrane, and intracellular domains.

A *de Novo* Mutation in the Coding Sequence for Neurophysin-II (Pro^{24}→Leu) Is Associated With Onset and Transmission of Autosomal Dominant Neurohypophyseal Diabetes Insipidus

Repaske DR, Browning JE (Children's Hosp Med Ctr, Cincinnati, Ohio)
J Clin Endocrinol Metab 79:421–427, 1994   112-95-2-14

Background. —Autosomal dominant neurohypophyseal diabetes insipidus (ADNDI) is an inherited form of diabetes insipidus (DI) caused by an inadequate serum concentration of arginine vasopressin (AVP). Those affected usually have polyuria and polydipsia in the first years of life but a normal renal response to AVP. Linkage studies indicate that the genetic locus of ADNDI is the AVP–neurophysin-II (AVP-NPII) gene or a closely linked gene.

Objective. —The molecular basis of ADNDI was studied in 7 members of a family in which a novel exon II mutation was identified in 3 generations. The disease appeared in the second generation coincidentally with a de novo mutation in the NPII-coding region of one allele of the AVP-NPII gene. All third-generation members who inherited the mutant allele developed ADNDI, whereas the one who did not inherit the allele was unaffected.

Findings. —Nucleotide sequence analysis of the AVP-NPII gene revealed a C→T mutation at nucleotide 1761 in 1 allele of the gene. The mutant gene encoded a normal AVP peptide but predicted a substitution of leucine for proline at amino acid 24 of NPII. Fifty control subjects lacked the mutation. The chromosome 20 carrying the mutation was identified by microsatellite haplotype analysis in the first affected individual, who had inherited the affected chromosomal segment from her unaffected mother.

Interpretation. —One explanation of how AVP is clinically deficient despite a normal AVP-NPII allele is that the binding of AVP to NPII that contains the mutation is disrupted. Another is that the mutant precursor peptide is incompletely processed and that the abnormal precursor that accumulates leads to degeneration of the affected hypothalamic nuclei.

▶ It just had to be. We again find the power of molecular biological techniques to show us exactly where the disordered physiology lies. Both central and nephrogenic diabetes insipidus must have multiple genotypes for the same disease phenotype. As with any multistep pathway, one should expect lesions along that pathway to produce similar syndromes. That is precisely the situation with diabetes insipidus.

The V_2 vasopressin receptor is the one that regulates water balance in the renal tubule. As one might expect in familial disorders, each family would have its own "private" mutation within the critical protein. Both families described had disorders within the coding region of the gene for the V_2 receptor. The phenotype co-segregated with the gene mutation and presents strong evidence for this mutation being the cause for resistance to arginine vasopressin in those affected. Proof of this hypothesis awaits expression of the mutated gene in an appropriate cell line. In addition, the identification of the specific mutation provides a mechanism for the very early diagnosis of nephrogenic diabetes insipidus, before clinical evidence for hypernatremic dehydration.

The second report (Abstract 112-95-2-14) gives equal time to the "upstream" arm of the vasopressin–renal tubule loop. Vasopressin is synthesized as a prohormone with its carrier protein, NPII, a 10-kDa protein that carries it along axons to terminate in the pars nervosa of the pituitary. Failure of production of vasopressin from any cause produces the syndrome of central diabetes insipidus, more usual in our practice as a result of infiltrative or destructive lesions of the hypothalamus. In the present family with central DI, a single base mutation in the AVP-NPII gene was detected. The investigators concluded that this mutation was the pathophysiologic mechanism for the disorder, because the genotype and the phenotype co-segregated.

Both of these problems are predictable, although the genetics are not. However, whatever the cause of central DI, it is far easier to manage DI with long-acting V_2 agonists, e.g., dDAVP, than it is to manage fluid and electrolyte balance in patients with nephrogenic DI.—A.D. Rogol, M.D., Ph.D.

Suggested Reading

The following articles are recommended to the reader:

Ogilvy-Stuart AL, Wallace WHB, Shalet SM: Radiation and neurosecretory control of growth hormone secretion. *Clin Endocrinol (Oxf)* 41:163–168, 1994.
▶ Cranial irradiation reduces but does not abolish somatostatin tone. It does more severely reduce GHRH; therefore, manipulating somatostatin tone may augment GHRH analogue therapy in children with radiation-induced GH deficiency.
Theintz G: Endocrine adaptation to intensive physical training during growth. *Clin Endocrinol (Oxf)* 41:267–272, 1994.
▶ Training for competitive sports usually requires high volume and intensity

of exercise. The effects of such exercise on growth and adolescent development are discussed with emphasis on the GH and gonadal axes.

Kirk JMW, Trainer PJ, Majrowski WH, et al: Treatment with GHRH (1-29) NH$_2$ in children with idiopathic short stature induces a sustained increase in growth velocity. *Clin Endocrinol (Oxf)* 41:487–493, 1994.

▶ As expected, the growth velocity in short stature, non-GH deficient children increased with GHRH analogue therapy. Although predicted height increased after 1 year of therapy, catch-down growth followed cessation of therapy. Actual final height data are the only significant measure of efficacy, so one must be cautious in the interpretation of these data.

Burstein S: Growth disorders after cranial radiation in childhood. *J Clin Endocrinol Metab* 78:1280–1281, 1994.

▶ A concise review of the effects of various types of radiation therapy on the GH and gonadal axes.

Conte FA, Grumbach MM, Ito Y: A syndrome of female pseudohermaphroditism, hypergonadotropic hypogonadism, and multicystic ovary associated with missense mutations in the gene encoding aromatase (P450 arom). *J Clin Endocrinol Metab* 78:1287–1292, 1994.

▶ A complete clinical description and location of precise genetic defect in a patient with aromatase deficiency.

Ogilvy-Stuart AL, Clayton PE, Shalet SM: Cranial irradiation and early puberty. *J Clin Endocrinol Metab* 78:1282–1286, 1994.

▶ Girls irradiated before age 4 have a high incidence of early puberty, although boys may also show such a trend.

Carlsson LMS, Attie KM, Compton PG, et al: Reduced concentration of serum growth hormone–binding protein in children with idiopathic short stature. *J Clin Endocrinol Metab* 78:1325–1330, 1994.

▶ Children with short stature have reduced GHBP levels that may be a marker for a reduced complement of GH tissue receptors.

Chatelain P, Job JC, Blanchard J: Dose-dependent catch up growth after 2 years of GHRH in IUGR children. *J Clin Endocrinol Metab* 78:1454–1460, 1994.

▶ Although highly variable responses to GHRH were noted in this heterogeneous group of children, higher doses of GH were associated with greater growth ratio.

Magiakou MA, Mastorakos G, Chrousos GP: Final stature in patients with endogenous Cushing Disease. *J Clin Endocrinol Metab* 79:1082–1085, 1994.

▶ Incomplete catch-up growth in treated patients does not permit them to reach midparental target height.

Allen DB, Brook CGD, Bridges NA, et al: Therapeutic controversies: Growth hormone (GH) treatment of non-GH deficient subject. *J Clin Endocrinol Metab* 79:1239–1248, 1994.

▶ An excellent summary from multiple points of view of an ongoing controversy.

Smith EP, Boyd JP, Frank GR, et al: Estrogen resistance caused by a mutation in the estrogen receptor gene in a man. *N Engl J Med* 331:1056–1061, 1994.

▶ A complete clinical description of a single patient with a pinpointing of a base mutation in the estrogen receptor shows that estrogen action is critical to bony epiphyseal fusion.

3   Aging

This Year's SQUAWKs (Something Quite Unusual and Worthwhile Knowing)

Ugwusnadu and Harding (*Eur J Obstet Gynecol Reprod Biol* 54:153, 1994) reported that 2 postmenopausal women who were receiving tamoxifen for estrogen-receptor–positive breast cancer experienced uterine fibroid growth and postmenopausal bleeding. Glueck et al. (*J Lab Clin Med* 123:59, 1994) reported 4 women who had triglyceride levels greater than 1,500 mg/dL and acute pancreatitis develop when placed on estrogen replacement therapy. Triglyceride levels greater than 750 mg/dL are an absolute contraindication and those greater than 300 mg/dL are a relative contraindication to estrogen replacement therapy. Tayal et al. (*Age Ageing* 23:320, 1994) reported 12 individuals older than 60 years of age with hypopituitarism and nonspecific presentations including weakness, hypotension, weight loss, falls, cognitive decline, and urinary incontinence. Levels of TSH were normal in 7 of 12 patients. Hormone replacement therapy improved quality of life. Abs et al. (*Eur Neurol* 33:416, 1993) reported 7 patients who had both a pituitary adenoma and a meningioma. A patient had penile curvature deformity and Peyronie-like plaque develop after intracorporeal self-injection of prostaglandin E$_1$ (Chen et al: *J Urol* 152:961, 1994). Inhaled beclomethasone dipropionate suppresses dehydroepiandrosterone levels in postmenopausal women with chronic obstructive airways disease, suggesting that this may play a role in the accelerated osteoporosis seen in these patients (Smith et al: *Aust N Z J Med* 24:396, 1994).

Introduction

> *A human being would certainly not grow to be seventy or eighty years old if his longevity had no meaning for the species to which he belongs. The afternoon of human life must also have a significance of its own and cannot be merely a pitiful appendage of life's morning.*
>
> *Carl Gustav Jung*

The past year was predominantly one of consolidation in the field of geriatric endocrinology. The major features were the beginning of papers on dehydroepiandrosterone administration (Abstract 112-95-3–18) and a flurry of activity concerning inhibin measurements and inhibin's possible role in modulating ovarian and adrenal tumors (Abstract 112-95-3-12). This momentary lull in new activity allows us to speculate about the future. Clearly, we are poised to see a series of studies on the effects of testosterone on the aging process. Sih et al. (*J Am Geriatr Soc* 42:SA7, 1994) have reported in abstract form that testosterone continues to increase strength through 6 months (and this effect appears to be maintained at 1 year) with no side effects. Studies on the effects of GHRH (Vittone et al: *Clin Res* 42:216A, 1994), IGF-I (Ghiron et al: *Clin Res* 42:48A, 1994), and the nonpeptide GH releasing compound, L692,492 (Aloi et al: *J Clin Endocrinol Metab* 79:943, 1994) have appeared, and we can expect a series of articles attempting to determine whether these agents perform better than GH (Abstract 112-95-3-1) in reversing age-related frailty. The big picture of the role of local growth factors (Nicolas et al: *J Clin Endocrinol Metab* 78:1011, 1994) and cytokines (Khosla et al: *J Clin Endocrinol Metab* 79:707, 1994) in the pathogenesis of osteoporosis has begun to emerge. However, it should be recognized that our FUTURESCOPE has a limited vision, for, as pointed out by Arthur C. Clarke, "One fact about the future of which we can be certain is that it will be utterly fantastic!"

Evidence continues to accumulate about the importance of undernutrition in the development of frailty in older persons. Serum albumin was demonstrated to be an independent risk factor for mortality in men and women older than 70 years of age (Corte et al: *JAMA* 272:1036, 1994). Cytokine production is increased in persons with rheumatoid arthritis and is associated with loss of body cell mass and decreased serum albumin levels secondary to the cytokine effects on energy metabolism and intake (Roubenoff et al: *J Clin Invest* 93:2379, 1994). In a nursing home study, we found that one third of residents losing weight were depressed and that appropriate treatment of depression reversed weight loss (Morley and Kraenzle: *J Am Geriatr Soc* 42:583, 1994). Depression may produce anorexia and weight loss secondary to increasing corticotropin releasing factor activity in the hypothalamus. Depression is a major treatable cause of premature aging.

Sleep disorders are commonly associated with aging. Melatonin levels in the circulation decrease with aging (Sharma et al: *Biol Psychiatry* 25:305, 1989). Older persons with sleep disturbances have decreased secretion of the major urinary metabolite of melatonin 6-sulphatoxy-melatonin (Harmov et al: *BMJ* 309:167, 1994). It is possible that melatonin therapy may be beneficial in correcting sleep disturbances in older persons.

A study from Japan suggested that the DCCT trial may apply to older patients with type 2 diabetes (Morisaki: *J Am Geriatr Soc* 42:142, 1994). They followed 114 patients with NIDDM older than 60 years (mean age, 68 years) for 5 years. Progression rates for retinopathy were directly related to mean glycosylated hemoglobin levels. Those whose HbA$_1$C was lower than 7% had a 2% retinopathy; 7% to 8%, 20%; 8% to 9%, 40%;

and greater than 9%, 61%. This strongly suggests that tight diabetic control will slow progression of retinopathy in older individuals.

John E. Morley, M.D.

Pituitary

Effects of Recombinant Human Growth Hormone on Metabolic Indices, Body Composition, and Bone Turnover in Healthy Elderly Women
Holloway L, Butterfield G, Hintz RL, Gesundheit N, Marcus R (Palo Alto Veterans Affairs Med Ctr, Calif; Stanford Univ, Calif; Genentech Inc, South San Francisco)
J Clin Endocrinol Metab 79:470–479, 1994   112-95-3-1

Objective.—The clinical application of GH in the elderly should be associated with significant long-term anabolic effects without deleterious side effects. A double-blinded, placebo-controlled, randomized, 6-month intervention trial was conducted to assess the effects of daily ad-

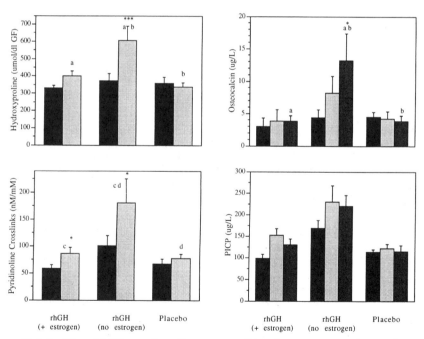

Fig 3–1.—Effect of rhGH on markers of bone turnover. Urinary bone resorption markers are shown in **lefthand graphs** and indicate results at baseline (*black*) and 6 months (*light shaded*). Serum bone formation markers are shown in **righthand graphs** and indicate results at baseline (*black*), 3 months (*light shaded*), and 6 months (*dark shaded*). Asterisks indicate significance of changes from baseline: *P < .05; ***P < .001. *Bars showing similar letters differ significantly (P < .05). Abbreviation*: PICP, type I procollagen extension peptide. (Courtesy of Holloway L, Butterfield G, Hintz RL, et al: *J Clin Endocrinol Metab* 79:470–479, 1994.)

ministration of recombinant human GH (rhGH) on metabolic indices, body composition, and bone turnover in healthy elderly women.

Treatment.—Twenty-seven healthy women, with a mean age of 66.7 years, received rhGH or placebo as a single daily injection. Initially, 19 women received rhGH at a dose of .043 mg/kg of body weight. However, the dose was reduced by 50% after several weeks because of side effects that included unacceptable fluid retention and edema in 58% and symptoms of carpal tunnel syndrome in 2 women. The remaining 7 elderly women began treatment at the reduced dose. Thirteen women who received rhGH and 14 women assigned to placebo completed 6 months of treatment, including 6 women in the rhGH group who took estrogen.

Results.—With rhGH, circulating IGF-I and IGF-I–binding protein-3 (IGFBP-3) increased in women taking estrogen and those not taking estrogen; no changes in IGF-I and IGFBP-3 occurred in the placebo group. In addition, rhGH decreased fat mass by 11% and relative adiposity by 9%, and increased endogenous creatine clearance by 9.2%. Moreover, rhGH dramatically increased markers of bone turnover, especially in women not taking estrogen. Hydroxyproline excretion increased by 20% in women who took estrogen and by 80% among women who did not, and pyridinoline excretion increased by 44% and 75%, respectively (Fig 3–1). Women not taking estrogen had significantly greater osteocalcin concentrations, but there were no significant changes in circulating type I procollagen extension peptide in either group. However, all these changes were not accompanied by consistent changes in lean body mass, energy metabolism, or nitrogen balance. Except for a transient increase in serum T_3 levels, rhGH did not affect blood pressure, thyroid status, or fibrinogen concentration. In addition, rhGH had no effect on circulating lipoproteins, and actually reduced LDL cholesterol levels in women not taking estrogen. In 8 women who remained on rhGH for 12 months, the 6-month changes in IGF-I, IGFBP-3, and markers of bone turnover persisted, but there was no significant increase in axial or appendicular bone mass.

Conclusion.—Recombinant human GH can be given to healthy elderly women without obvious adverse effects on major cardiovascular risk factors. It is a powerful initiator of bone remodeling but is unlikely to achieve major improvement in bone mass when used alone. These effects should be balanced against a high prevalence of side effects, particularly fluid retention and carpal tunnel syndrome.

▶ This study provides further evidence that GH is not a contender as a hormonal fountain of youth. Another study found that GH failed to enhance the muscle strength response that elderly males have during resistance exercise training (Taafe et al: *J Clin Endocrinol Metab* 79:1361, 1994). A 12-week treatment period with GH in women with osteoporosis increased biochemical markers of bone formation and resorption but did not alter bone density (Clemmesen et al: *Osteoporos Int* 3:330, 1993). Growth hormone enhanced protein synthesis efficiency in trauma victims (Petersen et al: *J Trauma* 36:726, 1994) and improved nitrogen balance in patients undergoing gastrointestinal surgery (Tacke et al: *Infusionsther Transfusionsmed* 21:24, 1994). Thus, as first pointed out in the 1990 YEAR BOOK OF ENDOCRINOLOGY (pp 61–64), the major use of GH appears to be to treat severe malnutrition in older patients.

Hexarelin, a GH-secreting peptide with no homology to GHRH, has blunted GH-releasing activity in older persons that can be partially reversed by arginine and GHRH (Arvat et al: *J Clin Endocrinol Metab* 79:1440, 1994). The GHRH-6 increases GH to a greater extent than GHRH in older persons, and its effect is maintained for at least 4 days after oral administration (Ghigo et al: *Eur J Endocrinol* 131:499, 1994). A nonpeptide GH-releasing agent, L692,429, increases GH in older persons, in part by inhibiting somatostatin release (Aloi et al: *J Clin Endocrinol Metab* 79: 943, 1994). The GH response to GHRH is enhanced by the acetylcholinesterase inhibitor, pyridostigmine, which enhances cholinergic tone and decreases somatostatin release. This effect is less marked in older individuals (Coiro et al: *Gerontology* 38:217, 1992). The future is sure to be filled with multiple treatment strategies that attempt to reverse the changes of aging.—J.E. Morley, M.D.

Water Metabolism

Body Fluid Balance in Dehydrated Healthy Older Men: Thirst and Renal Osmoregulation

Mack GW, Weseman CA, Langhans GW, Scherzer H, Gillen CM, Nadel ER (Yale Univ School of Medicine, New Haven; New Britain Gen Hosp, Conn)
J Appl Physiol 76:1615–1623, 1994   112-95-3-2

Background.—Older individuals are known to be more susceptible to dehydration than are younger persons. Studies comparing young men with men aged 65–75 years found that thirst perception was reduced in the older group after a period of dehydration. Aging is also associated with changes in renal function. Thus, the maintenance of water homeostasis in older individuals appears to be influenced by impairments in the physiologic control of water input and output. The hypothesis that a shift in the operating point for control of body fluid volume and composition exists in healthy older individuals was tested.

Methods.—Study participants were 10 men, aged 65–78 years, and 6 men, aged 18–28 years. Both groups fasted and refrained from alcoholic and caffeine beverages for 12 hours before the experiment. Thirst was assessed on a visual-analogue rating scale after a period of dehydration induced by heat and exercise. Blood and urine samples were obtained after the study subjects were allowed to rehydrate with tap water during a 3-hour rehydration period. Total body water (TBW) loss and total sweat loss were calculated, as were changes in extracellular fluid and intracellular fluid.

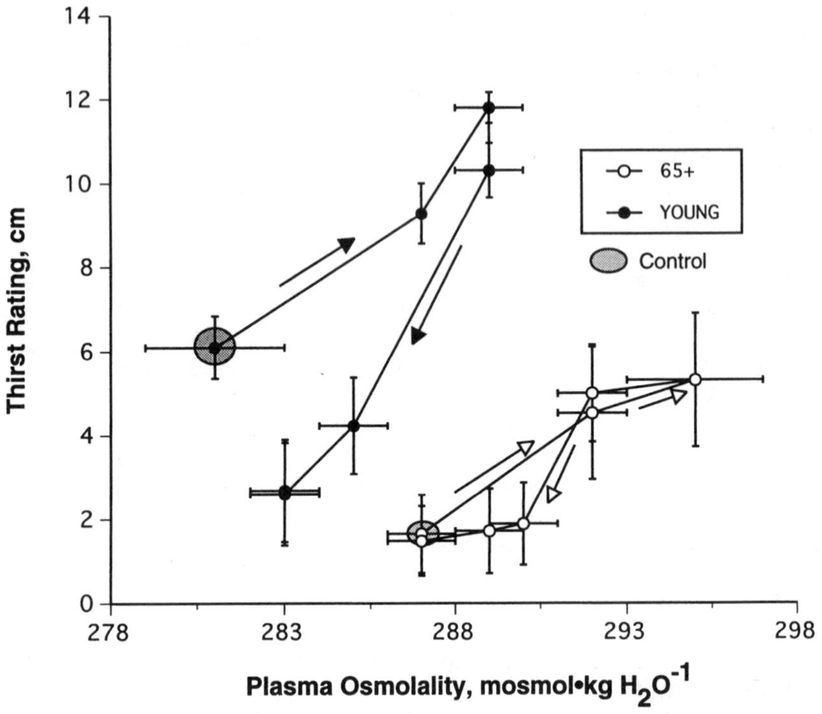

Fig 3–2.—Relationship between plasma osmolality and perceived thirst. Data points represent means ± SE for each group at rest before dehydration; after 1 hour of dehydration, 2 hours of dehydration, and 30 minutes recovery from dehydration (no fluid ingested); and at 1, 2, and 3 hours of rehydration. (Courtesy of Mack GW, Weseman CA, Langhans GW, et al: *J Appl Physiol* 76:1615–1623, 1994.)

Results.—In the older men, baseline plasma volume was lower, plasma osmolality was higher, and perceived thirst was lower than in the young men. The 2 age groups had similar TBW losses during dehydration, but the osmotic threshold for increased thirst was shifted to a higher plasma osmolality value in the older group. Dehydration produced a significantly higher subjective thirst rating in the younger group. Total fluid intake was 16.6 mL/kg in young men vs. 8.9 mL/kg in older men. The relation between thirst and the rate of fluid intake was identical, however, for the 2 age groups. The stimulus-response relationship between plasma osmolality and sense of thirst in younger and older men is shown in Figure 3–2.

Conclusion.—Many previous reports of chronic dehydration in older individuals examined elderly patients confined to bed. In this study, healthy active older men were found to be hyperosmotic and hypovolemic compared with younger men. The older group demonstrated appropriate osmotic control of thirst and renal osmoregulatory function, but there appeared to be a shift in the operating point for control of body fluid volume and composition. This shift may represent an adaptive mechanism to protect against hyponatremia.

▶ The original description of impaired thirst recognition was made by Phillips et al. (*N Engl J Med* 311:753, 1984). Studies in human beings (Silver et al: *J Am Geriatr Soc* 40:556, 1992) and animals (Silver et al: *J Gerontol* 46:117, 1191) have shown that the age-related deficit in thirst perception is related predominantly to a decrease in the mu opioid central drinking drive. Older people live in a water desert, with the inability to recognize the need to drink adequate amounts of fluid to maintain their intravascular volume. This regularly results in orthostatic hypotension and orthostatic dizziness (which can occur without blood pressure changes) in older patients and occasionally in syncopal episodes. For this reason, it is essential to measure the blood pressure in all older individuals while they are standing!—J.E. Morley, M.D.

Ozone Increases Atrial Natriuretic Peptides in Heart, Lung and Circulation of Aged vs. Adult Animals
Vesely DL, Giordano AT, Raska-Emery P, Montgomery MR (Univ of South Florida, Tampa; James A Haley VA Med Ctr, Tampa, Fla)
Gerontology 40:227–236, 1994   112-95-3-3

Background.—Ozone has become a primary health concern in 96 cities in the United States that failed to meet the U.S. Ambient Air Quality Standard for ozone of .12 ppm as a 1-hour maximum concentration once per year. Ozone can cause pulmonary edema and simultaneously decrease blood pressure, and these changes may be mediated by atrial natriuretic peptides. Animals were studied to examine this possibility and to determine whether aged animals respond differently to ozone.

Methods.—The concentration of atrial natriuretic peptides recognized by atrial natriuretic factor (ANF), proANF 1–30, and proANF 31–67 radioimmunoassays in the lung, heart, and circulation were measured in adult (4–6 months old) and aged rats (24–26 months old) exposed to .5 ppm of ozone for 8 hours.

Results.—Ozone significantly increased the content of atrial natriuretic peptides in the lungs of both adult and aged animals. Similarly, ozone increased the content of these peptides by 2–5 times in the heart and doubled the concentration of these peptides in the circulation. The increases in these peptides were of equal magnitude in aged and adult rats. As previously reported, levels of atrial natriuretic peptides in the aged animals at room air were higher in the hearts and circulation, but not in the lungs, compared with those in younger animals, and the addition of ozone enhanced the atrial natriuretic peptide concentrations to the same extent as that observed in adult rats.

Discussion.—Ozone increases atrial natriuretic peptides in the lungs, heart, and circulation to the same extent in aged and adult animals, indicating an equal response to ozone with aging. Because atrial natriuretic peptides increase pulmonary capillary permeability and are potent vasodilating peptides, these peptides may mediate the decreased blood pressure and pulmonary edema associated with ozone exposure.

▶ It would appear that as chlorofluorocarbons reduce ozone concentrations in the stratosphere, ozone levels have been increasing in our cities! As physicians, we need to be aware of the environmental toxins to which our patients are exposed and to play a role in the development of sensible environmental policies if our species is to survive.

Reviewing the literature can be perplexing at times. Two studies examined arginine vasopressin (AVP) levels in healthy elderly patients; the first concluded that "age does not influence AVP" (Duggan et al: *Age Ageing* 22:332, 1993) and the second that "aging is accompanied by an increase in plasma VP concentrations" (Johnson et al: *J Am Geriatr Soc* 42:339, 1994). Because one of these studies was done in Ireland and the other in Australia, one could conclude that this is the result of the ozone hold in the southern hemisphere. In the 1992 YEAR BOOK OF ENDOCRINOLOGY (pp 65–66), it was pointed out that AVP levels fail to rise at night as they do in younger individuals, perhaps accounting for the nocturia commonly complained of by older patients.—J.E. Morley, M.D.

Diabetes Mellitus

Medical Conditions and Motor Vehicle Collision Injuries in Older Adults

Koepsell TD, Wolf ME, McCloskey L, Buchner DM, Louie D, Wagner EH, Thompson RS (Univ of Washington, Seattle)
J Am Geriatr Soc 42:695–700, 1994   112-95-3–4

Background.—The number of injuries and deaths resulting from motor vehicle collisions increases substantially after age 60 years. Part of the excess mortality seen in this age group can be attributed to sharply higher case fatality rates, but the greater number of both fatal and nonfatal injuries seen implies that age-related deterioration of driving skills may also contribute. Whether medical conditions that impair sensory, cognitive, or motor function are associated with risk of driving accidents was investigated in an older adult population.

Method.—Members of Group Health Cooperative of Puget Sound aged 65 and older and who were licensed drivers in 5 counties participated in the study. Cases were those who were injured while driving during 1987 and 1988. Controls were matched to cases on age, sex, and county of residence, but had experienced no injury during the study period. Outcome included injury requiring medical care related to a police-investigated motor vehicle collision. The risk factors evaluated included selected medical conditions active within the previous 3 years as shown by medical records.

Relative Risk of Motor Vehicle Collision Injury Among Patients With Diabetes in Relation to Features of Diabetes

Characteristic	Percent Prevalence among		Odds Ratio*	
	Cases (n = 234)	Controls (n = 446)	Est.	(95% CI)
Diabetes mellitus (any)	11.1	4.5	2.6	(1.4–4.7)
Treated with insulin	2.6	0.4	5.8	(1.2–28.7)
Treated with oral hypoglycemics	5.3	1.3	3.1	(0.9–11.0)
Treated with diet alone	2.6	2.9	0.9	(0.4–2.4)
Diagnosed within last 5 years	3.0	2.2	1.4	(0.5–3.7)
Diagnosed over 5 years ago	8.1	2.2	3.9	(1.7–8.7)
Neither diabetes nor coronary heart disease	72.8	81.5	1.0	(Reference)
Diabetes only	7.2	3.8	2.0	(0.9–4.3)
Coronary heart disease only	16.2	14.1	1.2	(0.8–1.9)
Both diabetes and coronary heart disease	3.8	0.7	8.0	(1.7–37.7)

* From matched analysis. Reference category is individuals without diabetes, except as noted for last 4 rows.
(Courtesy of Koepsell TD, Wolf ME, McCloskey L, et al: J Am Geriatr Soc 42:695–700, 1994.)

Results.—The study group consisted of 235 cases along with 448 controls. The 2 groups had similar age and sex characteristics. A slightly larger proportion of cases were nonwhite, and a smaller proportion were currently married. Injury risk was found to be higher than that in controls in patients with the following medical conditions: diabetes (95% confidence interval [CI]: 1.4–4.7), particularly those treated with insulin (odds ratio [OR] = 5.8, 95% CI: 1.2–28.7) or oral hypoglycemic agents (OR = 3.1, 95% CI: 0.9–11.0); those with a history of diabetes of more than 5 years (OR = 3.9, 95% CI: 1.7–8.7); and those with both diabetes and coronary heart disease (OR = 8.0, 95% CI: 1.7–37.7) (table). More injuries were also found in older drivers with coronary artery disease (OR = 1.4), depression (OR = 1.7), alcohol abuse (OR = 2.1), or who had fallen (OR = 1.4), although these conditions were of borderline statistical significance.

Conclusion.—The most striking observation is the increased risk of motor vehicle collision injury among older persons with diabetes. Past studies have shown conflicting results in this regard: some have found elevated risk among all ages of drivers with diabetes, whereas others have found significant association between diabetes and vehicle collision rate. Overall, the results show that a higher risk of driving accidents is largely associated with diabetes treated with insulin or oral hypoglycemic agents. Although the findings reported here need to be replicated in other studies, their clinical plausibility and agreement with other research suggests that they should be taken seriously by physicians in a position to advise their patients on whether to continue driving.

▶ This article creates a major ethical dilemma for physicians dealing with older patients with diabetes. This study suggests that patients should be advised to not drive and possibly should be reported to the Department of Motor Vehicles as high-risk drivers. We have previously demonstrated that physicians have little knowledge concerning the management of older persons' driving. Many do not even take a history of whether the person is still driving! (Miller and Morley: *J Am Geriatr Soc* 41:722, 1993.) A minimum approach to older patients with diabetes would appear to be to ask their driving status; check their mental status and exclude depression using standardized geriatric instruments; check their vision, including color vision; discuss with them the possible dangers of driving; and consider sending them for a computerized driving evaluation or encouraging them to take the American Association of Retired Persons refresher driving course.

The reasons for the higher crash rate in older drivers with diabetes appears to be multifactorial. As previously chronicled in the 1989 YEAR BOOK OF ENDOCRINOLOGY (p 61) and the 1991 YEAR BOOK OF ENDOCRINOLOGY (pp 64–65), hyperglycemia is associated with impaired cognitive function. Recurrent hypoglycemia can also lead to deterioration in cognitive function and personality disorders (Gold: *Diabetic Med* 11:499, 1994). Cerebral atrophy occurs more commonly in diabetic than nondiabetic patients (Araki et al: *Neuroradiology* 36:101, 1994). Elderly individuals have reduced awareness of the autonomic but not neuroglycopenic symptoms of hypoglycemia (Meneilly: *J Clin Endocrinol Metab* 78:1341, 1994). This appears to be related to a reduced epinephrine response to hypoglycemia. Patients with diabetes also have been shown to have poorer balance and decreased sensorimotor function than do age-matched individuals with other diseases (Lord: *Diabetic Med* 10:614, 1993).—J.E. Morley, M.D.

Hormonal Changes in Elderly Men With Non-Insulin-Dependent Diabetes Mellitus and the Hormonal Relationships to Abdominal Adiposity

Chang T-C, Tung C-C, Hsiao Y-L (Natl Taiwan Univ, Taipei, Republic of China; Taipei Municipal Chung-Hsiao Hosp, Taipei, Taiwan, Republic of China)

Gerontology 40:260–267, 1994   112-95-3–5

Objective.—In elderly men with NIDDM, changes in serum hormone levels and the hormonal relationships to abdominal adiposity were studied.

Subjects.—Forty elderly men aged 60 years and older, 20 elderly men with NIDDM older than 60 years, and 30 control individuals aged 21–40 years were examined. In elderly men with NIDDM, mean plasma HbA_{1c} was 7.5%, mean fasting blood sugar was 145.7 mg/dL, and 2-hour postprandial blood sugar level was 209.4 mg/dL.

Results.—Elderly men, with and without NIDDM, had lower serum T_3, testosterone, and IGF-I levels, and higher serum LH and FSH levels compared with controls. Elderly men with NIDDM had even lower serum testosterone levels (median, 4.9 ng/mL) than did elderly men without NIDDM (median, 5.6 ng/mL). Elderly men had a higher waist/hip circumference (W/H) ratio than did controls. Elderly men with NIDDM had a higher body mass index (BMI), skinfold thickness, and W/H ratio than did elderly men without NIDDM. The W/H ratio correlated positively with age and serum LH and FSH levels, and correlated negatively with serum IGF-I, T_3, and testosterone levels. Age, serum IGF-I, T_3, T_4, TSH, LH, and FSH levels were not related to BMI or skinfold thickness, whereas only serum testosterone levels correlated negatively with BMI and skinfold thickness. Age correlated positively with serum LH and FSH levels and negatively with serum IGF-I and testosterone levels.

Summary.—Elderly men with NIDDM have markedly reduced serum testosterone levels and an increased W/H ratio, in addition to the age-related decrease of serum T_3, IGF-I, and testosterone levels and the increase in W/H ratio and serum LH and FSH levels. The S/H ratio, a parameter of abdominal adiposity, is associated with changes in serum IGF-I, testosterone, LH, FSH, and T_3 to a greater degree than BMI or skinfold thickness. It appears that degenerative changes of the testes and an increase in abdominal adiposity may both play a role in the decrease in serum testosterone levels and influence gonadotropin secretion secondarily.

▶ The authors' data, as opposed to their conclusions, lend further support to the concept that older persons develop a hypothalamic-pituitary hypogonadism, as previously shown in the 1991 YEAR BOOK OF ENDOCRINOLOGY (pp 79–81). Insulin-like growth factor binding protein-I levels were demonstrated to increase with age and to not be inhibited by insulin in older persons to the same extent as they are in younger persons (*J Clin Endocrinol Metab* 77:1152, 1993).

A Finnish study found that the prevalence of diabetes in persons older than age 70 years was 22% for men and 28% for women, and the presence of diabetes was not diagnosed in one third of the subjects (Hiltunen et al: *Diabetic Med* 11:241, 1994). Persons with diabetes who are older than 65 years of age have 4.5 times the chance of dying than do those without diabetes (Croxson et al: *Diabetic Med* 11:250, 1994). Nearly 40% of patients with new onset type 2 diabetes who are older than age 65 years are not obese (Pagano et al: *Diabetic Med* 11:425, 1994). Magnesium supplementation for 4 weeks improved insulin-mediated glucose disappearance, total body glucose disposal, and glucose oxidation in elderly patients with type 2 diabetes (*J Clin Endocrinol Metab* 78:1510, 1994).—J.E. Morley, M.D.

Male Hormones

Reversal of Sexual Impotence in Male Patients With Chronic Obstructive Pulmonary Disease and Hypoxemia With Long Term Oxygen Therapy
Aasebø U, Gyltnes A, Bremnes RM, Aavaag A, Slørdal L (Univ Hosp of Tromsø, Norway; Haukeland Hosp, Bergen, Norway; The Norwegian Radium Hosp, Oslo, Norway)
J Steroid Biochem Mol Biol 46:799–803, 1993   112-95-3-6

Background.—Erectile impotence is frequent in men with respiratory failure and has been ascribed to hypoxia. Many patients have reported regaining penile erection when placed on long-term oxygen therapy (LTOT).

Study Plan.—The effects of oxygen therapy were examined in 19 men who were sexually impotent and had hypoxic chronic obstructive pulmonary disease; all were eligible for LTOT because of arterial oxygen tension pO_2 less than 7.3 kPa. Twelve patients received LTOT for 1 month, and 7 received it for 24 hours.

Results.—Five of the 12 patients given LTOT for 1 month regained morning erections. The arterial pO_2 increased significantly in these patients, as did the serum testosterone level. The patients who failed to respond had significantly lower levels of pO_2 and serum testosterone and higher levels of sex hormone–binding globulin. None of the patients treated for only 24 hours had a reversal of sexual impotence despite a significant increase in pO_2. Baseline serum testosterone levels were significantly higher in the patients treated for 24 hours than in the patients treated for 1 month. Levels of sex hormone–binding globulin remained high.

Conclusion.—An adequate period of oxygen therapy may reverse sexual impotence in some men with chronic obstructive pulmonary disease.

▶ Erythropoietin therapy appears to improve sexual performance in patients on hemodialysis (Steffensen and Clunsholt: *Nephrol Dial Transplant* 9:1215, 1993). Both serum inhibin and free testosterone levels decline with aging. Levels of FSH increase at 40 years of age. Levels of FSH correlated inversely with inhibin levels (Haji et al: *Maturitas* 18:143, 1994). Two studies have suggested that trazodone (150–300 mg) can improve potency in males with organic impotence (Chiang et al: *Kao Hsiung I Hsveh Ko Hsveh Tsa Chi* 10:287, 1994; Kurt et al: *J Urol* 152:407, 1994).—J.E. Morley, M.D.

Three-Year Safety and Efficacy Data on the Use of Finasteride in the Treatment of Benign Prostatic Hyperplasia
Stoner E (Merck Research Lab, Rahway, NJ)
Urology 43:284–294, 1994   112-95-3–7

Background.—Finasteride is a synthetic 4 azasteroid that inhibits steroid 5α-reductase [5α-R], an intracellular enzyme that converts testosterone to dihydrotestosterone. The goal of therapy was to decrease prostate volume, increase urinary flow rate, improve symptoms, and halt the disease's progression.

Methods.—For 12 months, 543 patients were randomly assigned to a placebo or to a treatment of finasteride, 1 or 5 mg. After 12 months of

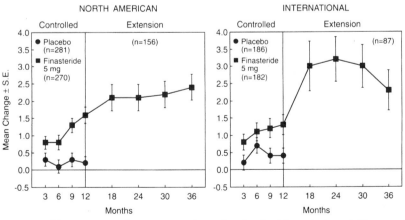

Fig 3–3.—Maximum urinary flow rate: mean change from baseline (± standard error). (Courtesy of Stoner E: *Urology* 43:284–294, 1994.)

therapy, patients invited to continue an open-label extension study extended their original treatment of 5 mg of finasteride. Results in these patients, who took 5 mg of finasteride for the initial 12 month double-blinded therapy and again during the 24-month open-extension study, were reported.

Results.—After 36 months of treatment with 5 mg of finasteride, 297 patients of the original 543 were analyzed on the key efficacy variables. Overall, serum dihydrotestosterone decreased on average 65%; prostate volume decreased from baseline by approximately 27%; maximum urinary flow improved by approximately 2.3 mL/sec (Fig 3–3); symptom scores improved 3.6 points. With regard to prostate volume, 42% of all patients had a 30% or greater reduction. At least 40% of all patients exhibited a 3 mL/sec increase in maximum urinary flow rate. In symptom scores, at least 48% of patients showed a 50% increase. Finasteride was well tolerated, with no further evidence of adverse experiences.

Conclusion.—Daily treatment with 5 mg of finasteride offered an excellent safety profile and sustained clinical efficacy. This treatment, with its low incidence of side effects, is recommended as an extremely favorable, low-risk medical option for treatment of BPH.

▶ Unfortunately, in times of diminished research funding, drug companies have gained excessive control over new drug studies and have made it difficult to interpret the validity of the statistical manipulations undertaken. This study has many such problems.

Nearly half of the patients had withdrawn after 36 months of finasteride therapy. Benign prostatic hypertrophy is a lifelong condition; this study does not answer the effects of 10–20 years of treatment. It seems to me that surgery remains the superior option for this disease. I find it amazing that the Food and Drug Administration allows finasteride on the market but has kept highly efficacious and clearly safe metformin out of the United States for decades.—J.E. Morley, M.D.

Menopause

Estrogen Replacement Therapy and Memory in Older Women

Robinson D, Friedman L, Marcus R, Tinklenberg J, Yesavage J (Veterans Affairs Med Ctr, Palo Alto, Calif; Stanford Univ, California)
J Am Geriatr Soc 42:919–922, 1994   112-95-3–8

Objective.—Studies on the effects on cognitive function of estrogen replacement therapy in older women yield varied results. These inconsistencies may be caused by differences in the type of instruments used to measure cognitive function, the level of cognitive functioning among study participants, and age. The relation between estrogen replacement therapy and recall of proper names and words in older women was assessed in a case-control study.

Subjects.—From a group of 278 community-dwelling women aged 55–93 years, 72 older women receiving estrogen replacement therapy were matched for age and education with a group of 72 women not receiving estrogen. All women had scores of 27 or greater in the Folstein Mini-Mental State Examination and had approximately equivalent scores in the Geriatric Depression Scale and Quick Vocabulary Test. Of 58 women with a complete history of replacement therapy, 54 received conjugated equine estrogen, including 26 who also received medroxyl progesterone acetate. Forty women took the estrogen at .625 mg/day, and the rest received between 0.3 and 1.25 mg/day. Twenty-eight women received the medication 30 days per month, and 18 received it 25 days per month. Estrogen was used for a mean of 13.37 years.

Results.—Older women receiving estrogen replacement therapy had significantly better scores on the proper name recall test than women who did not receive estrogen. There was significantly greater variance among women receiving estrogen than among those who did not. The groups did not significantly differ on the word recall task.

Summary.—Contrary to previous reports, estrogen use in postmenopausal women who do not have dementia is associated with enhanced recall of proper names. The increased interindividual variability of performance among women receiving estrogens may account for the mixed results on the cognitive effects of estrogen in older women.

▶ Another cross-sectional epidemiologic study also demonstrated improved verbal memory in healthy postmenopausal women (Kampen and Sherwin: *Obstet Gynecol* 83:979, 1983). Two previous studies from this group showed that verbal memory improved after estrogen replacement in women who had a surgical menopause (Sherwin: *Psychoneuroendocrinology* 13:343, 1988; Phillips and Sherwin: *Psychoneuroendocrinology* 17:483, 1992). Estrogen therapy has also been shown to improve subjective memory in postmenopausal memory (Campbell et al: *Clin Obstet Gynecol* 4:31, 1977) and memory in nursing home residents (Caldwell et al: *J Gerontol* 7:228, 1952). Other studies have failed to find a salutary effect of estrogen on memory (Barrett-Connor et al: *JAMA* 269:2637, 1993; Kaiser et al: *J Am Geriatr Soc* 42:SA39, 1994). Overall, the studies suggesting that estrogen may improve memory are tantalizing. However, possible effects of estrogen on general well-being and the possibility that women who select estrogen have better basal cognitive function represent potential confounding factors. At best, it seems likely that estrogen may have minor effects on only one or two forms of memory function. It will also be important to separate estrogen effects from those of progesterone, because our FUTURESCOPE tells us that animal studies have suggested an amnestic effect of progesterone on visuospatial memory (Farr S: *Physiol Behav* In press, 1995). This is a complex area whose study and interpretation is fraught with difficulties, not the least of which will be whether one can in a politically correct world suggest that sex hormones modulate cognitive function. It should be noted that females perform better than males in 4 of 7 memory tasks where this has been appropriately tested!—J.E. Morley, M.D.

Is Sexual Life Influenced by Transdermal Estrogen Therapy: A Double Blind Placebo Controlled Study in Postmenopausal Women

Nathorst-Böös J, Wiklund I, Mattsson L-Å, Sandin K, von Schoultz B (Karolinska Inst, Stockholm, Sweden; Danderyd Hosp, Sweden; Östra Hosp, Göteborg; Västra Frölunda, Stockholm, Sweden)

Acta Obstet Gynecol Scand 72:656–660, 1993   112-95-3-9

Background.—A number of studies have observed a decline in sexual interest and activity at the time of menopause. Estrogen therapy is known to combat vaginal dryness and dyspareunia in postmenopausal women, but whether it affects other aspects of sexuality is uncertain.

Objective.—In the course of a clinical trial of quality of life for postmenopausal women, the effects of an estradiol patch on sexual function were studied in women 45–65 years of age who required hormonal replacement for menopausal symptoms.

Methods.—A total of 239 women were randomized to receive estradiol, in the form of an Estraderm patch providing 50 µg per 24 hours, or a placebo patch. The patches were changed twice per week for 12

Differences Between Pre- and Post-Treatment Values for Each Item in the "McCoy Sex Scale" in Women Receiving Placebo (P) and Women Receiving Transdermal Estradiol Therapy (E)

	P	E	*p*-value
1. Are you satisfied with your present frequency of sexual activity?	0.33	0.63	0.04
2. How many times a day have you had sexual thoughts or fantasies during the last month?	−0.09	0.24	0.003
3. How enjoyable is sex for you?	−0.15	0.22	0.02
4. How often during sex do you feel aroused or excited (for instance increased heart beat/ flushing / vaginal wetness / heavy breathing)?	−0.05	0.26	0.30
5. How often do you have an orgasm during sex?	0.06	0.19	0.60
6. How often do you suffer from lack of vaginal lubrication (wetness) during sex?	−0.02	1.11	0.0004
7. How often do you suffer from pain during intercourse?	−0.01	0.90	0.0003
8. How satisfied are you with your partner as lover?	−0.10	0.08	0.15
9. How satisfied are you with your partner as fellow and friend?	−0.06	−0.05	0.82

(Courtesy of Nathorst-Böös J, Wiklund I, Mattsson L-Å, et al: *Acta Obstet Gynecol Scand* 72:656–660, 1993.)

weeks. At the end of the study, the women received medroxyprogesterone acetate in a daily dose of 10 mg for 2 weeks. The McCoy Sex Scale Questionnaire was given at the outset and after treatment was completed.

Results.—Five of 117 women randomized to receive estradiol (4%) were withdrawn, most of them because of poor compliance. One was a suicide that appeared unrelated to treatment. The withdrawal rate from the placebo group was 8%. Baseline sexual function was comparable in the 2 groups. Women in both groups reported an increased frequency of sexual activity during the study period. In addition, those given estradiol noted more enjoyment of sexual activity, better lubrication, and less dyspareunia. The frequency of sexual fantasies increased markedly, but arousal and orgasm were no more frequent than before the study began (table). Other aspects of the quality of life improved in the estradiol-treated women but not in placebo recipients.

Conclusion.—Transdermal estradiol therapy not only relieves local symptoms in postmenopausal women but also enhances pleasure in sexual activity. However, estrogen therapy is not indicated for primary disorders of sexual desire.

▶ Although estrogen appears to be one factor related to the quality of sexuality at the time of menopause, physicians need to search for other treatable problems. Menopause was not associated with an increase in depression risk in the Massachusetts Women's Health Study, but a prolonged symptomatic perimenopause did produce a transitory increase in depressive symptoms (Avis et al: *Ann Epidemiol* 4:214, 1994). However, Hay et al: (*Br J Psychiatry* 164:313, 1994) found that women attending a menopause clinic had a high likelihood of being depressed. Women who seek treatment for osteoarthritis (Dexter and Brandt: *J Rheumatol* 21:279, 1994) and sleep disturbances in the perimenopausal period (Shaver et al: *Family Pract Res J* 13:373, 1993) should be screened for depression.

In addition to improving sexual life, other positive claims for estrogen were made this year. Meta-analysis suggested that estrogen therapy produced a subjective improvement in postmenopausal incontinence (Fantl et al: *Obstet Gynecol* 83:12, 1994). Little objective effect of estrogen therapy could be demonstrated. Estrogens may be protective against the development of lens opacities (*Arch Ophthalmol* 112:85, 1994). Breast tenderness may either get better or worse after hormone replacement therapy, suggesting that it is not a contraindication to this therapy (Marsh et al: *Maturitas* 19:97, 1994).—J.E. Morley, M.D.

Menopausal Status Influences Ambulatory Blood Pressure Levels and Blood Pressure Changes During Mental Stress

Owens JF, Stoney CM, Matthews KA (Univ of Pittsburgh, Pa; Brown Univ, Providence, RI)
Circulation 88:2794–2802, 1993   112-95-3-10

Background.—Ovarian hormones, particularly estrogen, appear to protect women from coronary heart disease (CHD) in middle life. The relative absence of these hormones after menopause may contribute to accelerated rates of CHD in later life. Frequent and large cardiovascular and neuroendocrine responses to mental or psychological stress may influence an individual's risk for cardiovascular diseases, and preliminary data suggest that reproductive hormones may affect the amplitude of these responses. Whether postmenopausal women exhibit greater blood pressure and catecholamine responses to mental stress than do premenopausal women was investigated.

Study Design.—In the laboratory, 15 male and 34 premenopausal and postmenopausal female volunteers, aged 40–55 years, performed 3 standardized mental and physical challenges while blood pressure, heart rate, plasma catecholamines, lipids, and lipoproteins were measured. The 2 mental tasks consisted of mirror image tracing and public speaking, and the physical stress involved performing a 2.5-minute isometric handgrip

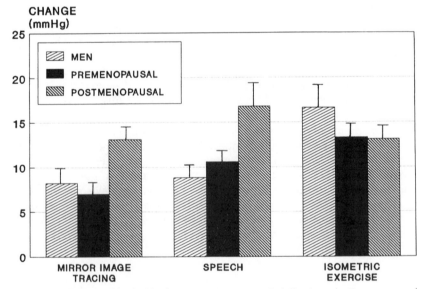

Fig 3–4.—Change in diastolic blood pressure in response to 3 challenging tasks. Data are mean ± SEM for men, premenopausal women, and postmenopausal women. (Courtesy of Owens JF, Stoney CM, Matthews KA: *Circulation* 88:2794–2802, 1993.)

task. The participants then wore an ambulatory blood pressure monitor during 2 consecutive workdays.

Results.—For both mental stressors, postmenopausal women had greater blood pressure responses and tended to have greater norepinephrine responses than did premenopausal women (Fig 3–4). For all women, the greater the changes in norepinephrine responses to public speaking, the lower the levels of estradiol; the greater the changes in blood pressure responses to both mental stressors, the greater the FSH and LH levels and the lower the estradiol level (for mirror image tracing only). Postmenopausal women exhibited higher ambulatory diastolic blood pressure levels during the workday than premenopausal women, even after controlling for body mass index, resting blood pressure during the laboratory testing, and age. Both premenopausal and postmenopausal women had similar responses to the physical stressor.

Postmenopausal women had larger blood pressure responses to the speech task and mirror image tracing task than did men, but both postmenopausal women and men exhibited similar norepinephrine responses to mental stress. Postmenopausal women and men had similar and higher ambulatory diastolic blood pressure levels compared with premenopausal women. In public speaking, larger blood pressure responses correlated with higher total cholesterol level and lower educational attainment.

Implications.—Menopause is associated with enhanced stress-induced cardiovascular response and elevated ambulatory blood pressure during the workday. These heightened responses may play a critical role in the risk of cardiovascular morbidity and mortality in postmenopausal women.

▶ Lindheim et al. *(J Soc Gynecol Invest* 1:79, 1994) reported that both the pressor and norepinephrine responses to behavioral stress tests were blunted by estrogen replacement alone but not when it was given together with a progestogen.

Although still controversial (Posthuma et al: *BMJ* 308:1268, 1994), there is a strong belief that hormone replacement reduces the risk of ischemic heart disease by about 50%. The effects of estrogen on lipids account for only half of this effect. Estrogens have also been shown to reduce the impedance to flow in the internal carotid and middle cerebral arteries (Granger et al: *Lancet* 338:839, 1992; Penotti et al: *Am J Obstet Gynecol* 169:1226, 1993) and the uterine artery (Bowrne et al: *Lancet* 335:1470, 1990). These effects may be partially reversed by progestogens (Marsh et al: *Fertil Steril* 62:771, 1994). These effects of estrogens may be the result of the release of prostacyclins (Steinleitner et al: *Am J Obstet Gynecol* 161:1677, 1989) and nitric oxide (Gisclard et al: *Pharmacol Exp Ther* 244:19, 1988). Ethinyl estradiol attenuated the paradoxical acetylcholine-induced coronary artery vasoconstriction response seen in postmenopausal women (Reis et al: *Circulation* 89:52, 1994). Overall, these studies on hormonal replacement therapy suggest that the addition of progestogens may decrease the beneficial effect of estrogen on the prevention of atherosclerotic disease.—J.E. Morley, M.D.

Hormonal Status and Clinical Relevance of Hirsutism in Elderly Women

Pepersack T, Rossi C, Dupuis F, Lefevre A, Vanhaeverbeek M, Dekoninck W (Centre Hospitalier André Vésale, Montigny-le-Tilleul, Belgium)
Acta Endocrinol 129:307–310, 1993   112-95-3-11

Introduction.—Hirsutism often occurs in elderly women, but its etiology in these patients is not established. To clarify the etiology of hirsutism in this population, serum androgen concentrations were related to anthropometric determinations, bone mass, and serum lipids.

Methods.—Ten hirsute women and 10 age-matched nonhirsute women between the ages of 65 and 92 years were studied. The hirsutism was mainly facial, had been present for at least 2 years, and was not accompanied by other signs of virilization. Androgen levels were measured at baseline, after ACTH stimulation, and after dexamethasone suppression. Other measurements included serum lipids, skinfold thickness, body density, body mass index, and bone density.

Results.—The women with hirsutism had significantly elevated serum testosterone, dihydrotestosterone, and free testosterone levels compared with the nonhirsute women. The serum cortisol response after ACTH stimulation was similar in both groups, but the hirsute women had a nonsignificantly greater androgen response than the control subjects. Dexamethasone inhibition produced similar inhibition of serum cortisol and circulating androgens in the 2 groups, but the hirsute women had higher levels of 17-hydroxyprogesterone before and after the test than did the control subjects, suggesting a partial 21-hydroxylase deficiency. There were no differences in serum cholesterol levels or vertebral bone density. Hirsute women had lower subscapular and suprailiac skinfold thicknesses, and although height and weight did not differ, the body mass index was significantly lower in the hirsute women than in the control subjects. There were no correlations between androgen levels and anthropometric measures or bone mineral density.

Conclusion.—Hirsutism in elderly women was associated with higher androgen levels, which were likely caused by adrenal activity, possibly an adrenal steroidogenic block. The hirsute patients also exhibited anthropometric findings that are characteristic of the anabolic effects of androgens.

▶ The role of androgens in older women has been poorly studied. Although their potential positive effects on bone, muscle strength, libido, and memory have all been alluded to in the literature, there is no strong evidence to support its effects. The study reported here suggests one clear negative effect of androgens: hirsutism.

Valenzuela et al. (*Int J Gynecol Obstet* 43:313, 1993) defined the characteristics of postmenopausal women most likely to show withdrawal bleeding after a progestin challenge test. Features associated with bleeding include a high body mass index, an estradiol level above 40 pg/mL, an estrogenic vaginal cytologic pattern, and less than 5 years from menopause. Women who bled also had higher dehydroepiandrosterone sulfate, androstenedione, and testosterone levels. The progestin challenge test may be useful in identifying women at high risk for endometrial cancer developing.—J.E. Morley, M.D.

Elevated Serum Inhibin Concentrations in Postmenopausal Women With Ovarian Tumors
Healy DL, Burger HG, Mamers P, Jobling T, Bangah M, Quinn M, Grant P, Day AJ, Rome R, Campbell JJ (Monash Univ, Melbourne, Victoria, Australia; Prince Henry's Inst of Med Research, Melbourne, Victoria, Australia; Royal Women's Hosp, Melbourne, Victoria, Australia; et al)
N Engl J Med 329:1539–1542, 1993   112-95-3-12

Introduction.—Inhibin is secreted by the granulosa cells of the ovary before menopause; it inhibits the secretion of FSH. Women with granulosa-cell tumors have been found to have elevated serum inhibin levels. The usefulness of inhibin as a biochemical marker of early ovarian cancer was evaluated in postmenopausal women with epithelial ovarian cancer.

Methods.—Serum inhibin was measured before and 1 week after surgery in 210 postmenopausal women with suspected ovarian cancer and in 23 postmenopausal women with nongynecologic cancer. Of the 210 women, 143 had ovarian cancer.

Results.—Preoperative serum inhibin concentrations were elevated in 25% of the 210 women and in 29% of the 143 women who did have ovarian cancer. Women who had mucinous carcinomas and granulosa-cell tumors had higher mean values of serum inhibin than did women with other types of cancers. Elevated values were found in 89% of the women with mucinous cystadenocarcinomas, 77% of those with mucinous borderline cystic tumors, 100% of those with granulosa-cell tumors, 18% of those with serous cystadenocarcinomas, none of those with serous borderline cystic tumors, and 17% of those with other types of ovarian cancer. Elevated values were also found in 2 of the 28 women with nonovarian cancer, 11 of the 41 women with benign ovarian diseases, and 1 woman with colon cancer. Serum inhibin concentrations decreased after surgery in all of the women with elevated values. There were negative correlations between inhibin and FSH values and between estradiol and FSH values in the women with granulosa-cell tumors but not in women with mucinous carcinomas or other types of ovarian cancer. There were no correlations between serum inhibin and serum CA-125 concentrations.

Discussion.—The rapid recovery of normal serum inhibin concentrations after surgery suggest that inhibin monitoring could have use as a tumor marker. However, it does not appear that inhibin measurement would be more effective than annual pelvic examination, ultrasonography, and serum CA-125 measurement as a screening procedure for early ovarian cancer.

▶ Inhibin-deficient mice have gonadal tumors and a cachexia syndrome develop (Matzuk et al: *Proc Natl Acad Sci U S A* 91:8817, 1994). The cachexia appears to be the result of elevated activin levels that produce hepatocellular necrosis. Inhibin deficiency also results in adrenal cortical tumors. This may be a factor that contributes to the large number of adrenal incidentalomas found in older patients.

Blaakaer et al. (*Eur J Obstet Gynecol Reprod Biol* 52:105, 1993) found elevated inhibin levels in 60% of women with malignant epithelial ovarian tumors. Levels of FSH were reduced and correlated to inhibin levels. Inhibin production was associated with prolonged survival, suggesting that inhibin may play a protective (tumor-suppressive) role. Inhibin levels, but not CA-125, were elevated in a patient with recurrent sex cord ovarian cancer (Puls et al: *Gynecol Oncol* 654:396, 1994). Inhibin appears to be a key hormonal modulation for ovarian cancers and an excellent tumor marker for the gynecologic cancer that kills more women than do all other cancers.

Follicle aspiration in women undergoing in vitro fertilization demonstrated a decreased inhibin level in the fifth decade (Pellicer et al: *Fertil Steril* 61:63, 1994). Perimenopausal women have been demonstrated to have abrupt decreases in inhibin levels with a concomitant increase in FSH followed by a return to normal levels (Hse: *Maturitas* 18:9, 1993).—J.E. Morley, M.D.

Thyroid

Complex Alteration of Thyroid Function in Healthy Centenarians

Mariotti S, Barbesino G, Caturegli P, Bartalena L, Sansoni P, Fagnoni F, Monti D, Fagiolo U, Franceschi C, Pinchera A (Univ of Pisa, Italy; Univ of Parma, Italy; Univ of Modena, Italy)
J Clin Endocrinol Metab 77:1130–1134, 1993   112-95-3-13

Objective.—Thyroid function during physiologic aging was studied, taking advantage of 2 groups of selected aged individuals: 41 healthy centenarians (9 men, 32 women) aged 100–110 years; and 33 healthy elderly individuals, aged 65–80 years, selected by the criteria of the EUR-AGE SENIEUR protocol. The control groups included 98 healthy younger adults, aged 20–64 years, and 52 patients, aged 28–82 years, with miscellaneous nonthyroidal illnesses.

Results.—There was a low prevalence of autoantibodies to thyroglobulin and thyroid peroxidase in centenarians as well as in the highly selected healthy elderly group. Three (7.3%) centenarians had subclinical primary hypothyroidism, and their data were excluded from analysis.

Median serum free T_4 levels in centenarians (mean, 11.7 pmol/L) did not differ significantly from those in younger adult controls, whereas median serum free T_3 (FT_3) levels were significantly lower in centenarians (mean, 3.68 pmol/L) compared with those in the elderly and younger adult groups. Similarly, the median serum TSH levels were significantly lower in centenarians (mean, 0.97 mU/L) than in elderly and younger adults, but serum TSH was significantly lower in elderly adults than in younger adults. Both serum FT_3 and TSH concentrations showed a significant inverse correlation with age. In spite of lower FT_3 in centenarians compared with patients with nonthyroidal illness, median circulating rT_3 was significantly lower in centenarians than in patients with nonthyroidal illnesses but significantly higher than those in elderly and younger adults.

Conclusion.—Thyroid function appears to be well preserved until the eighth decade of life in healthy individuals, but a complex derangement develops with extreme aging (i.e., a reduction in serum FT_3). This derangement appears to be the consequence of both reduced thyroid activity, resulting from decreased serum TSH concentration, and impaired peripheral 5′-deiodinase activity.

▶ This study extends the concept that circulating thyroid hormone levels show little change with advancing age. The gradual, small decrease in T_3 levels in healthy persons is most probably the result of the failure of T_3 clearance to decline in concert with T_3 production. For T_4, both clearance and production are decreased. This emphasizes the fact that dynamic changes can occur in hormones with aging, with minimal differences in circulating levels.

Doucet et al. (*J Am Geriatr Soc* 42:984, 1994) found that older patients had fewer signs or symptoms of hypothyroidism than did younger individuals. In particular, older persons were less likely to complain of cold, cramps, or paresthesias or demonstrate weight gain. Szabolics et al. (*Eur J Endocrinol* 131:462, 1994) again reported that subnormal TSH levels are not rare in older persons, questioning the use of the super-sensitive TSH test as a screening test for hyperthyroidism. They also attempted to use elevated thyroglobulin levels to diagnose autonomous thyroid function in older persons. Thyroglobulin levels were not altered by age or nonthyroidal illness and fluctuated less than TSH levels. However, some euthyroid patients had increased thyroglobulin levels. It is possible that thyroglobulin should be added to the diagnostic armamentarium to help elucidate the significance of low TSH levels in older individuals. Radioactive iodine has become the treatment of choice for hyperthyroidism in older patients. Yamadas et al. (*J Am Geriatr Soc* 42:513, 1994) provided evidence that older persons, compared with younger persons, with Graves' disease require a shorter methimazole treatment period to normalize thyroid hormone levels and thyrotropin receptor antibody levels and to restore normal thyroidal T_3 suppressibility. The recurrence rate after discontinuation of methimazole was more than 20% in those younger than 30 years and 0% in those older than 60 years. Unfortunately, the rates of side effects for different ages were not reported. This study does, however, suggest that methimazole may be a rational therapeutic choice in older persons with Graves' disease!—J.E. Morley, M.D.

Bone

Age-Associated Bone Loss in Men and Women and Its Relationship to Weight

May H, Murphy S, Khaw K-T (Addenbrooke's Hosp, Cambridge, England)
Age Ageing 23:235–240, 1994   112-95-3-14

Introduction.—Loss of bone mass appears to be a major factor in the increased risk of fracture that accompanies aging. Most elderly individuals who sustain hip fractures have low bone mineral density (BMD) measurements. The relationship of BMD with age and weight was determined in a group of men and women 65 to 75 years of age.

Methods.—Study participants were community-dwelling men and women who were not selected with reference to their health status. Dual-energy x-ray absorptiometry (DXA) was used to measure BMD in the neck and trochanteric area and Ward's triangle of the femur and lumbar spine (L2–L3). Weight and height of the 434 men and 508 women were recorded and body mass index (BMI) calculated as weight in kg/(height in meters)^2.

Results.—Characteristics of the elderly men and women were broken down by 5-year age groups: 65–69 years and 70–74 years. For both men and women, mean heights were significantly lower in the older age groups. In women, but not in men, mean weights and BMI were significantly lower for those 70–74 years of age. There was a significant reduction in mean BMDs at all femoral sites for women aged 70–74 years vs. women aged 65–69 years. In older men, mean BMDs were significantly lower only at Ward's triangle. Mean BMD values in the hip and spine were significantly higher in men than in women after adjusting for differences in weight. But approximately one third of the decline in BMD with age, for both men and women, could be explained by the associated age-related decline in weight.

Conclusion.—Both men and women show a similar rate of decline in BMD after age 65 years. At all measured sites, BMD was strongly associated with weight, and differences in weight explained about one third to one half the differences in BMD between men and women. Some of the age-related loss of bone may be prevented by maintaining weight later in life.

▶ It would appear that one factor predicting BMD in women older than 60 years of age is milk consumption as an adolescent (Soroko et al: *Am J Pub Health* 84:1319, 1994). Grip strength in older women who exercise regularly is also a determinant of BMD (Kritz-Silverstein and Barrett-Connor: *J Bone Miner Res* 9:45, 1994). Thiazide use was associated with increased

BMD in older men and women in a community-based sample (Morton et al: *Am J Epidemiol* 139:1107, 1994). The major factors predicting hip fracture in older persons besides femoral BMD density are falling to one side, potential energy of the fall, and a decreased BMI (Greenspan: *JAMA* 271:128, 1994). This suggests that trochanteric padding may be a key preventive measure to reduce hip fractures in persons at high risk of falling.

A study in African-American women demonstrated that low BMI, stroke, use of walking aids, and alcohol consumption increased the propensity to fracture a hip (Griso et al: *N Engl J Med* 330:1555, 1994). African-American women aged 55–75 years have significantly greater BMD, lower 25(OH)$_2$ vitamin D levels, and higher PTH and calcitriol levels (Kleerekoper et al: *J Bone Miner Res* 9:1267, 1994). About one quarter of African-American women are at high risk for hip fracture, making them an important population in which BMD should be assessed at menopause.—J.E. Morley, M.D.

Calcitriol Corrects Deficient Calcitonin Secretion in the Vitamin D-Deficient Elderly
Quesada JM, Mateo A, Jans I, Rodriguez M, Bouillon R (Hosp Reina Sofia, Cordoba, Spain; Katholieke Universiteit, Leuven, Belgium)
J Bone Miner Res 9:53–57, 1994   112-95-3–15

Introduction.—Thyroid C cells that produce calcitonin also have vitamin D receptors and synthesize calbindin D$_{28k}$, which suggests that calcitriol may regulate calcitonin production. The influence of calcitriol deficiency and treatment on calcitonin production were studied in elderly, vitamin D–deficient patients.

Methods.—Blood samples were collected before and at .5, 10, and 30 minutes after infusion of calcium gluconate in 9 normal young adults and 8 elderly, vitamin D–deficient adults with normal renal function. After the infusion, the patients were given calcitriol intravenously every other day for 3 treatments; the calcium infusion was repeated on the 7th day.

Results.—The young and elderly patients had similar baseline serum concentrations of creatinine, calcium, and phosphate. Baseline serum 25-hydroxy-vitamin D (25-OHD$_3$) was lower, calcitonin was significantly lower, and PTH and alkaline phosphatase were higher in the elderly patients. The increases in ionized calcium with the calcium infusion were similar in the young and elderly groups. The calcitriol injections did not significantly change total or ionized calcium concentrations but did increase serum phosphate and decrease PTH. Calcitonin increased to the level seen in the young patients. During the calcium infusion, calcitonin concentration rose and fell quickly in the young group. The calcitonin increase was slower during calcium infusion in the elderly group but significantly faster after the calcitriol injections. When measured in relation to ionized calcium changes, the increase in calcitonin was similar to that seen in young patients after the calcitriol therapy.

Discussion.—Calcitriol therapy in a dose that does not change serum total or ionized calcium concentrations can dramatically improve calcitonin secretion to nearly normal levels in elderly patients with mild vitamin D deficiency. This normalization of calcitonin concentrations may have a beneficial effect on bone resorption in elderly patients.

▶ Sheraki et al. (*Bone Miner* 20:223, 1993) found that 1α-hydroxyvitamin D₃ treatment for 5 years produced a 6% increase in radial mineral density, compared with an 11% decline in the control group. Orimo et al. (*Calcif Tissue Int* 54:370, 1994) reported that this treatment increased trochanteric bone mineral density and decreased vertebral fractures. Chapuy et al. (*BMJ* 308:1081, 1994) found that 800 IU of cholecalciferol and 1.2 g of calcium per day decreased the risk of hip fractures for a 3-year treatment period. Walking at anaerobic threshold level for 7 months decreased urinary calcium and improved bone mineral density in postmenopausal women (Hatori et al: *Calcif Tissue Int* 52:411, 1993). Endogenous potassium bicarbonate improved calcium balance, reduced bone resorption, and increased bone formation (Sebastion et al: *N Engl J Med* 330:1776, 1994). Slow-release sodium fluoride, in combination with calcium, inhibited new vertebral fractures during a 2.5-year period (Pak et al: *Ann Intern Med* 120:625, 1994). Three years of intermittent cyclic etidronate treatment decreased the vertebral fracture rate (Harris et al: *Am J Med* 95:557, 1993). Although there is a Pandora's box of effective therapies for osteoporosis, there are not yet clear-cut guidelines for which subsets of older patients with osteoporosis will benefit from treatment.—J.E. Morley, M.D.

Prediction of Bone Density From Vitamin D Receptor Alleles
Morrison NA, QI JC, Tokita A, Kelly PJ, Crofts L, Nguyen TV, Sambrook PN, Elsman JA (Garvan Inst of Med Research, Sydney, Australia)
Nature 367:284–287, 1994   112-95-3-16

Purpose.—Osteoporotic fracture risk is largely determined by an individual's bone density in early adulthood. Low bone density is under significant genetic control via effects on bone turnover. Common allelic variants in the gene encoding the vitamin D receptor (VDR) can predict differences in bone turnover.

Findings.—In monozygotic and dizygotic twins, VDR genotype was the strongest predictor of bone density at both the lumbar spine and trochanteric region. A study of unrelated women revealed that postmenopausal women with bone densities more than 2 SD below the values of normal young women had overrepresentation of the genotype associated with lower bone density, the *BB* type. Women with the more favorable genotype, the *bb* type, did not reach this bone density level until age 71 years, compared with age 63 years for those with the *BB* genotype. The mechanisms by which the VDR gene influences bone density were unclear, although messenger RNA levels may have been altered by allelic differences in the 3' untranslated region.

Discussion.—Allelic variants in the VDR gene may account for up to three fourths of the total genetic effect on bone density in healthy individuals. Identification of this genetic marker may be important for early intervention in persons at increased risk of osteoporosis, for understanding the mechanisms of variability in bone density, and for development of specific targeted therapy.

▶ The concept that a simple allelic alteration in the receptor for 1,25-dihydroxyvitamin D could strongly predict the development of osteoporosis was highly appealing and received worldwide media coverage. Unfortunately, it appears that the prophecy of this paper, like Chicken Little's belief that the sky was falling, may be logically underenhanced. Hustmyer et al. (*J Clin Invest* 94:2130, 1994) have already reported an inability to find a relationship between vitamin D receptor gene polymorphisms and bone mineral density. This genetic wishbone appears to have no more substance than the Emperor's new clothes.—J.E. Morley, M.D.

Surgery for Sporadic Primary Hyperparathyroidism in the Elderly
Öhrvall U, Åkerström G, Ljunghall S, Lundgren E, Juhlin C, Rastad J (Uppsala Univ, Sweden)
World J Surg 18:612–618, 1994   112-95-3-17

Objective.—The symptoms, histopathologic findings, morbidity, and mortality in elderly patients with primary hyperparathyroidism (HPT) treated surgically were studied.

Patients.—Between 1963 and 1990, 90 women and 18 men aged 75–85 years (mean, 79 years) had a primary operation for sporadic HPT. Most patients (78%) had other significant diseases, including cardiovascular diseases (hypertension, cardiac insufficiency, cerebrovascular lesions, angina pectoris, and atrial fibrillation) in 69% and diabetes mellitus in 13%. One fourth of the patients were institutionalized before surgery.

Clinical Features.—The average preoperative serum calcium concentration was 2.99 mM (range, 2.60–4.65 mM). Six patients had a hypercalcemic crisis. Psychogenic symptoms were overrepresented (56% of patients), including dementia (22%), and relatively few patients (13%) had had renal stone disorder. Skeletal complaints were common (29%). Seven patients (6.5%) were overtly asymptomatic.

Outcome.—Bilateral neck exploration showed a single adenoma in 69% of patients and multiglandular disease in 27%. The average weight of the adenomas was 1,183 g; 60% of adenomas were of the chief cell type, and 9.3% were of the oxyphil cell type. Other histopathologic diagnoses were chief-cell hyperplasia in 24% and water–clear cell hyperplasia in 2.8%. Perioperative 30-day mortality after 1980 involved only one patient (1.4%) with myocardial infarction. Complications developed in 8.7% of the 69 patients operated on after 1980, including infections, vocal cord paralysis, and incisional hematomas. At a mean of 3.1 years after surgery, 95% of all patients achieved normocalcemia. Persistent HPT developed in only 2.8% of patients operated on after 1980. Symptoms were alleviated in 62% of patients, including 59% of patients with dementia. Overall, 56% died a mean of 4.2 years after surgery, mainly from cardiovascular disorders. Patients who died during the first year after surgery were affected primarily by diabetes mellitus and heart disease.

Summary.—Primary HPT in individuals aged 75 years or older is associated with prevalent psychogenic disturbances, oxyphil adenomas, and multiglandular parathyroid disease. The favorable outcome of surgery permits a rather liberal attitude toward parathyroid exploration among very elderly patients.

▶ Primary hyperparathyroidism is an important treatable condition in older persons. In our experience, anorexia and weight loss are common presentations of primary hyperparathyroidism in the elderly. Larsson et al. (*J Intern Med* 234:585, 1993) could show no added risk of hip fracture in persons with hyperparathyroidism. Percherstarfer et al. (*J Clin Endocrinol Metab* 78:1268, 1994) found that cancer patients with a raised PTH-related protein have a poor hypocalcemic response to bisphosphonates, a more advanced tumor state, and a poor prognosis.—J.E. Morley, M.D.

Adrenal

Effects of Replacement Dose of Dehydroepiandrosterone in Men and Women of Advancing Age
Morales AJ, Nolan JJ, Nelson JC, Yen SSC (Univ of California, La Jolla; Nichols Inst Reference Labs, San Juan Capistrano, Calif)
J Clin Endocrinol Metab 78:1360–1367, 1994   112-95-3–18

Introduction.—The changes in body composition that are characteristic of aging are accompanied by a progressive decline of adrenal secretion of dehydroepiandrosterone (DHEA) and its sulfate ester (DS), paralleling that of the GH–IGF-I axis. Epidemiologic data support beneficial effects of DHEA and DS, but their biological role in humans remains elusive. The hypothesis that the decline in DHEA contributes to the shift from anabolism to catabolism associated with aging was tested.

Methods.—A replacement dose of 50 mg of DHEA was administered orally at bedtime to 17 women and 13 men ranging in age from 40 to 70 years. All participants in the double-blind, placebo crossover trial were nonobese, nonsmokers, had stable dietary and exercise regimens, and were taking no medications. Fifteen of the women were menopausal and 8 were receiving estrogen replacement. Each participant was randomly given 3 months of DHEA and 3 months of placebo. Concentrations of androgens, lipids, apolipoproteins, IGF-I, IGF-binding protein-1 (IGFBP-1), IGFBP-3, insulin sensitivity, percent body fat, libido, and sense of well-being were measured during each treatment period. Eight of the men and 5 of the women underwent 24-hour sampling at 20-minute intervals for GH determination.

Results.—Within 2 weeks of DHEA administration, serum levels of DHEA and DS were elevated from placebo values in both men and women, reaching the levels typically found in young adults. These levels were maintained throughout the 3-month treatment period and were normalized within 2 weeks after DHEA was discontinued. Serum levels of androgens increased twofold in women; men showed only a small rise in androstenedione. Neither men nor women exhibited changes in circulating levels of sex hormone–binding globulin, estrone, or estradiol. There was a slight decline in high density lipoprotein levels in women, but no other lipid changes. No alterations were observed in percent body fat or insulin sensitivity. Serum IGF-I levels increased significantly and IGFBP-1 decreased significantly for both sexes, despite a lack of change in mean 24-hour GH and IGFBP-3 levels, suggesting an increased bioavailability of IGF-I to target tissues. No change in libido was reported, and the majority of both men (67%) and women (84%) noted an improved sense of well-being on DHEA. Less than 10%, however, reported any change after placebo administration.

Conclusion.—The hypothesis that DHEA has a biological function in human beings was supported by these findings. A replacement dose of DHEA restored DHEA and DS levels in men and women older than age 40 years, inducing an increase in bioavailable IGF-I. Catabolic processes and physical and psychological well-being may be enhanced with DHEA replacement.

▶ Further evidence for a positive effect of DHEA came from the findings of Casson et al. (*Am J Obstet Gynecol* 169:1536, 1993) that oral administration decreased CD4+ (helper) T cells and increased CD8+/CD56+ (natural killer) cells with a marked increase in natural killer cytotoxicity. Nordin et al. (*J Endocrinol* 81:131, 1981; *J Steroid Biochem Mol Biol* 15:171, 1981) showed that DHEA treatment increases testosterone and estradiol levels. These studies continue to support the concept that DHEA deficiency may play a role in the physiologic changes associated with aging.—J.E. Morley, M.D.

Nutrition

Differences Between Young and Old Females in the Five Levels of Body Composition and Their Relevance to the Two-Compartment Chemical Model

Mazariegos M, Wang Z, Gallagher D, Baumgartner RN, Allison DB, Wang J, Pierson RN Jr, Heymsfield SB (St Luke's-Roosevelt Hosp, New York; Univ of New Mexico, Albuquerque)
J Gerontol 49:M201–M208, 1994   112-95-3–19

Background.—Although young and old females are known to differ in body composition, the extent of age-related changes remains uncertain. The methods used in earlier studies involved assumptions that themselves may be age-dependent, and the studies included young and old individuals who may have differed substantially with respect to body size and health status.

Objective and Methods.—Body composition was evaluated at a number of levels in 19 pairs of females, 19–35 years of age (mean age, 30 years), and older than 65 years (mean age, 74 years), matched for body weight and height. All participants were whites who were in good health. The methods used included isotope dilution measurements, dual photon absorptiometry, whole-body counting, hydrodensitometry, and anthropometric observations.

Findings.—The older females had a greater absolute fat mass and percentage of body weight as fat, larger total circumferential and skinfold measurements, and lower body density than did the young females. In the older group, fat was especially increased in the area of the trunk. Skeletal muscle mass was less in the older group, as were bone mineral mass and extracellular solids. Total body water values also were lower in the elderly group, but the ratio of body water to fat-free body mass (FFM) did not differ significantly from that in young females. Absolute values of extracellular fluid did not differ significantly with age, but elderly females had lower values for total body potassium and intracellular fluid. Body cell mass was significantly less in older females, and it comprised a lower fraction of FFM. The hydration and density of FFM were similar in the 2 groups, but the potassium content of FFM was lower in the elderly group.

Discussion.—These results agree well with those obtained by Cohn et al. for the density and hydration of FFM, but Cohn's findings suggested that the oldest females have higher FFM hydration and lower FFM density. Both studies found that old women have less skeletal muscle than young women of similar body size.

▶ Although this study finds that older individuals have a greater percentage of body fat than younger persons, it does not answer the question raised by both Cohn et al. (*J Lab Clin Med* 105:305, 1985) and Silver et al. (*J Am Ge-*

riatr Soc 41:211, 1993) of whether the major increase in body fat occurs at the time of the menopause and then declines in later life.

Roberts et al. (*JAMA* 272:1601, 1994) reported that older persons, after overfeeding, failed to experience the same degree of spontaneous hypophagia that younger persons did. After underfeeding, older patients failed to show the hyperphagia seen in younger persons. These studies support the contention that aging is associated with a physiologic impaired ability to regulate energy intake. Martinez et al. (*Regul Pept* 49:109, 1993; *Life Sci* 53:1643, 1993) reported on a group of older individuals who had an idiopathic pathologic anorexia of aging. These subjects had increased plasma cholecystokininoctapeptide levels and decreased CSF levels of beta-endorphin. They also had increased CSF levels of tryptophan and histidine. These are the precursors for serotonin and histamine, both of which have been suggested to play a role in producing anorexia.—J.E. Morley, M.D.

Suggested Reading

Mooradian AD, Wong NCW: Age-related changes in thyroid hormone action. *Eur J Endocrinol* 131:451–461, 1994.

▶ This highly recommended review suggests that aging is associated with resistance to thyroid hormone action. A number of biochemical changes in response to T_3 have been demonstrated to be decreased with aging, e.g., malic enzyme, $Na^+K^+ATPase$, S_{14}, and Ca^{2+} ATPase. It is suggested that this resistance to thyroid hormone is responsible for the occurrence of apathetic hyperthyroidism and some of the clinical signs of hypothyroidism seen in euthyroid elderly individuals.

Blumenthal HT, Perlstein IB: The biopathology of aging of the endocrine system: The parathyroid glands. *J Am Geriatr Soc* 41:1116, 1994.

▶ This is a detailed review of the age-related changes of the parathyroid gland. The authors suggest that hyperparathyroidism represents a part of the continuum of aging changes.

Villareal DT, Morley JE: Trophic factors in aging: Should older people receive hormonal replacement therapy? *Drugs Aging* 4:492–509, 1994.

▶ An overview of the ability of various hormones to reverse the aging process. The place of estrogen is fairly well established. Testosterone in men is becoming a major contender.

4 Calcium Regulating Hormones and Bone Metabolism

Introduction

Early in 1994, a study from Sydney, Australia, appeared in the *Wall Street Journal* (among other publications) with the title "Single Gene Is Linked to Osteoporosis, Hinders Delivery of Calcium to Bones." The actual title of the article was "Prediction of Bone Density From Vitamin D Receptor Alleles" (Morrison et al: *Nature* 367:284, 1994), in which it was found that subjects with a *bb* genotype had the highest average bone density, those with a *BB* genotype had the lowest, and those with *bB* were intermediate. Presumably this genetic variability translates to variations in the vitamin D receptor, which could account for variability in the ability of vitamin D to influence calcium (and perhaps phosphorous) absorption and/or delivery to bones. If so, conceivably one could identify individuals at risk early in life, give them vitamin D supplementation, and thereby perhaps build a greater bone density and lessen bone loss after attainment of peak bone mass.

The above study was the outgrowth of several years of work relating to variability in the gene for the vitamin D receptor and markers of bone turnover, of which one was osteocalcin levels that were found to have a positive correlation with bone formation (Morrison et al: *Proc Natl Acad Sci U S A* 89:6665, 1992). Other factors reflecting bone formation (type I procollagen peptide, bone alkaline phosphatase) have been or probably will be studied.

Markers of bone resorption (urinary hydroxyproline, total and free pyridinoline, and deoxypyridoline cross-links, type I collagen cross-linked N telopeptides, and serum C terminal cross-linked telopeptide) also have been or likely will be studied. Thus, subjects with markers indicating higher bone turnover have a lower bone density.

This all makes a very nice story that, if it were true, would probably lead to major advances in our ability to deal with osteoporosis. However, there are some flies in the ointment, namely, the variability in the ability to reproduce these results. Although investigators in Japan and Britain (Spector et al: *J Bone Miner Res* 9:1435, 1994) have confirmed these results, 3 groups of investigators in the United States have been unable to do so (Hustmyer et al: *J Clin Invest* 94:2130, 1994; Gallagher et al: *J Bone Miner Res* 9:143S, 1994; Looney et al: *J Bone Miner Res* 9:148S, 1994).

Why the discrepancies? Dr. Michael Parfitt, to whom I have referred previously in these pages as the "Aristotle of the skeleton and its disorders," has suggested the following resolution (Parfitt: *Lancet* 344:1581, 1994). Although the study populations in Sydney and in Indianapolis consisted of descendants of immigrants from Europe, their patterns of migration differed, with a higher proportion from Britain in Australia and a higher proportion from continental Europe in the United States. Also, another negative report from Sweden (*Lancet* October 1, 1994, p 949) supports this analysis because Swedish immigrants were more strongly represented in the United States than in Australia. It suggests that polymorphism for the vitamin D receptor gene might be associated with polymorphism for an independent bone density gene in one geographic region but not in another. If this hypothesis is correct, then Morrison and co-workers' observation, although not quite as exciting as it originally seemed, might yet prove to be the initial step in the eventual discovery of a new gene that has a major influence on bone density. It will be interesting to see how this plays out.

Will G. Ryan, M.D.

Psychologic Symptoms Before and After Parathyroid Surgery

Solomon BL, Schaaf M, Smallridge RC (Walter Reed Army Med Ctr, Washington, DC; Walter Reed Army Inst of Research, Washington, DC)
Am J Med 96:101–106, 1994   112-95-4–1

Background.—Primary hyperparathyroidism, which is being increasingly diagnosed, is classically characterized by metabolic bone disease, renal stones, gastrointestinal complaints, and nonspecific neuromuscular and neuropsychiatric changes. Psychological symptoms ranging from mild personality changes to severe depression and psychosis have been reported, but the type and number of psychological symptoms in patients with primary hyperparathyroidism has not been previously investigated.

Methods.—Eighteen patients with primary hyperparathyroidism were compared with 20 patients with benign thyroid disease. Psychological symptoms were assessed using the Symptom Checklist-90-Revised. Serum total calcium, ionized calcium, PTH, albumin, alkaline phosphatase, urea nitrogen, creatinine, protein, and phosphate were measured before surgery and at 1, 3, and 6 months after surgery.

Findings.—The patients with hyperparathyroidism had significantly greater levels of total and ionized serum calcium and PTH before surgery. Biochemical normalization occurred 1 month after surgery. These patients displayed multidimensional psychological symptom distress before surgery in the areas of obsession-compulsion, interpersonal sensitivity, depression, anxiety, hostility, and psychoticism. They also had a greater number and intensity of symptoms of distress. The hyperparathyroid group had significantly higher levels of paranoid ideation compared with the control group, although these levels did not quite reach the clinical range. The greatest symptom improvement occurred within 1 month after surgery, at which time the hyperparathyroid group approached the normative mean. Somatization and phobic anxiety did not differ between groups before or after surgery.

Conclusion.—In patients with primary hyperparathyroidism, psychological symptom distress is multidimensional. Symptoms are improved substantially by 1 month after parathyroidectomy. The Symptom Checklist-90-Revised is a simple, quick, cost-effective tool for quantitatively assessing the psychological symptoms of patients with primary hyperparathyroidism.

▶ A brave attempt at a knotty problem. Are hyperparathyroid patients really psychologically symptomatic before surgery, as often suspected, and are they helped by surgery? This study would appear to answer in the affirmative (see also Kleerekoper: *Am J Med* 96:99, 1994).—W.G. Ryan, M.D.

Value of Technetium 99m Sestamibi Iodine 123 Imaging in Reoperative Parathyroid Surgery

Weber CJ, Vansant J, Alazraki N, Christy J, Watts N, Phillips LS, Mansour K, Sewell W, McGarity WC (Emory Univ, Atlanta, Ga)
Surgery 114:1011–1018, 1993   112-95-4-2

Introduction.—None of the imaging techniques used to localize elusive parathyroid tumors before reoperation are consistently diagnostic. A new agent, technetium-99m sestamibi (T/S), has been recently introduced to enhance parathyroid scintigraphy. Its usefulness in preoperative and intraoperative imaging of elusive parathyroid tumors was evaluated in patients with persistent hyperparathyroidism.

Methods.—The T/S imaging studies were performed on 10 patients in preparation for reoperative parathyroid surgery, 2 patients with primary hyperparathyroidism, and 2 patients considered poor operative risks. Some of the patients also underwent other localizing studies, including thallium technetium scanning (6 patients), CT scanning (12), MRI (2), arteriography (2), and venous sampling (1).

Results.—Fourteen of 16 parathyroid tumors surgically identified were correctly localized by T/S imaging. The T/S imaging studies produced 2 false negatives and no false positives. Of the other localizing procedures, thallium technetium scanning identified 1 of 6, CT scans identified 3 of 12, venous sampling identified 1, and MRI and arteriography identified no tumors. The T/S imaging was able to localize all 4 mediastinal tumors, which were not identified by thallium technetium or CT scans. It also localized 1 lesion at the aortic arch and 1 adenoma in the aortopulmonary window; both lesions were undetected by numerous other imaging studies. Unusual neck lesions, including an undescended left inferior parathyroid near the mandible, could also be localized with T/S imaging.

Discussion.—Imaging with T/S is more useful than thallium technetium or CT scanning in localizing elusive parathyroid tumors. Localization with T/S was false negative in 13% and false positive in 0% of lesions.

▶ There were several articles this year about this technique for parathyroid scanning. As indicated here, it appears to be a decided improvement over previous techniques for parathyroid tumor localization, with only about 13% false negatives and no false positives.—W.G. Ryan, M.D.

Prospective Evaluation of Selective Venous Sampling for Parathyroid Hormone Concentration in Patients Undergoing Reoperations for Primary Hyperparathyroidism
Sugg SL, Fraker DL, Alexander HR, Doppman JL, Miller DL, Chang R, Skarulis MC, Marx SJ, Spiegel AM, Norton JA (Natl Cancer Inst, Bethesda, Md; Natl Inst of Diabetes and Digestive and Kidney Diseases, Bethesda, Md; Henry H Jackson Found, Rockville, Md; et al)
Surgery 114:1004–1010, 1993   112-95-4-3

Introduction.—The operative success rate for hyperparathyroid surgery is 85% to 95%. Complication rates are more frequent during reoperations. Preoperative testing using selective venous sampling (SVS) for PTH has been unsatisfactory because of a high percentage of false negative or false positive results. The results of using SVS as part of a prospective series of localizing procedures in patients undergoing reoperation for hyperparathyroidism were reported.

Methods.—A total of 223 patients with primary hyperparathyroidism underwent ultrasonography, technetium thallium scanning, CT, and MRI of the neck. Patients with 2 or more positive test results underwent reoperation. The rest had SVS if angiography was equivocal. Parathyroid hormone was measured.

Results.—In 76 of 86 patients undergoing SVS, there were significant gradients in levels of PTH obtained from the left and right sides of the neck and the thymus. When these measurements were compared with operative findings, the results showed 69 true positive, 11 false positive, and 9 false negative findings for a sensitivity of 88% and a specificity of 86%. In false positive patients, the PTH gradient was not helpful in identifying the side on which the abnormal gland was located. In false negative patients, 80% had venous gradients and 20% had no gradient. In 28 patients who underwent SVS only, 82% had positive gradients and an operative success rate of 93%. In 7 patients with no positive preoperative test results, the success rate was 71%.

Conclusion.—In this study, there were only 3 false positive SVS results that misled surgeons. The technique is sensitive and selective for PTH and is the test of choice for reoperative procedures where parathyroid abnormalities have not been detected by other imaging techniques.

▶ This is a study to be done when "your back is against the wall," so to speak. Or when, as Harry Truman said, "The buck stops here." With the recent salutary results with technetium-99m sestamibi scanning, perhaps at least some of these can be avoided. Time will tell which will prove to be the "gold standard."—W.G. Ryan, M.D.

Reexploration and Angiographic Ablation for Hyperparathyroidism
McIntyre RC Jr, Kumpe DA, Liechty RD (Univ of Colorado Health Sciences Ctr, Denver)
Arch Surg 129:499–505, 1994   112-95-4-4

Background.—Many reviews have defined the causes of failed initial surgery for primary hyperparathyroidism. Although the reasons for failure are well-documented, persistent and recurrent hyperparathyroidism continues to be a clinical problem. The causes of initial failure, the accuracy of preoperative localization tests, the role of angiographic parathyroid ablation, and the safety and efficacy of reexploration for hyperparathyroidism were investigated.

Methods.—Forty-two patients undergoing reexploration or angiographic ablation for hyperparathyroidism were assessed retrospectively. Follow-up ranged from 1 month to 13 years. In preoperative localization studies, the cervical approach was used when the abnormal gland was suspected of being in the neck or mediastinum superior to the aortic arch. Sternotomy was used for deeper mediastinal glands unresectable through a cervical approach. Angiographic ablation of mediastinal glands was done with contrast administration after a catheter was wedged into the selective feeding artery.

Findings.—Initial failure resulted from mediastinal glands in 18 patients, surgeon inexperience in 12, supernumerary glands in 6, and other anatomical anomalies. Hyperplasia accounted for hyperparathyroidism in 26% of the patients and adenomas in 74%. Preoperative localization studies included technetium-99m sestamibi scanning, with a sensitivity of 86%; technetium-thallium scanning, with a sensitivity of 67%; arteriography, with a sensitivity of 63%; and venous sampling, with a sensitivity of 52%. Computed tomography, MRI, and ultrasonography were also used, with sensitivities of 42%, 33%, and 27%, respectively. In 89% of 37 patients undergoing reexploration, hypercalcemia resolved. Localization results were negative in all 4 patients in whom failures occurred. Angiographic ablation succeeded in 67% of 6 patients. One patient in whom ablation failed had successful mediastinal exploration. Hypoparathyroidism occurred in 14.3%. There were no cases of recurrent nerve injury.

Conclusion.—In this series, the most common causes of initial failure were ectopic mediastinal glands and incomplete surgical exploration. The technetium-99m sestamibi scan is the most sensitive preoperative localization study. Angiographic ablation of parathyroid tissue is most effective for patients who are poor surgical candidates and for avoiding mediastinum sternotomy. Reexploration and angiographic ablation were associated with a high success rate with acceptable morbidity and mortality.

▶ The concluding paragraph gives the meat of the article.—W.G. Ryan, M.D.

Results of Ultrasonically Guided Percutaneous Ethanol Injection Into Parathyroid Adenomas in Primary Hyperparathyroidism
Vergès BL, Cercueil JP, Jacob D, Vaillant G, Brun JM, Putelat R (Univ Hosp, Dijon, France)
Acta Endocrinol 129:381–387, 1993   112-95-4–5

Introduction.—Surgery may sometimes be unadvisable in high-risk patients with primary hyperparathyroidism. An alternative treatment for patients unable to undergo surgery consists of ultrasonically guided ethanol injection. The advantages and limitations of this new procedure were evaluated in a group of 13 patients.

Patients and Methods.—Patients selected for ultrasonically guided percutaneous injection of ethanol into parathyroid adenomas ranged in age from 66 to 98 years. Volumes of the parathyroid tumors ranged from .11 to 4.18 mL. Local anesthesia was used, and a 20-gauge needle was inserted into the tumor under complete ultrasound control. The solution (.5 to 1 mL of 95% ethanol) was injected when the needle-tip was seen inside the parathyroid tumor. One to 8 injections were performed in each patient. The injections were given 3–8 days apart when 2 or more were required. Total success after treatment consisted of complete normalization of calcium and PTH levels.

Results.—The ultrasound-guided ethanol injection treatment was totally successful in 7 patients who had undergone 1–3 injections. Plasma calcium and PTH levels were normal during a median follow-up of 28 months. Four patients had a partial success, showing significant clinical improvement and normal plasma calcium levels yet persistent elevated PTH levels during a median follow-up of 20 months. The ethanol injection treatment failed in 2 patients, both of whom subsequently underwent surgery.

Conclusion.—Ultrasonically guided percutaneous injection of ethanol was found to be a useful alternative for patients with primary hyperparathyroidism who have contraindications for surgery. The treatment was generally well tolerated. Transient dysphonia, observed in 4 patients, was the only side effect. Necrosis of the tumor must be total for a successful outcome. Plasma calcium and phosphorus levels are significantly reduced 48 hours after successful injections. Tumor size does not appear to affect outcome.

▶ This is an alternative method of parathyroid ablation in patients who are poor surgical risks. I'm not aware of any experience with this at our institution, but it may be useful to keep in one's "hip pocket."—W.G. Ryan, M.D.

Surgical and Medical Management of Patients With Pulmonary Metastasis From Parathyroid Carcinoma
Obara T, Okamoto T, Ito Y, Yamashita T, Kawano M, Nishi T, Tani M, Sato K, Demure H, Fujimoto Y (Tokyo Women's Med College; Mitsui Mem Hosp, Tokyo; Natl Med Ctr, Tokyo)
Surgery 114:1040–1049, 1993   112-95-4–6

Background.—Medical treatment with bisphosphonate, a potent inhibitor of osteoclast-mediated bone resorption, has recently been identified as a promising way to control intractable hypercalcemia caused by parathyroid cancer recurrence. The surgical and medical management of patients with pulmonary metastasis from parathyroid carcinoma was evaluated, and their responses to bisphosphonate treatment were described.

Methods.—Between 1980 and 1992, 7 patients with pulmonary metastasis of parathyroid carcinoma were treated at 1 center. Resection was performed in 6 patients. The last had long-term bisphosphonate therapy alone. Bisphosphonate was also administered to 3 patients before or after surgery.

Findings.—Two patients had a unilateral thoracotomy for a single pulmonary lesion. Four patients with multiple lesions had staged bilateral thoracotomies. In 3 patients who were alive and well 3, 8, and 12 years after their first thoracotomy, postoperative serum calcium levels normalized after each thoracotomy. In the other 3 patients, hypercalcemia persisted. Bisphosphonate treatment in 2 patients was also unable to control hypercalcemia. The serum calcium level was maintained in the 13 mg/dL range in 1 patient by bimonthly bisphosphonate treatment alone for 3 years.

Conclusion.—In some of these patients with pulmonary metastasis of parathyroid carcinoma, aggressive surgery was definitively effective. Although bisphosphonate therapy offers an alternative to resection, its efficacy is limited.

▶ Parathyroid carcinoma, fortunately rare, is a knotty problem at best. The most effective approach is resection of as much malignant parathyroid tissue as possible. The usefulness of bisphosphonates is limited, although later-generation, very potent ones may be more helpful.—W.G. Ryan, M.D.

Assessment of the Serum Levels of Bone Alkaline Phosphatase With a New Immunoradiometric Assay in Patients With Metabolic Bone Disease
Garnero P, Delmas PD (INSERM Unit 234, Hôpital E Herriot, Lyon, France)
J Clin Endocrinol Metab 77:1046–1053, 1993   1 12-95-4-7

Introduction.—Circulating bone alkaline phosphatase (B-ALP) is used as a measure of bone turnover. Monoclonal antibody immunoassays are more sensitive to liver ALP than to B-ALP and actually determine B-ALP indirectly. The results of a new direct immunoradiometric assay for B-ALP were studied.

Methods.—Serum samples from 353 normal adults, aged 20–88 years, and 57 patients with Paget disease, including 12 with liver disease, were assayed for B-ALP, PTH, γ-glutamyl transferase (γGT), osteocalcin, and pyridinoline. Total ALP (T-ALP) was determined colorimetrically, and ALP isoenzymes were determined by agarose-gel electrophoresis.

Results.—The cross-reactivity between liver ALP and B-ALP was 16%. Bone ALP and T-ALP correlated with each other and with age in both sexes. Bone ALP increased significantly in premenopausal and postmenopausal women, and the increase was significantly higher than that of T-ALP. Bone ALP in patients with metabolic disease was significantly higher than that in normal controls, and B-ALP values correlated with T-ALP values in patients with Paget disease. Bone ALP values decreased significantly in patients with Paget disease treated with IV bisphosphonate pamidronate.

Conclusion.—The normal range of B-ALP as measured by immunoradiometric assay has been determined. The assay is sensitive and can be used to detect bone regression caused by menopause and as a marker in other metabolic bone diseases.

▶ Although considerable progress has been made in differentiating B-ALP from liver ALP in serum, the assay is still imperfect because of a 15% overlap. Until this can be overcome, it is likely that in the assessment of a single individual with a small increase of either, the assay will still not be clinically useful. In situations where the changes are large, as in some patients with Paget's disease or liver disease, it should be more helpful.—W.G. Ryan, M.D.

Determinants of Remission of Paget's Disease of Bone

Patel S, Stone MD, Coupland C, Hosking DJ (Queens Med Centre, Nottingham, England; Cardiff Royal Infirmary, Wales; City Hosp, Nottingham, England)
J Bone Miner Res 8:1467–1473, 1993   112-95-4-8

Introduction.—Studies have shown the effectiveness of treatment with bisphosphonates in decreasing bone turnover in patients with Paget's disease. However, there has been little research documenting the duration and factors influencing remission with this treatment. These issues were addressed in this study, which is unique because of its long-term follow-up.

Methods.—Sixty patients with Paget's disease were treated with disodium pamidronate between 1986 and 1992 and were evaluated every 6 to 8 weeks. Serum alkaline phosphatase (ALP) levels were used to identify remission and relapse. Bone turnover, the treatment dose, and bone cell response were evaluated as possible remission determinants.

Results.—All patients had a remission; 50 relapsed. Initially, all patients had elevated ALP levels; these were reduced to normal with treatment in 57% of the patients. Fasting urinary hydroxyproline levels were reduced to normal in 41%, and most patients reported symptomatic improvement. The duration of remission ranged from 3 to 25 months (mean, 9.5 months). The treatment dose was not related to the duration

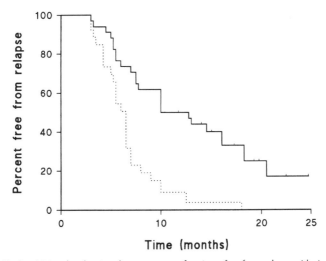

Time (months)

Fig 4–1.—Kaplan–Meier plot showing the percentage of patients free from relapse with time. *Solid and dotted lines* represent patients with a minimum post-treatment alkaline phosphatase below and above the upper limit of normal, respectively. There was a highly significant difference between the 2 groups (P < .001) using the log-rank test. Patients with a minimum alkaline phosphatase level above the upper limit of normal were 3.6 times more likely to have relapsed at any given time point (95% confidence limits 1.9–6.4). (Courtesy of Patel S, Stone MD, Coupland C, et al: *J Bone Miner Res* 8:1467–1473, 1993.)

of remission. Univariate analysis of patient and treatment variables revealed that the initial ALP, the proportional decrease in ALP 6 weeks after the first disodium pamidronate infusion, and the lowest ALP reached significantly predicted remission duration. Multivariate analysis identified the 6-week decrease in ALP as the most important influence on remission duration. Patients with a normal post-treatment ALP were significantly more likely to still be in remission at 1 year than were patients who maintained an abnormally high ALP (Fig 4-1). However, even among patients with a post-treatment ALP in the normal range, the duration of remission was widely varied.

Discussion.—Both initial and minimum ALP levels correlated negatively with the duration of remission, as could be expected. However, the great variation in remission duration in patients with minimum ALP levels in the normal range may reflect the difficulty in applying population-based normal ranges in individuals. The early response of ALP to treatment was the most useful predictor of the duration of remission, which may indicate the importance of bone cell sensitivity to bisphosphonates.

▶ There appears to be individual resistance to etidronate, which also is seen with pamidronate. In this study, the 6-week post-treatment ALP response appeared to best predict duration of remission. My own approach to treatment is to give relatively modest doses (30 to 60 mg × 1) to patients with relatively low ALP and go up from there depending on response. Patients with higher serum ALP levels tend to be more resistant, and I have given 60 mg/day × 5 on sequential days to one of these patients. Complete remission cannot be predicted from a normal serum ALP, because often residual disease is still seen on bone scan.—W.G. Ryan, M.D.

Osteoporosis and Bone Morbidity in Cardiac Transplant Recipients
Lee AH, Mull RL, Keenan GF, Callegari PE, Dalinka MK, Eisen HJ, Mancini DM, DiSesa VJ, Attie MF (Univ of Pennsylvania, Philadelphia)
Am J Med 96:35–41, 1994   112-95-4-9

Introduction.—Osteopenia and spinal compression fractures are serious problems in some cardiac transplant patients. This study was conducted with 31 male cardiac transplant patients (mean age, 56 years) and 14 male patients (mean age, 58 years) with severe congestive heart failure (CHF) to examine the incidence of osteopenia and pathologic fractures.

Methods.—Bone mineral content and bone mineral density (BMD) determinations were made of patients' lumbar spine and hip. Radiographs were taken of the lateral thoracic and lumbar spine.

Results.—Cardiac transplant patients had undergone transplantation an average of 26 months before testing, had used immunosuppressive drugs for an average of 2 years, and had undergone an average of 2.5 rejection episodes. Although proximal femur BMD was below normal, and 6 transplant patients and 1 patient with CHF had vertebral BMDs below the fracture threshold, the results were not significant. No clinical measurements were prognostic. Eight of the transplant patients, but only 2 of the patients with CHF, had vertebral compression fractures. Here the difference between the 2 groups was significant. Parathyroid hormone and 1,25-dihydroxyvitamin D were elevated in patients with CHF, and serum osteocalcin was elevated in both groups, but the results were not significant. Transplant patients with fractures had twice as many rejection episodes as did their counterparts without fractures.

Conclusion.—Although cardiac transplant patients and patients with CHF had below-normal femoral BMD, the condition did not appear to be related to immunosuppressive drug therapy, although corticosteroid therapy for rejection episodes may have increased the incidence of spinal fractures. Increased PTH and diuretic use in patients with CHF may contribute to bone loss. Additional studies need to determine whether osteopenia is related to CHF or whether it occurs over time as a result of cardiac transplantation.

▶ Femoral neck bone density changes more slowly than vertebral bone density, and this may be the reason that there was not a significant difference between the transplanted group (average post-transplant duration, 2 years) and the one not yet transplanted. The results pertaining to the vertebral spine suggest that immunosuppressive therapy indeed had an adverse effect there.—W.G. Ryan, M.D.

Noninvasive Testing in the Diagnosis of Osteomalacia
Bingham CT, Fitzpatrick LA (Mayo Clinic and Found, Rochester, Minn)
Am J Med 95:519–523, 1993   112-95-4–10

Introduction.—Osteomalacia is difficult to diagnose except by bone biopsy. Several investigators have attempted to develop a noninvasive test for the condition. Whether identifying vitamin D deficiency or hyperparathyroidism could be useful in diagnosing osteomalacia was determined.

Methods.—Seventeen patients with osteomalacia diagnosed by bone biopsy were studied radiographically and had serum calcium, phosphate, 25-hydroxycholecalciferol [25-$(OH)D_3$], and 1,25-dihydroxycalcitriol [1,25-$(OH)_2D_3$] determined.

Results.—Eight patients had low calcium levels, 9 had low phosphate levels, and 2 had low levels of both. Sixteen patients had elevated alkaline phosphatase and isoenzyme concentrations. Urinary calcium concentrations were low in 3 patients. Serum 25-$(OH)D_3$ levels were low in 5 patients, and 1,25-$(OH)_2D_3$ levels were low in 4. Three of these 4 patients had normal 25-$(OH)D_3$ values. Levels of PTH were elevated in 7 patients. Nine patients had osteopenia, 3 patients had pseudofractures, and 6 patients had abnormal bone scans.

Conclusion.—Although clinical, biochemical, and radiologic findings were inconclusive, all patients had at least 1 physical symptom suggestive of osteomalacia on physical examination. Determination of 1,25-$(OH)_2D_3$ levels may be helpful in detecting vitamin D deficiencies, but prospective studies need to be conducted to evaluate the efficacy of this test. Although clinical and radiologic tests may be useful for screening purposes, bone biopsy remains the diagnostic tool in inconclusive cases.

▶ According to this article, noninvasive testing is relatively insensitive in the diagnosis of osteomalacia. I would think the more florid the condition, the more likely this approach would be positive. Whether it is necessary to establish the presence of mild degrees of osteomalacia by biopsy is moot, at least to my thinking. One can juice up the 25-$(OH)D_3$ levels with appropriate quantities of vitamin D.—W.G. Ryan, M.D.

Rates of Cancellous Bone Remodeling and Turnover in Osteopenia Associated With Primary Biliary Cirrhosis

Hodgson SF, Dickson ER, Eastell R, Eriksen EF, Bryant SC, Riggs BL (Mayo Clinic and Found, Rochester, Minn)
Bone 14:819–827, 1993   112-95-4-11

Introduction.—Primary biliary cirrhosis (PBC) mainly affects women and frequently results in bone fractures. The incidence of fractures and the mechanism of bone loss has not been determined. This histologic study was conducted to determine bone turnover in premenopausal women with PBC and osteopenia and to examine the relationship between the extent of liver disease and bone turnover.

Methods.—Twelve normal women and 12 women with PBC and osteopenia, all premenopausal, were followed for 42 months. Calcium absorption studies, radiocalcium kinetic studies, biochemical measurements, and bone histomorphometry studies were conducted on all patients.

Results.—Ten of 12 patients with PBC had advanced liver disease. The amount of bone being remodeled was significantly decreased in patients with PBC. Wall thickness decreased. There was a significant correlation between true fractional calcium absorption and 1,25-dihydroxyvitamin D. Bone turnover increased as hepatic disease worsened. The same factors that suppress osteoblast function also cause bone loss.

Conclusion.—Bone loss is related to suppressed osteoblast function. Bone remodeling increases as hepatic disease worsens. It is hypothesized that agents that suppress bone remodeling and liver transplantation can stop bone loss, and it is suggested that clinical trials should be initiated to study this hypothesis.

▶ The first 2 sentences of the concluding paragraph seem paradoxical. How can bone remodeling increase as osteoblast function decreases? If resorption is the culprit, then net bone loss occurs. These authors later reported that calcitonin was ineffective in preventing bone loss. I tried to convince the liver transplant team at our institution to try IV pamidronate before transplantation, but I wasn't successful. It seemed to be a bigger battle than I wanted to fight.—W.G. Ryan, M.D.

Osteopenia in Adults With Cystic Fibrosis
Bachrach LK, Loutit CW, Moss RB (Stanford Univ, Calif)
Am J Med 96:27–34, 1994   112-95-4-12

Background.—The prolonged survival times of patients with cystic fibrosis have been accompanied by the emergence of medical complications such as diabetes and infertility. Osteopenia has also been reported. The frequency and severity of osteopenia in young adults with cystic fibrosis were investigated.

Methods.—Bone mineral measures obtained from 22 white patients with cystic fibrosis, aged 18-42 years, were compared with normative data collected from healthy white control subjects at a university medical center. The group with cystic fibrosis included 14 women. Sites assessed included the lumbar spine, femoral neck, and whole body bone mineral.

Findings.—The patients with cystic fibrosis had bone mineral values significantly below those expected for age and sex at all sites using all expressions of bone mass. Mean Z-scores for the lumbar spine bone density, femoral neck, and whole body were -2.8, -2.5, and -2, respectively. Bone mineral apparent density was also significantly decreased in patients at the lumbar spine and femoral neck; thus, bone mineral deficits seen in patients with cystic fibrosis were not attributable to bone size differences. Bone mineral was significantly correlated with age, weight, height, and body mass index. Pulmonary status, glucocorticoid use, and gonadal function did not predict bone mineral status.

Conclusion.—Osteopenia and osteoporosis are common in young adults with cystic fibrosis. Age and body mass predict bone mineral, although the pathogenesis of this bone mineral deficit is probably multifactorial.

▶ This article confirms that adults with cystic fibrosis, not unexpectedly, have osteopenia, presumbably resulting from malabsorption. Levels of 25-hydroxyvitamin D tended to be borderline low or low, but PTH levels were normal. No mention was made of serum calcium or alkaline phosphatase, but presumably these were okay as well. Surprisingly, there was no correlation between osteopenia and the use of glucocorticoids.—W.G. Ryan, M.D.

Osteoporosis, Metabolic Aberrations, and Increased Risk for Vertebral Fractures After Partial Gastrectomy
Mellström D, Johansson C, Johnell O, Lindstedt G, Lundberg P-A, Obrant K, Schöön I-M, Toss G, Ytterberg B-O (Univ of Gothenburg, Sweden; Univ of Lund, Sweden; Univ of Linköping, Sweden)
Calcif Tissue Int 53:370–377, 1993   112-95-4-13

Background.—Partial gastrectomy is commonly done for peptic ulcer disease in elderly men in Sweden. A higher prevalence of fractures in the proximal end of the femur and reduced bone density has been reported. Partial gastrectomy has been considered an important cause of secondary osteoporosis. In this case-control study, bone mineral density (BMD), prevalence of vertebral fractures, and metabolic indicators of bone turnover were studied.

Methods.—One hundred twenty-nine men undergoing surgery between 1952 and 1961 were compared with 216 men from a community-based population study. The mean patient age was 72 years; all were born between 1910 and 1915.

Findings.—Vertebral fractures occurred in 19% of men with previous partial gastrectomy and in 4% of the control population. Bone mineral density measured in the right calcaneus was 20% lower in men who had a Billroth II procedure and 8% lower in those who had a Billroth I. Compared with control subjects, men with partial gastrectomy had greater serum levels of osteocalcin and alkaline phosphatase activity, a lower serum level of 25-hydroxyvitamin D (25OHD), and a lower body mass index (BMI). No differences were noted in serum levels of free calcium, intact PTH, or free T_4. More men with partial gastrectomy were smokers than were control subjects. Smokers had significantly lower serum levels of intact PTH and 25OHD as well as lower BMD and BMI than nonsmokers. However, the relationships between intact PTH and ionized calcium and osteocalcin were preserved. Gastroscopy was done in 78 men with multiple biopsies in the gastric remnant and the small intestine. Chronic gastritis was present in all but 2 men. An assessment of sternal bone marrow smears indicated that 40% of the men undergoing a Billroth procedure lacked bone marrow reticular iron. Iliac bone biopsies were done in several patients with low BMD and vertebral fractures, but there was no evidence of osteomalacia.

Conclusion.—Partial gastrectomy in men results in decreased BMD and an increased prevalence of vertebral fractures. Although osteoporosis was associated with signs of increased bone turnover, it was not significantly associated with secondary hyperparathyroidism. No evidence of osteomalacia was found in the limited number of patients with bone mineral reduction and increased vertebral fractures.

▶ These findings are similar to those in the previous abstract about cystic fibrosis. Although PTH levels were not increased as in the preceding study, serum osteocalcin and alkaline phosphatase (measures of bone formation) were increased, an apparent paradox. Until we know more, the take-home message from these 2 studies would seem to be to pay careful attention to vitamin D and calcium intake. The amount should likely be titrated by whatever means available or appropriate.—W.G. Ryan, M.D.

Clinical Trial of Fluoride Therapy in Postmenopausal Osteoporotic Women: Extended Observations and Additional Analysis
Riggs BL, O'Fallon WM, Lane A, Hodgson SF, Wahner HW, Muhs J, Chao E, Melton LJ III (Mayo Clinic and Mayo Found, Rochester, Minn)
J Bone Miner Res 9:265–275, 1994   112-95-4-14

Background.—In patients with osteoporosis, sodium fluoride works by stimulating bone formation rather than by inhibiting bone resorption. It is capable of yielding significant increases in cancellous bone mass, but the true test of efficacy is its ability to increase bone mineral density (BMD) and decrease risk of fracture. Further follow-up of a previously reported clinical trial of sodium fluoride in osteoporosis is reported.

Methods.—The original 4-year clinical trial included 202 women with postmenopausal osteoporosis and one or more vertebral fractures. They were randomized to receive sodium fluoride, 75mg/day, or placebo. In addition, both groups received calcium, 1,500 mg/day, in the form of calcium carbonate. The women were evaluated every 6 months for 4 years. Fifty of the 66 women in the sodium fluoride group consented to an additional 2 years of treatment and follow-up. Follow-up included monitoring of new fractures in the vertebrae from T4 through L5. The definition of a new fracture was a 15% or greater decrease in baseline vertebral height since the last measurement.

Results.—In women receiving sodium fluoride, lumbar spine BMD (LS-BMD) increased by nearly 9% per year, compared to .3% per year in the placebo group. Radial BMD decreased by 2% per year in the NaF group. Thirty-one percent of women in the sodium fluoride group failed to respond to treatment in ways that were not explained by failure to achieve adequate serum fluoride levels.

Vertebral fracture rate (VFR) was no different between the sodium fluoride and placebo groups during the first 4 years of the study, although they decreased somewhat in the 2-year extension. The women in the extension group also had a decrease in nonvertebral fractures, but the rate was still higher than in the placebo group during the first 4 years. Vertebral fracture rate increased by 11% for each 1-μM increase in serum fluoride over baseline and decreased with increasing LS-BMD. If higher LS-BMD values were associated with only moderate increases in serum fluoride or with moderate rates of change in LS-BMD, then VFR decreased with increasing BMD. As long as the rate of change in LS-BMD was under 17% of baseline, VFR decreased as LS-BMD increased; more rapid changes in LS-BMD were associated with increasing VFR. As long as mean serum fluoride remained no more than 8 μM above baseline, VFR decreased with increasing LS-BMD.

Conclusion.—According to the outcome criteria of this study, sodium fluoride is not effective in the treatment of osteoporosis. However, achieving moderate but not large increases in serum fluoride level and LS-BMD may yield 30% to 35% decreases in VFR. The decreases in VFR achieved by antiresorptive drugs may work through some mechanism different than that of sodium fluoride and other formation stimulating drugs. Some patients do not respond to sodium fluoride treatment.

▶ How the dose of 75 mg/day of sodium fluoride was arrived at in this study is something of a mystery, because it has been published previously that doses in excess of 60 mg/day resulted in morphologically abnormal bone. Here it appears that patients who took a lesser dose fared better. Perhaps the use of fluoride in osteoporosis will be resurrected with further study.—W.G. Ryan, M.D

Abnormal Bone Mineralization After Fluoride Treatment in Osteoporosis: A Small-Angle X-Ray-Scattering Study
Fratzl P, Roschger P, Eschberger J, Abendroth B, Klaushofer K (Ludwig Boltzmann-Inst for Osteology, Vienna; Universität Wien, Vienna; Friedrich Schiller-Universität Jena, Germany)
J Bone Miner Res 9:1541–1549, 1994   112-95-4–15

Introduction.—Clinical studies have shown the efficacy of sodium fluoride in increasing bone mass and bone mineral density in patients with osteoporosis. However, the fracture prevention of fluoride-treated bone has not been proven, prompting doubts about its biomechanical properties. To determine whether new bone after fluoride treatment may have a higher density of mineral crystals in the collagen matrix, the mineral ultrastructure was examined in both normal and fluoride-treated bone.

Methods.—Bone biopsies were taken from the iliac crests of 3 patients with postmenopausal osteoporosis before and after fluoride treatment, from 1 patient with iatrogenic fluoride overdose, and from 3 control patients. The bone sections were examined using back-scattered electron imaging (BEI) and small-angle x-ray scattering (SAXS).

Results.—The typical thickness of the mineral crystals was similar in the controls and in the patients with osteoporosis before fluoride treatment, whereas the mineral crystals were significantly thicker in the patient with severe fluorosis. The ultrastructure of bone in the fluorotic patients (Fig 4–2) was completely different from that in the control patients (Fig 4–3) because of the presence of very large crystals in addition to the normal smaller crystals. The osteocytic lacunae were hypo-

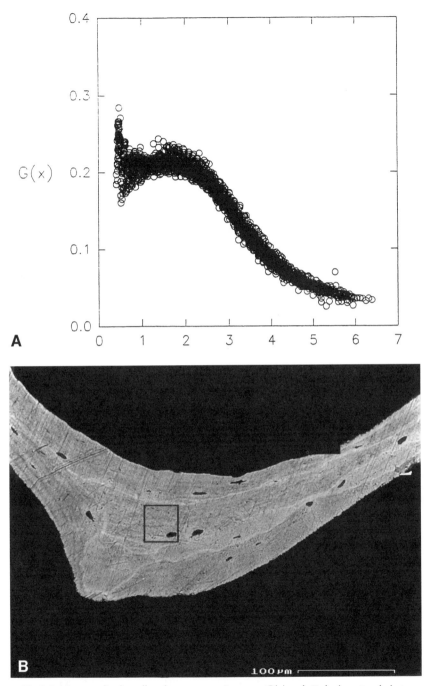

Fig 4–2.—A, normalized small-angle x-ray scattering curve $G(x)$ and, **B,** back-scattered electron image from normal bone. **A,** superposition of 60 measurements from samples A, B, C, D1, E1, and F1; **B,** typical trabecula from sample D1. (Courtesy of Fratzl P, Roschger P, Eschberger J, et al: *J Bone Miner Res* 9:1541–1549, 1994.)

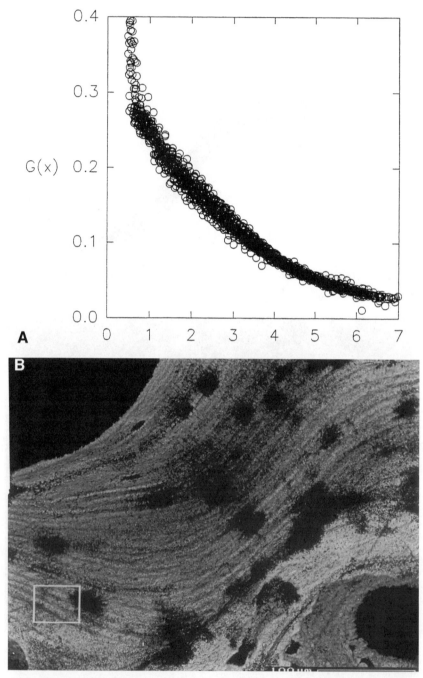

Fig 4–3.—A, normalized small-angle x-ray scattering curve G(x) (superposition of 24 measurements); **B,** back-scattered electron image from fluorotic bone sample (sample G). (Courtesy of Fratzl P, Roschger P, Eschberger J, et al: *J Bone Miner Res* 9:1541–1549, 1994.)

mineralized in fluorotic bone, whereas the lamella had a normal arrangement of collagen fibrils. Although the mineralization pattern was consistent in normal bone and in the bone from the severely fluorotic patient, it was quite variable in bone biopsies from osteoporotic patients after fluoride treatment, with patterns similar to both normal bone and fluorotic bone. Radiographic microanalysis revealed that fluorine was present in the areas with a fluorotic mineralization pattern and was undetectable in the areas with a normal mineralization pattern.

Discussion.—The ultrastructure of bone in patients treated with fluoride consists of old bone tissue with normal mineralization and of new bone tissue with pathologic mineralization similar to that seen in patients with fluorine toxicity. This extrafibrillar mineralization increases the hardness and also increases the brittleness of the bone. Therefore, further research should study the risk-benefit ratio of the increased bone strength accompanying fluoride-induced new bone growth with the decreased bone strength accompanying subsequent replacement of old normal bone with low-quality bone.

▶ Based on these observations, one might question whether any dose of fluoride would be beneficial to bone. However, the proof will be in the definitive demonstration of a reduction in fracture rate (or lack thereof).—W.G. Ryan, M.D.

Reversal of Vertebral Deformities in Osteoporosis: Measurement Error or "Rebound"?
Nelson DA, Kleerekoper M, Peterson EL (Wayne State Univ, Detroit; Henry Ford Hosp, Detroit)
J Bone Miner Res 9:977–982, 1994   112-95-4-16

Background.—In the past decade, marked variability has been reported in vertebral fracture rates in spinal osteoporosis, depending on the criterion used for defining fractures. Vertebral deformities and fractures can be identified by digitized morphometry of vertebral bodies on lateral spine films. However, this method has been associated with the phenomenon of "disappearing fractures," resulting from the apparent increase in vertebral body heights of previously deformed vertebrae on subsequent radiographs. Although this phenomenon is considered biologically implausible and a result of measurement error, some deformity disappearances on morphometry may be real events.

Methods and Findings.—Two hypotheses were tested in the current study: that the "rebound" phenomenon results from measurement error and that some deformed vertebrae rebound toward their original shape and size, showing an elastic response to deformation. The measured heights of nondeformed vertebrae increased about half the time as a result of random variation, whereas deformed vertebrae rebounded more than half the time. Three heights, anterior, midline, and posterior, changed independently of one another in the deformed cases. Analysis of vertebral heights that increased at least 10% from one film to the next in deformed and nondeformed vertebrae showed that an increase in this magnitude is much more common in deformed than nondeformed cases. Analysis of the scatter of observations of anterior height over time in a representative vertebrae showed increases and reductions in vertebral body height using both the 10% and 15% criteria. Results were similar for all 3 height measurements in all vertebrae studied.

Conclusion.—The variability inherent in morphometric data from serial spine radiographs results in both disappearing fractures and a high false positive fracture rate. These problems can be minimized by using more stringent criteria for defining significant deformities or true fractures. The question of whether some vertebral deformities are transient events remains unanswered.

▶ I would have some difficulty swallowing the notion that some vertebral deformities are transient events.—W.G. Ryan, M.D.

Genetic Influences on Type I Collagen Synthesis and Degradation: Further Evidence for Genetic Regulation of Bone Turnover
Tokita A, Kelly PJ, Nguyen TV, Qi J-C, Morrison NA, Risteli L, Risteli J, Sambrook PN, Eisman JA (St Vincent's Hosp, Sydney, Australia; Univ of Oulu, Finland)
J Clin Endocrinol Metab 78:1461–1466, 1994   112-95-4-17

Background.—In normal populations, osteocalcin levels are genetically determined. There are additional markers of bone turnover: carboxyterminal propeptide of type I procollagen (PICP) correlates with bone formation; pyridinoline cross-linked carboxyterminal telopeptide of type I collagen (ICTP) correlates with bone resorption; and the aminoterminal propeptide of type III procollagen (PIIINP) correlates with nonosseous connective tissue synthesis. Whether these markers reflect genetic influences on bone turnover was examined.

Methods.—Serum PICP, ICTP, and PIIINP were measured in 42 pairs of female monozygotic twins (mean age, 48.4 years) and in 40 pairs of dizygotic female twins (mean age, 45.6 years). Bone mineral density was determined at the lumbar spine and femoral neck by dual-photon absorptiometry.

Results.—Neither age nor menopausal status correlated with serum PICP or ICTP, although serum levels were higher before menopause and declined in the first 10 postmenopausal years. Monozygotic twin intraclass correlation coefficients were significantly higher than those in dizygotic twins for both serum PICP and ICTP. Based on Falconer's index of heritability, genetic factors contributed to 95% of variance in serum PICP, 64% in ICTP, and 35% in PIIINP. The significant correlation between PICP and ICTP indicated common genetic influences on both peptides. Serum PICP correlated inversely with both lumbar spine and femoral neck bone mineral densities. A similar but nonsignificant trend was observed for ICTP levels and these bone mineral densities. Differences in lumbar spine bone mineral density negatively and independently correlated with differences in serum osteocalcin, ICTP, and PICP. The difference in femoral neck density negatively correlated with the within-pair difference in serum osteocalcin only.

Conclusion.—Both the synthesis and degradation of type I collagen are genetically determined. This phenomenon is related to the genetic regulation of bone mineral density.

▶ This article helps to "flesh out" some of the ideas presented in the introduction.—W.G. Ryan, M.D.

The Bone-Remodeling Transient: Implications for the Interpretation of Clinical Studies of Bone Mass Change
Heaney RP (Creighton Univ, Omaha, Neb)
J Bone Miner Res 9:1515–1523, 1994   112-95-4–18

Background.—A bone-remodeling transient, a complex series of events in the cell-based remodeling apparatus of bone, occurs when the remodeling rate changes. A computer simulation of the bone-remodeling transient was described.

Methods and Findings.—In this computer simulation, the focus is explicitly on changes in clinically measurable bone mass or density. Quantitative remodeling data were collected by histomorphometry and calcium tracer kinetics. The simulation showed that a great deal of the apparent gain in bone produced by several agents currently used to treat osteoporosis can be explained as a remodeling transient, rather than as a fundamental change in remodeling balance. Gains as great as 30% or more can be produced by nothing more than the remodeling transient, under certain possible combinations of basal remodeling rate, remodeling period, and degree of bone loss. The importance of separating response across the first remodeling period from bone changes that may occur thereafter for assessing bone-active agents was evident.

Conclusion.—The simulations done suggest that even some of the more dramatic responses associated with various bone-active agents may consist of little more than a transient. Transients of great enough magnitude to perturb bone measurable mass must occur as part of treatment response.

▶ The author of this article is one of my heroes in the area of metabolic bone disease. Here he cautions about interpretations in magnitude of change in bone mass based on early or short-term data.—W.G. Ryan, M.D.

Suggested Reading

The following articles are recommended to the reader:

Bilezikian JP: Management of hypercalcemia. *J Clin Endocrinol Metab* 77:1445–1449, 1993.

Kleerekoper M: A cure in search of a disease: Parathyroidectomy for nontraditional features of primary hyperparathyroidism. *Am J Med* 96:99–106, 1994.

Inzucci SE, Robins RJ: Effects of growth hormone on human bone biology. *J Clin Endocrinol Metab* 78:691–694, 1994.

5 The Adrenal Cortex

Introduction

January 11, 1995. It has been a mild Chicago winter (so far). The weather is a balmy 35°, but fog has enveloped the city and literally draped it with a black veil of mist. The major news story is the weather and how it has paralyzed travel because of the closing of both of this great city's airports. Even network news was weather related.

Yet, amid all the news that was not fit to see, all 3 networks carried 1 bit of health news. In the typical fashion of media hyperbole, the headline teaser proclaimed, "French scientist discovers the fountain of youth!" As I am veering to the other side of fifty, this, of course, caught my attention. There on the screen was the familiar and majestic image of the great French scientist, Dr. Emile-Etienne Baulieu. For those of you who may not know Dr. Baulieu, he is the inventor of RU-486, more popularly known as the French "abortion pill." Dr. Baulieu also is credited with, among many other discoveries, the isolation of dehydroepiandrosterone (DHEA) some 30 years ago while working on testosterone and estrogen. His stature is such that when he speaks, the world listens. And what he is now speaking about is a hormone that may ease aging. He cites evidence that DHEA can improve the quality of life for a longer period and could lessen some of the more unpleasant effects of aging, e.g., fatigue and muscle weakness. Dr. Baulieu cites the work of Dr. Samuel Yen and his group at the University of California in San Diego. In his study, middle-aged men (13) and women (17) received DHEA (50 mg/day) for 6 months and felt better, slept better, were more energetic, and could handle stress better than placebo-treated control subjects.

We have known for a long time that aging is associated with a drastic reduction in circulating levels of DHEA. There have also been data from animal studies that support the salutary effect of DHEA in older animals treated with the compound. As early as 1986, Dr. Yen's group provided evidence that DHEA-S concentration in the plasma is independently and inversely related to death from any cause and death from cardiovascular disease in men older than age 50 years (N Engl J Med 315:1519, 1986). Now, there is strong evidence suggesting that DHEA replacement might help reduce some of the physical limitations of aging. It is interesting to note that the American media gave very little attention to DHEA until the French and other European media had focused on Dr. Baulieu. In fact, the French news magazine *Le Point* dramatically announced his "fantastic discovery" with great fanfare. However, he has gone on record deploring journalists who have labeled DHEA as a panacea for all problems associated with aging. Thanks to his international stature and presence, he has, in turn, shifted the spotlight from Paris back to San Diego to Dr. Yen. With further controlled studies, we shall soon learn whether DHEA does reduce fatigue, osteoporosis, weight gain, and memory loss associated with aging. Now, that's exciting! The abstracts that follow can be no match for the DHEA story.

C.R. Kannan, M.D.

Physiology of Aldosterone Secretion

Effects of Magnesium on the Renin-Angiotensin-Aldosterone System in Human Subjects
Ichihara A, Suzuki H, Saruta T (Keio Univ, Tokyo)
J Lab Clin Med 122:432–440, 1993   112-95-5-1

Introduction.—Intravenous administration of magnesium or magnesium sulfate has been found to increase survival in patients with acute myocardial infarction. The renin-angiotensin-aldosterone (RAA) system is an important humoral and hemodynamic regulator in patients with acute myocardial infarction. The effects IV administration of magnesium have on the RAA system were studied.

Methods.—Six healthy volunteers with normal blood pressure received either IV glucose or IV glucose plus $MgSO_4$ solution. The other solution was infused in each patient 1 week later. After another week, the $MgSO_4$ or glucose was infused after oral administration of either diltiazem or indomethacin for 3 days. Serum and urinary electrolytes, plasma renin activity (PRA), plasma aldosterone concentration (PAC), plasma ACTH, and plasma cortisol were monitored regularly before and after infusion.

Results.—Glucose solution infusion did not change PRA, PAC, or serum or urinary electrolytes, with or without pretreatment. With the $MgSO_4$ solution, PRA increased significantly at 30 and 60 minutes after infusion, and PAC decreased significantly at 180 minutes after infusion. The only changes in electrolytes were increases in serum and urinary magnesium and urinary calcium. Blood pressure and urinary volume did not change. In patients given $MgSO_4$ and diltiazem, PRA increased, but PAC did not change. In patients given $MgSO_4$ and indomethacin, PAC decreased, but PRA did not change. Electrolyte changes were not affected by either diltiazem or indomethacin. Urinary excretion of prostaglandins was increased with $MgSO_4$, but this was partially controlled with indomethacin pretreatment. Plasma ACTH did not change with any treatment, and plasma cortisol decreased similarly with all infusions.

Discussion.—Magnesium induces renin release independently of changes in blood pressure, renal function, sodium, or chloride. The increased excretion of prostaglandins, which was partially inhibited by indomethacin, implicates them as mediators of magnesium-induced renin release. The decrease in PAC was dissociated from PRA elevation and was inhibited by diltiazem pretreatment, suggesting that intracellular calcium may mediate magnesium-induced changes in PAC. The benefits of magnesium infusion in patients with myocardial infarction may be caused by the reduction of aldosterone production.

▶ Finally, a role has been found for magnesium, the forgotten ion, in regulation of the RAA axis. This comes as no surprise, inasmuch as magnesium has been recognized to have a role in the release and action of PTH, 1,25-dihydroxycholecalciferol, arginine vasopressin, and insulin. Now, this paper provides evidence that magnesium infusion stimulates renin release and suppresses the production of aldosterone. The elegant use of indomethacin and diltiazem to illustrate the loci of action by these workers is indeed impressive. The article supposes that the beneficial effects of magnesium administration in patients with acute myocardial infarction (MI) are a result of the alteration in the RAA system. This, to me, is a leap of faith because no one, to my knowledge, has convincingly proven that abnormalities in the RAA system play a pathogenetic role in the acute MI setting.

Nonetheless, the article opens up some exciting commentary. First, the similarities between the effects of hypokalemia on the RAA system and those of magnesium infusion are striking. Hypokalemia can also stimulate PRA, while suppressing aldosterone production and release. It is now believed that hypokalemia inhibits the enzyme activity of corticosterone methyl oxidase, required in the formation of aldosterone. Second, if magnesium infusion raises PRA but decreases aldosterone synthesis, could these dual effects raise angiotensin II levels, a potentially vasotonic effect that is undesirable when one's coronaries are being blocked? Third, does the reverse, i.e., magnesium depletion, cause the opposite effect? Suffice it to say that this article will stimulate interest in the role of magnesium on the RAA system.

The list of secretagogues involved in aldosterone synthesis and release is continually growing. This list includes hormones (angiotensin-II, ACTH, and endothelin), ions (potassium and, now, magnesium), and neurotransmitters (dopamine, epinephrine, acetyl choline). In the past year, serotonin was added to this list when workers from France demonstrated that the 5-hydroxytryptamine (HT)-evoked aldosterone secretion involves the activation of 5-HT4 receptors (*J Clin Endocrinol Metab* 77:1662, 1993). Also, the role of the type I angiotensin receptor, as well as its response to sodium and potassium, received attention this past year (*Endocrinology* 134:776, 1994). In fact, Cook et al. have demonstrated the existence of different A-II receptor subtypes in patients with primary hyperaldosteronism caused by adenoma (*J Am Soc Nephrol* 4:111, 1994). The role of angiotensin-II receptor subtypes, I believe, is about to move from understudy to star in the next few years.

The next 3 abstracts deal with hyperaldosteronism as it applies to the clinician.—C.R. Kannan, M.D.

Hypermineralocorticism

Evaluation of Diagnostic Tests in the Differential Diagnosis of Primary Aldosteronism: Unilateral Adenoma Versus Bilateral Micronodular Hyperplasia

Gleason PE, Weinberger MH, Pratt JH, Bihrle R, Dugan J, Eller D, Donohue JP (Indiana Univ, Indianapolis)
J Urol 150:1365–1368, 1993   112-95-5-2

Introduction.—The differentiation and localization of excessive aldosterone production in patients with primary aldosteronism are critical to the selection of effective therapy. Unilateral adenoma is best treated by surgical intervention, whereas bilateral micronodular hyperplasia responds best to management with antihypertensive medications. The results of localization studies in patients with biochemically and pathologically confirmed primary aldosteronism were reported.

Methods.—A retrospective chart review identified 69 patients with unilateral adrenal adenoma and 11 with adrenal hyperplasia. The localization studies ordered for these patients were evaluated. Many patients had uncontrolled blood pressure despite aggressive antihypertensive therapy. The effects of adrenalectomy on hypertension were recorded as normalized, improved, or little changed.

Findings.—The mean patient age at diagnosis was 44.3 years. Mean systolic blood pressure was 190 mm Hg, and mean diastolic blood pressure was 120 mm Hg. The patients were unable to suppress aldosterone secretion with normal saline infusion or to stimulate plasma renin activity by provocative measures. Unilateral vs. bilateral localization of excessive aldosterone production was predicted accurately in 70% vs. 71% of cases, respectively, by adrenal venography. Corresponding percentages were 100% vs. 63% by adrenal vein hormone sampling, 46% vs. 56% by adrenal nuclear sampling, and 69% vs. 13% by anomalous postural decline of aldosterone. Adrenal CT correctly localized 86% vs. 80% of the lesions. Unilateral adrenalectomy normalized blood pressure in 79% of patients with unilateral adenomas but in only 18% of those with adrenal hyperplasia.

Conclusion.—Because aldosterone-producing adenomas and adrenal hyperplasia are not clinically distinguishable, localization studies are needed once primary hyperaldosteronism is biochemically confirmed. No single localization procedure is completely accurate; thus, 2 or more studies should be done.

▶ Any large study, even a retrospective one, that provides insight into the various localization tests used in the evaluation of patients with primary aldosteronism is worthy of review. This is doubly so when the experience reported is that of Dr. Myron Weinberger, a pioneer in this area, whose group has assessed the specificity and sensitivity of the 5 diagnostic tests used to establish this uncommon cause of hypertension. On a practical level, a full 5-procedure workup is not justified. For instance, scintigraphy is not readily available, venography can be dangerous, and selective venous catheterization of both adrenal veins is an expensive, invasive procedure that requires experience and expertise. The real question is, can one localize the etiology without invasive studies? In the authors' series of 29 patients with pathologically confirmed unilateral aldosterone-producing adenomas (APAs), 26 cases (86%) were correctly lateralized by CT. Similarly, in the 39 patients with surgically proven APA, the posture study identified the nature (but obviously not the side) of the lesion in 27 instances (69%). In practice, if an anomalous decline in plasma aldosterone concentration is demonstrable, and a unilateral lesion is visualized by CT imaging, I think most clinicians would be comfortable diagnosing unilateral APA. The 2 caveats that affect this comfort level are the limitations of the posture study and the occurrence of adrenal incidentalomas, i.e., false positives.

Let's take 2 worst-case scenarios: In one, the patient with no anomalous decline in aldosterone and a negative CT study can be mistakenly presumed to have hyperplasia when, in fact, the patient could have a small, renin-responsive unilateral adenoma. In the second scenario, the posture study is negative (as it can be in 30% of APA patients), but the CT shows "lateralization" resulting from an incidentaloma. The only sure thing is to perform venous effluent analysis by selective venous catheterization after ACTH administration. This is reaffirmed in the article, in which a 100% correct lateralization of unilateral adenoma was obtained by adrenal hormone sampling. Note that the same procedure was diagnostic only 63% of the time for bilateral localization. It is also interesting that scintigraphy correctly identified only 46% of patients with adenoma.

Do these data change the way we approach patients with proven aldosterone excess? I think not. Computed tomography will continue to be our first line of testing. The authors do note that CT correctly identified 80% of bilateral hyperplasia. Unfortunately, the study does not provide information on false positive results in patients with APA (unless none existed) or on the use of MRI in CT-negative patients with APA. The posture study to distinguish APA from bilateral hyperplasia is of little use if you are Japanese. Mune et al. (*J Clin Endocrinol Metab* 77:1020, 1993) studied 20 patients with surgically proven APA and found that the plasma aldosterone levels dropped with posture in only 2! Similarly, these patients demonstrated a reduced response to metoclopramide than had previously been reported in the literature. East is East, I guess!—C.R. Kannan, M.D.

A Case of Weak Mineralocorticoid-Producing Benign Adrenal Tumor
Matsumoto F, Kameoka H, Kokado Y, Iida S (Osaka Univ, Japan)
Urol Int 51:94–96, 1993   112-95-5–3

Introduction.—The hypermineralocorticoidism seen in patients with adrenal tumors typically is caused by an overproduction of aldosterone.

In a few patients with adrenal tumors, hypermineralocorticoidism may be caused by the overproduction of a weak mineralocorticoid, predominantly 11-deoxycorticosterone (DOC). However, a patient was seen whose hypermineralocorticoidism was caused by the overproduction of 18-hydroxydeoxycorticosterone (18-OH-DOC).

Case Report.—Man, 43, had been hypertensive for 3 years before an adrenal mass was incidentally discovered by ultrasonography. Physiologic and neurologic examinations, complete blood count, and urinary electrolytes were normal. Plasma aldosterone was reduced and plasma renin activity was suppressed. Plasma DOC, corticosterone, and 18-OH-DOC were elevated, and plasma 18-OH-DOC levels were extremely high. A right adrenal tumor was visualized with CT and MRI. Adrenal scintigraphy identified a focal area of increased uptake. After right adrenalectomy, the histologic findings were consistent with adrenocortical adenoma. Postoperatively, the weak mineralocorticoid levels normalized, as did the patient's blood pressure. In vitro studies of cultured tumor cells demonstrated higher production of both DOC and 18-OH-DOC than the other weak mineralocorticoids.

Discussion.—This is the first reported case of hypermineralocorticoidism caused by hyperproduction of 18-OH-DOC. Although the mechanism was unclear, the relative overproduction of both DOC and 18-OH-DOC in vitro implicates decreased 11β-hydroxylase activity. This patient did not exhibit typical symptoms of hypermineralocorticoidism, and the tumor was discovered incidentally. Clinical presentation may be subdued in patients with weak mineralocorticoid-producing tumors. Patients who have an adrenal tumor with atypical symptoms should be evaluated for weak mineralocorticoid production.

▶ Seek, and ye shall find! Here was a case of a routine "incidentaloma" measuring 3 × 3 cm in a hypertensive man without any unique features suggestive of endocrine hypertension. I would have screened him for pheochromocytoma, perhaps obtained an MRI to evaluate the signal intensity in a T_2-weighted image, and stopped there! The clues in this normokalemic, hypertensive man with an incidentally discovered adrenal mass were the low plasma renin activity and low aldosterone level—tests that most of us would not have performed in the managed (or mismanaged) care setting. Yet, these Japanese workers pursued this lead and went on to measure other "weak" mineralocorticoids, leading to the identification of the first case of adrenocortical adenoma secreting 18-OH-DOC.

The demonstration that ACTH administration resulted in marked increases in DOC, 18-OH-DOC, B and 18-OH-B when compared with cortisol indicates similarities between this tumor and its well-known but stronger counterpart of aldosterone-producing adenoma. The endocrinologic data in this case are strongly supported by the in vitro data obtained by studying the steroidogenic properties of the tumor cells grown in culture. So now we have an addition to the syndromes of tumorous mineralocorticoid excess. For another "twist" to the usual story of hyperaldosteronism, the next abstract will be of interest.—C.R. Kannan, M.D.

Unilateral Adrenal Hyperplasia
Pignatelli D, Falcão H, Coimbra-Peixoto A, Cruz F (Hospital de S João, Porto, Portugal)
South Med J 87:664–667, 1994   112-95-5-4

Introduction.—Primary hyperaldosteronism occurs in .1% to 2.0% of patients with hypertension. The most frequent causes are adenomas and bilateral hyperplasia. Serum potassium measurement is the most effective screening method, but the typical hypokalemia may not be present in some patients. A patient with primary unilateral adrenal hyperplasia without hypokalemia was described.

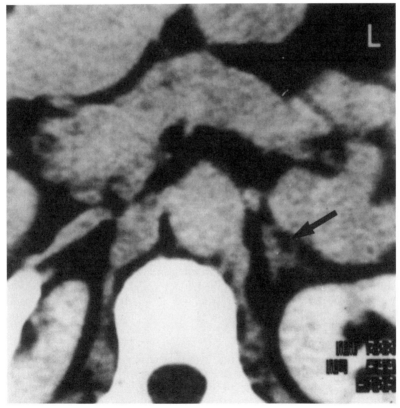

Fig 5–1.—Computed tomography scan reveals tumor in left adrenal gland (*arrow*). (Courtesy of Pignatelli D, Falcão H, Coimbra-Peixoto A, et al: *South Med J* 87:664–667, 1994.)

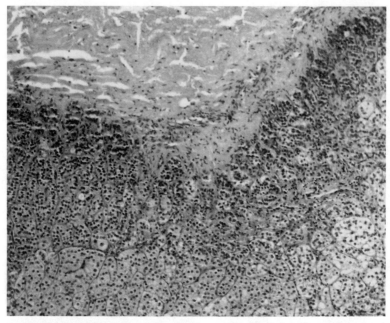

Fig 5–2.—Light microscopy of adrenal cortex shows diffuse thickening of zona glomerulosa layer and cellular nests extending to the capsule. (Courtesy of Pignatelli D, Falcão H, Coimbra-Peixoto A, et al: *South Med J* 87:664-667, 1994.)

Case Report.—Woman, 52, had arterial hypertension that was resistant to conventional therapy. Serum sodium was 138 mmol/L, serum potassium was 4.1 mmol/L, serum creatinine was 8.3 mg/dL, but urinary sodium was low at 73 mmol/day. The vanillylmandelic acid and urinary cortisol levels were normal. Serum aldosterone levels were high despite an unrestricted sodium diet (60.5 ng/dL) and decreased plasma renin activity levels after furosemide-induced volume depletion (.07 mg/mL/hr). The ratio of aldosterone to plasma renin activity was greater than 25:1, suggesting the presence of an aldosterone-producing adenoma. The dexamethasone-suppression test did not produce a significant reduction in serum aldosterone level or blood pressure. Computed tomography revealed a 7-mm tumor in the left adrenal gland (Fig 5–1), and a scintiscan confirmed the preferential uptake in the left adrenal gland. A left adrenalectomy was performed, and a complete remission was achieved. Pathologic examination showed diffused thickening of the zona glomerulosa layer with cellular nests that extended to the capsule (Fig 5–2).

Discussion.—Unilateral adrenal hyperplasia may, in fact, be more frequent than previously thought, as it can coexist with normokalemia. This condition may complicate the simple distinction between adenomas and hyperplasia as the cause of the aldosterone hypersecretion syndrome. It is hypothesized that primary unilateral adrenal hyperplasia is probably a new phase of the transformation between hyperplasia and adenomas that can also occur in the adrenal cortex similar to such transformations in other endocrine organs.

▶ Here is a case of hyperaldosteronism that had all the earmarks of a unilateral adenoma but histologically proved to be a case of unilateral hyperplasia. The patient was normokalemic (but with 36 mmol of potassium excretion daily) and had high concentrations of aldosterone in the plasma with suppressed plasma renin activity. Both the CT study and adrenal scinitigraphy with iodocholesterol demonstrated lateralization to the same side. The only surprise was that, histologically, the "tumor" demonstrated classic microscopic features of hyperplasia (Fig 5–2).

The authors' presumption that the case represented a phase of transition into adenoma is a valid one. This reminds me of a recent case at our institution. The patient was a 42-year-old woman with classic hypercortisolism: elevated 24-hour urine-free cortisol, nonsuppressible to 8 mg of dexamethasone, low plasma ACTH and dehydroepiandrosterone-S levels, and a 3.5-cm unilateral lesion in the right adrenal visualized by CT, along with a suppressed contralateral adrenal. The preoperative diagnosis was Cushing's syndrome because of a right-sided, cortisol-secreting adrenal adenoma. Much to our surprise (as well as the pathologist's!), the excised specimen revealed only hyperplasia with no evidence of a discrete tumor. Presumably, these cases represent "transitionalomas" and as such should be regarded as histologic curiosities.—C.R. Kannan, M.D.

Liddle's Syndrome

Brief Report: Liddle's Syndrome Revisited: A Disorder of Sodium Reabsorption in the Distal Tubule
Botero-Velez M, Curtis JJ, Warnock DG (Univ of Alabama, Birmingham; Veterans Affairs Med Ctr, Birmingham, Ala)
N Engl J Med 330:178–181, 1994   112-95-5–5

Background.—Liddle et al. described a disorder resembling primary aldosteronism but in which secretion of aldosteronism was negligible. They suggested that renal tubular ion transport might be so ineffective as to lead to a state simulating mineralocorticoid excess.

Case Report.—Girl, 16 years, who was hypertensive and hyperkalemic had a brother and sister, aged 14 and 19 years, respectively, with the same abnormalities. All of them had low urinary aldosterone levels, even when taking a low-sodium diet. Ratios of sodium to potassium in the saliva and sweat were high, and spironolactone failed to influence either the hypertension or the excretion of electrolytes. Urinary glucocorticoid levels were normal. Renal function declined, and dialysis was instituted 29 years after the patient had first been seen. A cadaver kidney was transplanted, and most recently, the patient had excellent renal function, was only mildly hypertensive, and had a normal serum potassium level. No relatives have had renal failure develop. A biopsy done 2 years after presenta-

Clinical Findings in a Family with Liddle's Syndrome*

VARIABLE	PROBAND	AFFECTED (N = 18)	UNAFFECTED (N = 15)	NOT AT RISK (N = 10)
Age (yr)	49	38±4	23±4	36±5
Blood pressure (mm Hg)				
Systolic	150	148±5	114±5†	112±6†
Diastolic	90	97±2	72±3†	78±3†
Serum potassium (mmol/liter)	4.4	3.6±0.1	4.2±0.1†	4.3±0.1†
Serum bicarbonate (mmol/liter)	19	28±1	27±1	26±1
Creatinine clearance (ml/min)‡	85	90±9	75±11	94±13
Urinary aldosterone excretion (ng/12 hr)‡	1059	369±388	1903±425§	2625±520§
Aldosterone:potassium ratio‡	62	22±23	171±26†	148±32¶

* Plus-minus values are mean ± standard deviation. The proband was studied as an outpatient in December 1991, 25 months after successful renal transplantation.
† $P < .001$ vs. affected family members.
‡ Determined in urine overnight. To convert creatinine clearance to milliliters per second, multiply by .017. To convert urinary aldosterone values to nanomoles per 12 hours and aldosterone:potassium ratios (expressed in terms of nanograms of aldosterone per millimole of potassium) to nanomoles per millimole, divide by 360.
§ $P = .01$ vs. affected family members.
‖ $P = .003$ vs. affected family members.
(Courtesy of Botero-Velez M, Curtis JJ, Warnock DG: N Engl J Med 330:178–181, 1994.)

tion had shown only slightly increased glomerular cellularity and occasional adhesions.

Further Observations.—Before transplantation, the proband's urinary sodium was not lowered maximally by sodium restriction, and hypertension and hypokalemia persisted during a sodium intake of 9 mmol daily. After transplantation, the plasma renin and aldosterone responses to sodium restriction were comparable to those of control recipients.

Heredity.—An expanded pedigree clearly demonstrated autosomal dominant inheritance. The 18 hypertensive family members had lower serum potassium levels than others who were unaffected, but there were no significant differences in renal function or urinary electrolyte excretion. The affected family members had decreased overnight rates of urinary aldosterone excretion when normalized for potassium content (table).

▶ Liddle's syndrome was first described in 1963, but this article gives it a new twist. The authors have done an admirable job of characterizing the tubular defect in the distal tubule of the kidney in the proband, as well as in her extended pedigree. Clearly, Liddle's syndrome belongs in the category of disorders in which the target organ behaves as if it were being stimulated by its trophic hormone when it actually is not. The abnormal transport of sodium across the distal renal tubule results in sodium retention, hypertension, volume expansion, and consequently, chronic suppression of aldosterone secretion. The potassium excretion is an obligatory counterpart to the enhanced sodium reabsorption at the distal tubule. Obviously, the cause of renal failure in the proband was unrelated to Liddle's syndrome. The authors establish the autosomal dominant mode of inheritance. The affected pedigree expresses itself with hypertension, suppressed plasma aldosterone concentrations, variable kaliuresis, low urine aldosterone excretion, and a low ratio of aldosterone to potassium in the urine. Thus, Liddle's syndrome enters into the clinical differential diagnosis of mineralocorticoid excess.

The nature and nomenclature of syndromes involving aldosterone can be quite confusing, even intimidating, to the novice in endocrinology. For the benefit of the "younger" readers of the YEAR BOOK, here is a quick review of the clinical syndromes of mineralocorticoid excess. The term "primary hyperaldosteronism" implies autonomous secretion of aldosterone and encompasses the following five entities: single aldosterone producing adenoma, bilateral micronodular or macronodular hyperplasia, glucocorticoid suppressible hyperaldosteronism, unilateral hyperplasia, and adrenocortical carcinoma. The mineralocorticoid secreted in excess in all of the above entities is aldosterone. Rarely, other mineralocorticoids, albeit weak, can be secreted as well. Thus, there may be mineralocorticoid excess from secretion of 11-deoxycorticosterone (DOC), 18-hydroxydeoxycorticosterone (18-OH-DOC), corticosterone, or 18-hydroxy (18-OH) corticosterone.

The next turn of the kaleidoscope brings into focus Bartter's syndrome, in which the mineralocorticoid excess is secondary to hyperreninemia from a tubular defect highlighted by chloruresis. Move the scope around a little more and you have the "syndromes of apparent mineralocorticoid excess." In these syndromes, a problem in the cortisol–cortisone shuttle leads to excessive exposure to cortisol of the mineralocorticoid receptor in the kidney. Examples of this phenomenon can be found in congenital cases, as with children, in cases of licorice ingestion, and perhaps in ectopic ACTH syndrome. Another twist of the kaleidoscope, and one has Liddle's syndrome, in which the problem is a target organ, in this case the distal renal tubule, transporting sodium at a frenzied pace, which leads to effects similar to stimulation by aldosterone. The final turn of the scope shows us pseudohypoaldosteronism, a genetic disorder caused by partial or complete resistance to aldosterone. The complexities of disorders involving aldosterone make it the most mysterious and intriguing of all adrenal hormones—C.R. Kannan, M.D.

Cushing's Syndrome

A Comparison of the Standard High Dose Dexamethasone Suppression Test and the Overnight 8-mg Dexamethasone Suppression Test for the Differential Diagnosis of Adrenocorticotropin-Dependent Cushing's Syndrome

Dichek HL, Nieman LK, Oldfield EH, Pass HI, Malley JD, Cutler GB Jr (Natl Inst of Child Health and Human Development, Bethesda, Md; Natl Inst of Neurological Disorders and Stroke, Bethesda, Md; Natl Cancer Inst, Bethesda, Md; et al)
J Clin Endocrinol Metab 78:418–422, 1994   112-95-5–6

Background.—The traditional gold standard for the differential diagnosis of Cushing's syndrome is the 6-day low-dose, high-dose dexamethasone suppression test (DST). The abbreviated overnight high-dose DST was recently developed as a more cost-effective approach to diagnosis. Because of the greater convenience of the abbreviated test, it was compared with the 6-day DST.

Methods.—Forty-one patients subsquently proven surgically to have Cushing's syndrome were enrolled in the study. Dexamethasone, 8 mg, was given orally at 11 PM. Blood samples for ACTH and cortisol measures were collected at 8, 8:30, and 9 AM the day before and at 7, 8, 9, and 10 AM the day after the treatment. The conventional 6-day test was also done.

6-Day Dexamethasone Suppression Test

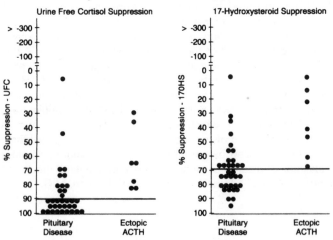

Fig 5–3.—Suppression of urinary free cortisol (**left panel**) and urinary 17-hydroxysteroid excretion (**right panel**) during the 6-day dexamethasone suppression test in 41 patients with surgically confirmed causes of Cushing's syndrome. *Abbreviations: 17-OHS,* 17-hydroxysteroid; *UFC,* urinary free cortisol. (Courtesy of Dichek HL, Nieman LK, Oldfield EH, et al: *J Clin Endocrinol Metab* 78:418–422, 1994.)

Findings.—The previously published criterion for the overnight 8-mg test had a sensitivity of 88% but a specificity of only 57% in diagnosing Cushing's disease. When the time of cortisol measurement and the diagnostic criteria for Cushing's disease were revised to obtain a specificity of 100%, the sensitivity of the overnight test was 71%. This was not significantly different from that of the 6-day test. Adding plasma ACTH concentrations to the test did not increase diagnostic accuracy compared with that of plasma cortisol level measurement alone. When the overnight test was combined with the 6-day test, the sensitivity and specificity were 91% and 100%, respectively, significantly better than that of the overnight test alone (Fig 5–3).

Conclusion.—The overnight DST has a low specificity for the diagnosis of Cushing's disease when performed as originally described. However, with revised sampling times and diagnostic criteria, it has a sensitivity and specificity comparable to those of the conventional DST. The diagnostic performance of a criterion that combines the findings of both tests is better than either test alone.

▶ It seems that the standard dexamethasone suppression test is continuously being refined. Readers may remember the article reviewed in the 1992 YEAR BOOK OF ENDOCRINOLOGY, which addressed "new and better" criteria for the interpretation of the standard 6-day, high-dose dexamethasone suppression test. The original criterion of 50% suppression as the great divide between pituitary- and non–pituitary-dependent and hypercortisolism (as defined by Liddle in the 1960s) apparently was not specific enough. The new criteria proposed that a 68% reduction in 17-hydroxycorticosteroids and/or a 90% reduction in urinary free cortisol provided more specificity in separating pituitary-dependent hypercortisolism (PDCD) from ectopic ACTH syndromes. Unfortunately, when the criteria were tightened, the specificity improved at the expense of a lowered sensitivity. Now, workers from the National Institutes of Health (NIH) have once again put another "standard" test in the crucible to see if it could stand improvement.

As our readers know, the modified 8-mg dexamethasone suppression test is now widely used in lieu of the 6-day standard test. The modified test has several advantages: It is simple, abbreviated, requires comparison of 2 plasma cortisol samples separated by an overnight oral bolus of 8 mg of dexamethsone, and, most important, it does away with cumbersome 24-hour urine collections. Above all, it is inexpensive. The criterion of 50% or greater suppression after an overnight 8-mg dose of dexamethasone indicated PDCD with a 92% accuracy and a 100% specificity (Tyrrell et al: *Ann Intern Med* 104:180, 1986). Thus, the common belief was that the modified 8-mg overnight dexamethasone test is as good, if not better, than the standard test. Well, not according to this article.

These workers have performed a head-to-head comparison of the old and new in 41 patients with hypercortisolism (34 with Cushing's disease and 7 with ectopic ACTH syndrome). When the 50% reduction in plasma cortisol was used as the criterion, the modified overnight test did not do as well as it should have. The test did yield a high sensitivity (88%) but, surprisingly, a low specificity (57%). This means that when a decline in plasma cortisol by 50% or greater after 8 mg of dexamethasone overnight was used as a criterion, the test "missed" only 12% of patients with PDCD. However, when suppression did happen, false positives were seen in almost half the patients who did not have PDCD. Of the 7 patients in this series with ectopic ACTH syndrome, 3 patients demonstrated "suppression" with the 50% criteria. Therefore, the authors tried modifying the test by revising sample time and test criteria. By this method, when the criterion of 68% was used to define suppression of plasma cortisol, virtually all patients with ectopic ACTH syndrome showed non-suppression, raising the specificity to 100%, i.e., no false positives. But, you guessed it. When the revised criteria were used, the sensitivity dropped to 71%. Of course, the authors found the greatest sensitivity (91%) and specificity (100%) when the 2 tests were combined. This does not make things easier.

The most compelling message from this brilliantly executed study is that the modified high-dose dexamethasone suppression test could stand modification of interpretive criteria; if the 68% decline in plasma cortisol is used and the result shows suppression, one does not have ectopic ACTH syndrome. If the patient does not suppress, one is out of luck and further testing is required. Isn't it frustrating! Just when you thought things got simpler, contradictions appear.

The same group from NIH is again in the spotlight in another of their impressive articles on the use of the metyrapone test and the 6-day, high-dose dexamethasone suppression test for the differential diagnosis of ACTH-dependent hypercortisolism (*Ann Intern Med* 121:318, 1994). The metyrapone test had a sensitivity and specificity identical to that of the standard 6-day, high-dose dexamethasone suppression test. Wonderful! But weren't we recently told by the drug companies that metyrapone will no longer be available for diagnostic or therapeutic use? So what are we left with? An old test that is cumbersome (and not the greatest when used alone), a good test using a drug that has been discontinued, and a modified, simple test that now appears murky. With these choices, no wonder the quest for the etiology of Cushing's syndrome has been likened to "searching for the Holy Grail!" (Orth: *Ann Intern Med* 121:377, 1994).

The main reason for the conundrum of Cushing's syndrome is the similarity between PDCD and some cases of ectopic ACTH syndrome. The next article (Abstract 112-95-5–7) provides an insight into that similarity.—C.R. Kannan, M.D.

Glucocorticoid Responsive ACTH Secreting Bronchial Carcinoid Tumours Contain High Concentrations of Glucocorticoid Receptors
Florkowski CM, Wittert GA, Lewis JG, Donald RA, Espiner EA (Christchurch Hosp, New Zealand)
Clin Endocrinol 40:269–274, 1994   112-95-5–7

Introduction.—It may be difficult to distinguish Cushing's syndrome secondary to an ACTH-secreting bronchial carcinoid tumor from a tumor caused by a pituitary microadenoma. In both cases, ACTH secretion may be responsive to glucocorticoids. It is not clear whether the bronchial carcinoids that do respond to glucocorticoid secrete corticotropin-releasing factor (CRF) as well as ACTH or whether they express glucocorticoid receptors.

Patients.—Two patients were encountered with Cushing's syndrome secondary to ACTH production by a small bronchial carcinoid tumor. In both patients, the ACTH secretion was suppressed by glucocorticoid, and the resected carcinoid tissue contained a high concentration of glucocorticoid receptors. The tumors contained 92 and 103 pmol/g protein, respectively, of glucocorticoid receptor binding capacity. Neither tumor contained CRF, and in neither patient did ACTH secretion respond to CRF administration.

Conclusion.—When an ACTH-secreting bronchial carcinoid tumor is responsive to glucocorticoid, the expression of glucocorticoid receptor in tumor tissue may be responsible.

▶ It has always been speculated that the reason for the similarities between pituitary-dependent hypercortisolism and some forms of ectopic ACTH syndrome is the expression of glucocorticoid receptors in the latter. Now there is proof. In this article, the authors found that bronchial carcinoid tumor tissue from 2 patients had glucocorticoid receptors. It is interesting to note that both patients responded to CRH, a clue that prompted these physicians to pursue the possibility of ectopic ACTH syndrome despite having no overt evidence to suggest its presence. It is also interesting that the excised tissue in the first patient showed immunopositivity to both ACTH and GH.

The data concerning the second patient are more complex. The CT scan of the pituitary, which was originally normal, later demonstrated a definite 8-mm mass in the center of the pituitary, leading to transsphenoidal surgery. When that failed, a bilateral adrenalectomy was done. Remarkably enough, the ACTH levels began to increase after the bilateral adrenalectomy, along with a mild increase in skin pigmentation, and the lung lesion literally "exploded" on the CT image as a 2-cm tumor. This is the classic behavior of Nelson's syndrome, except that it was happening in the lung and not in the pituitary! As expected, after removal of the carcinoid, the ACTH levels normalized, the pigmentation faded, and the hypoadrenalism was easily managed with conventional replacement. It seems we have come full circle since the description of amine precursor uptake decarboxylation (APUD) cells in the 1960s. Obviously, the neurosecretory APUD cells trapped in the lung had their message crossed and assumed pituitary-like properties, including the acquistion of glucocorticoid receptors. When a "microadenoma" developed in this tissue, it behaved exactly like the pituitary, including the evolution of a Nelson's-like picture after bilateral adrenalectomy. This article illustrates the remarkable crossover in the contents of ectopic and eutopic tissue.—C.R. Kannan, M.D.

Effective Reversibility of the Signs and Symptoms of Hypercortisolism by Bilateral Adrenalectomy

Zeiger MA, Fraker DL, Pass HI, Neiman LK, Cutler GB, Chrousos GP, Norton JA (Natl Cancer Inst, Bethesda, Md)
Surgery 114:1138–1143, 1993   112-95-5–8

Introduction.—Bilateral adrenalectomy has been shown to be a safe and effective treatment for patients with Cushing's syndrome caused by both primary adrenocortical disease and ectopic or metastatic disease. The long-term outcome of patients who underwent this procedure was examined.

Methods.—Of the 34 patients treated with bilateral adrenalectomy for Cushing's syndrome, 14 had ectopic ACTH syndrome; 10 had undergone previous unsuccessful treatment for Cushing's disease; 9 had primary adrenocortical hyperplasia, 5 micronodular and 4 macronodular; and 1 had Cushing's syndrome of unknown etiology. All had undergone at least 1 hypophysectomy. Survival and symptom resolution were assessed for each patient.

Results.—Of the 19 patients with hypertension, 15 (79%) required either no or less antihypertensive medication. Six of 7 (86%) patients with diabetes either discontinued insulin medication or changed from injected insulin to oral hypoglycemic agents. The symptoms of depression in 8 of 9 (88%) patients were resolved. Fatigue was reduced in 16 of 21 (76%) patients. Postoperative weight control was established in 23 of 29 (79%) patients. Normal menstruation returned in 6 of 8 (75%) amenorrheic patients. Hirsutism was resolved in 10 of 13 (77%) patients. There was no difference in symptom resolution between patients with primary or ectopic disease. The mean length of survival was 55 months, with a mean follow-up of 32 months (range, 3–67 months). Five of the 6 deaths occurred in patients with ectopic ACTH syndrome.

Discussion.—Bilateral adrenalectomy is a safe procedure that produces prolonged symptom resolution and improves survival in patients with primary Cushing's syndrome or ectopic ACTH syndrome.

▶ It is comforting to learn that when all else fails, there is always bilateral adrenalectomy to cure hypercortisolism, regardless of the etiology. This article is arguably the largest series from a single center (once again, the National Institutes of Health) that evaluates the outcome of bilateral adrenalectomy. The fact that the devastating effects of hypercortisolism are to a large extent reversible is reassuring. I believe that we often wait too long before recommending bilateral adrenalectomy. The inherent fear of Nelson's syndrome or the eventuality of Addison's disease probably contribute to the delay. The amelioration of hypertension, diabetes, obesity, psychopathy, and perhaps myopathy are strong reasons for recommending early surgical intervention when other recourses are no longer available. The most gratifying note is that no recurrence was noted in this series after a mean follow-up of

32 months. Similar findings have been reported by workers from Italy. Favia et al. (*World J Surg* 18:462, 1994) performed bilateral adrenalectomy in patients who had no response to or recurrence after transsphenoidal surgery for pituitary-dependent hypercortisolism and demonstrated that early intervention provided definitive control of hypercortisolism.—C.R. Kannan, M.D.

Addison's Disease

Early Adrenal Hypofunction in Patients With Organ-Specific Autoantibodies and No Clinical Adrenal Insufficiency
Boscaro M, Betterle C, Sonino N, Volpato M, Paoletta A, Fallo F (Univ of Padova, Italy)
J Clin Endocrinol Metab 79:452–455, 1994   112-95-5-9

Background.—Idiopathic Addison's disease frequently occurs in association with other organ-specific autoimmune diseases in which autoantibodies to adrenal cortex are markers of the condition. A variable subclinical period when the patient is asymptomatic with subtle adrenal dysfunction can precede the onset of clinical manifestations. The adrenal response to both standard ACTH and ovine CRH stimulation tests in patients with adrenal autoantibodies and no signs of adrenal insufficiency was investigated.

Method.—Nineteen women affected by organ-specific autoimmune disease and with adrenal autoantibodies were studied. All patients had normal adrenal steroid levels under baseline conditions and were normally responsive to a standard ACTH stimulation test (250 μg). Analysis of plasma ACTH, cortisol, and 17α-hydroxyprogesterone was carried out after administration of ovine CRH (100 μg as an IV bolus) stimulation.

Results.—In all patients, ovine CRH brought a maximum increase in plasma ACTH within 15 minutes. Plasma cortisol, which was normally responsive in 11 patients, showed little or no increase in the other 8 individuals. Two of these patients had overt adrenal failure develop after 1 year. The plasma 17α-hydroxyprogesterone response to ovine CRH, tested in 10 of 19 patients, paralleled that of plasma cortisol in all cases, excluding a steroidogenic block at the 21-hydroxylase site.

Conclusion.—The results of this study demonstrate the existence of a very early stage of Addison's disease in which adrenal function shows an impaired response to ovine CRH-stimulated ACTH.

▶ The evolution of autoimmune adrenal disease from the "marker stage" to the hypoadrenal state seems to be a long and winding road. In the 1994 YEAR BOOK OF ENDOCRINOLOGY, we reviewed a remarkable article on the natural history of autoimmune adrenal disease that speculated that immunotherapy with short-term glucocorticoid treatment might be interventional. In this article, Boscaro et al. provide us with diagnostic information on the hypothalamic-pituitary-adrenal axis in antibody-positive euadrenal patients.

The results are interesting for several reasons. First, the authors document the existence of a variable asymptomatic period with subtle adrenal dysfunction unmasked by the CRH test that precedes the onset of clinical manifestations. The fact that the cortisol response to CRH was suboptimal in 8 of 19 patients despite a perfectly normal ACTH response to CRH implies that the adrenal cortex in this subset of patients showed an attenuated response to endogenously released ACTH (in response to CRH) while responding perfectly to supraphysiologic doses of exogenously administered ACTH. The fact that the 17α-hydroxyprogesterone response was well preserved in all cases excludes steroidogenic blocks as a cause for the attenuated cortisol response to CRH. Second, the fact that 2 of the 8 patients progressed to overt clinical adrenal insufficiency may indicate the vulnerability of this subset. The authors found no significant change in antibody titers in this group when compared with the rest. Third, this paper adds to the growing belief that the supraphysiologic Cortrosyn stimulation test can overdrive minimal abnormalities in adrenal function and mask early subtle adrenal insufficiency. Although it is too early to say, the cortisol response to CRH may be a more sensitive index of adrenal function than ACTH stimulation. Regardless, such data as are provided in this article enhance our understanding of the evolution of adrenal failure in autoimmune adrenalitis.

Turning to other recent developments in the area of autoimmune adrenal disease, Song et al. (*J Clin Endocrinol Metab* 78:1108, 1994) have developed a technique for autoantibody epitope mapping of the 21-hydroxylase antigen in autoimmune Addison's disease. Taking this concept 1 step further, considerable attention has been focused on demonstrating autoantibodies to P450C17 and P450C21 in patients with Addison's disease, as well as those with pluriglandular failure syndromes (Uibo et al: *J Clin Endocrinol Metab* 78:323, 1994).

Finally, a recent report indicates that glucocorticoid deficiency can result from abnormalities in the ACTH receptor gene (Tsigos et al: *J Clin Invest* 92:2458, 1993).—C.R. Kannan, M.D.

Hyponatremia and Osmoregulation of Thirst and Vasopressin Secretion in Patients With Adrenal Insufficiency
Kamoi K, Tamura T, Tanaka K, Ishibashi M, Yamaji T (Nagaoka Red Cross Hosp, Japan; Niigata Univ, Japan; Teikyo Univ, Chiba, Japan; et al)
J Clin Endocrinol Metab 77:1584–1588, 1993   112-95-5-10

Background.—The mechanism underlying increased secretion of abnormal vasopressin (AVP) in glucocorticoid deficiency is unknown. To investigate further, 7 patients with adrenal insufficiency were studied to examine the response of AVP secretion to osmotic stimulus and to analyze the possible causative factors for persistent AVP secretion.

Clinical and Laboratory Features.—All patients had nausea or vomiting, 5 complained of thirst, 3 had hypotension, and 2 had hypoglycemia. All had severe hyponatremia with low plasma osmolality. Despite hypo-

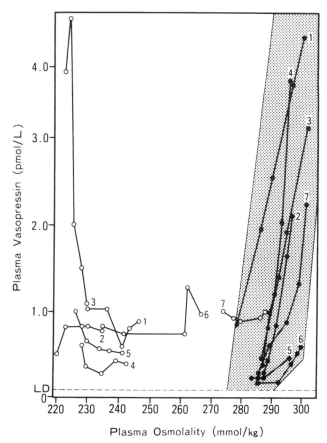

Fig 5–4.—Plasma vasopressin concentrations in relation to plasma osmolality during hypertonic saline infusion before (*open circles*) and after (*closed circles*) glucocorticoid replacement therapy in patients with adrenal insufficiency. Sequential values from individual patients are connected by *lines* and identified by *numbers*. The *shaded area* indicates normal ranges obtained in 62 healthy subjects. *Abbreviations:* LD, lowest vasopressin level that can be reliably detected in the assay. (Courtesy of Kamoi K, Tamura T, Tanaka K, et al: *J Clin Endocrinol Metab* 77:1584–1588, 1993.)

natremia, urinary sodium excretion persisted, with urine osmolality exceeding plasma osmolality. Plasma AVP levels were inappropriately elevated relative to plasma osmolality. Blood urea nitrogen, plasma creatinine, and plasma renin activity levels ranged from low to normal, and plasma and urinary potassium excretion were normal.

Findings.—Two patterns of change in plasma AVP were observed in response to osmotic stimulus produced by hypertonic 5% saline infusion: levels decreased with increasing plasma osmolality in 2 patients and fluctuated without a consistent pattern in the other 5 patients (Fig 5–4). However, in all patients, plasma AVP levels neither increased nor decreased to undetectable levels with a rise in plasma osmolality. Hypertonic saline infusion increased plasma sodium concentrations and osmolality to subnormal levels, and thirst persisted in 5 patients during the infusion. All patients were treated with 12.5–20 mg of hydrocortisone, and all improved clinically. The abnormality in AVP secretion and thirst was corrected with normalization of plasma sodium concentrations and osmolality.

Discussion.—Glucocorticoid deficiency in humans results in a clinical picture almost indistinguishable from that of inappropriate secretion of antidiuretic hormone. The persistent AVP secretion is caused by a loss in hypotonic suppression of the osmostat for AVP release, which may be occasioned primarily by the direct stimulatory effect of glucocorticoid deficiency per se on AVP secretion and aggravated secondarily by multiple nonosmotic stimuli including nausea, hypotension, and hypoglycemia. Inappropriate thirst may be caused by the same mechanism responsible for increased AVP secretion because both are controlled by the same osmotic and nonosmotic stimuli acting through the same closely related receptors and neuronal pathways.

▶ As every student of endocrinology knows, excluding adrenal insufficiency is an important criterion for the diagnosis of syndrome of inappropriate antidiuretic hormone. This is because the glucocorticoid-deficient state is associated with "appropriate" release of AVP. The authors' conclusion that glucocorticoid deficiency per se may contribute to persistent release of AVP is supported by available data that have demonstrated the presence of glucocorticoid receptors in the supraoptic nucleus of the rat. For the clinician, the sequence of events would seem to be that cortisol deficiency leads to desaturation of the glucocorticoid receptor, somehow resulting in persistent secretion of AVP as the result of loss of hypotonic suppression of the osmostats. The end result is continued secretion of AVP in spite of hypotonicity, leading to less than maximally dilute urine.—C.R. Kannan, M.D.

Effect of Glucocorticoid Replacement Therapy on Bone Mineral Density in Patients With Addison Disease
Zelissen PMJ, Croughs RJM, van Rijk PP, Raymakers JA (Univ Hosp, Utrecht, The Netherlands)
Ann Intern Med 120:207–210, 1994   112-95-5–11

Background.—Little is known about the occurrence of osteoporosis during replacement therapy with glucocorticoids in patients with hypocortisolism. The bone mineral density in a large group of patients with Addison's disease was investigated to determine the significance of their drug regimen in the development of osteoporosis.

Method.—A total of 91 patients with Addison's disease who had been receiving glucocorticoid replacement therapy for a mean of 10.6 years participated in the study. Measurements of bone mineral density of the lumbar spine and both femoral necks were made using a dual-energy x-ray absorptiometer. The results were compared with age-matched controls. Bone mineral density was considered to be decreased if it was less than 2 standard deviations of the mean value of the control population in at least 1 region.

Results.—Decreased bone mineral density was found in at least 1 of the measured regions in 10 of 31 men who participated and in 4 of 60 women. Five men experienced bone mineral density decline in 3 regions, 4 in the lumbar spine only, and 1 in the right femoral neck only. One woman had decreased bone mineral density in 3 regions; 1 in 2 regions (both femoral necks); and 2 in 1 region (lumbar spine). A significant correlation was seen between age and bone mineral density of the lumbar spine, left femoral neck, and right femoral neck. No significant differences were found between men and women with regard to age, duration of glucocorticoid treatment, or dose. However, men with decreased bone mineral density were seen to be taking a significantly higher dose of hydrocortisone per kilogram of body weight than men with normal bone mineral density. After correction for possible confounding variables, a significant linear correlation was confirmed between hydrocortisone dose per kilogram of body weight and bone mineral density of the lumbar spine in men but not in women.

Conclusion.—Decreased bone mineral density was found in more than 30% of male patients receiving long-term glucocorticoid replacement therapy for Addison's disease. The men receiving higher daily doses of hydrocortisone per kilogram of body weight experienced a significantly greater decrease in bone mineral density. Adjustment of glucocorticoid therapy to the lowest acceptable dose is vital, and regular measurement of bone mineral density may be helpful in indentifying men at risk for osteoporosis.

▶ Replacement glucocorticoid therapy for Addison's disease is clinically based, at best empirical, and lends itself poorly to scientific titration. The dose at which the patient feels good is presumed to be the correct one. Measuring cortisol or plasma ACTH levels to monitor and titrate replacement is very crude compared with that of sTSH for replacement thyroxine therapy. Yet, most clinicians are not bedeviled by problems with glucocorticoid replacement therapy. The clinical impression has been that glucocorticoid therapy at replacement doses, despite its lack of precision, does not increase the risk of steroid-related complications. The data in this article indicate that this is certainly not the case.

According to the authors, the male patients with normal bone mineral density (BMD) received 13.6 mg of hydrocortisone per square meter per day, whereas those with decreased lumbar BMD received 16.4 mg of hydrocortisone per square meter per day. Can this slight increment be responsible for the differences in bone density? Although the authors claim that other confounding variables were analyzed, this is unclear from the data provided. In contrast to the men, very few women in the study showed a decrease in lumbar BMD. Because of the small number of women who showed reduced

BMD, proper statistical comparisons were precluded. The data in this study are somewhat unexpected.

Another study by Valero et al. (*Bone Miner* 26:9, 1994) evaluated vertebral bone density as well as biochemical markers such as osteocalcin, procollagen type I, PTH, and 25-hydroxy vitamin D in 30 patients with Addison's disease on long-term replacement therapy. These workers found that the annual rate of bone loss was −.82%, similar to that in healthy controls. The conclusion in this study was that no significant trabecular bone loss or modification in markers on bone formation was seen in patients treated with replacement glucocorticoid therapy. In a study from New Zealand (*N Z Med J* 107:52, 1994), Florkowski et al. report that women, but not men, with Addison's disease who were receiving replacement therapy had a greater-than-expected reduction in bone density, and they postulated this to be a reflection of loss of adrenal androgens. One needs only to look back at the skepticism generated by the first articles in the early 1980s warning about bone loss resulting from subtle overtreatment with thyroid hormone replacement. Clearly, this is an area that needs further investigation.—C.R. Kannan, M.D.

Adrenal Tumors

Immunohistochemical Assessment of Proliferative Activity in Adrenocortical Neoplasms
Goldblum JR, Shannon R, Kaldjian EP, Thiny M, Davenport R, Thompson N, Lloyd RV (Univ of Michigan Hosps, Ann Arbor)
Mod Pathol 6:663–668, 1993   112-95-5–12

Background.—Many histologic criteria have been used to distinguish between benign and malignant adrenocortical tumors, but it is still difficult to assess the biological potential of a given tumor. The monoclonal antibody Ki-67 and proliferating cell nuclear antigen (PCNA) recognize nuclear proteins in proliferating cells in various tumors. Their usefulness in differentiating between benign and malignant adrenocortical neoplasms and as prognostic indicators was studied.

Methods.—Nineteen adenomas and 15 primary carcinomas were studied with immunostaining with the monoclonal antibodies MIB 1 and PC10 for recognition of Ki-67 and PCNA, respectively, and correlated with histologic diagnosis and clinical outcome.

Results.—Immunohistochemical staining for both PCNA and Ki-67 was predominantly localized within cell nuclei. Mitosing cells were also Ki-67 positive. Both the Ki-67 score and labeling index were significantly higher in malignant tumors than in benign tumors (Figs 5–5 and 5–6). Immunostaining of Ki-67 also correlated significantly with clinical outcome. During a mean follow-up of 25 months, patients who died of disease had significantly higher Ki-67 scores and labeling indices than those alive without disease. Immunostaining of Ki-67 was also highly correlated with mitotic counts, and mitotic counts also correlated with histologic diagnosis and clinical outcome. There was a strong correlation be-

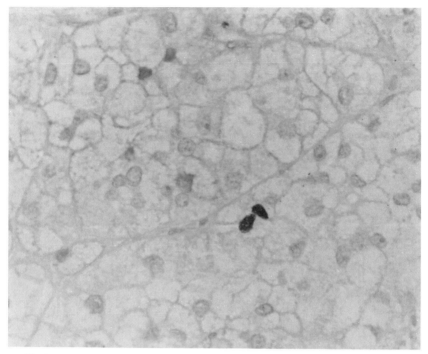

Fig 5–5.—The Ki-67 immunostaining of an adrenocortical adenoma. Only rare (1%) cells are stained with Ki-67 monoclonal antibody, MIB 1. (Courtesy of Goldblum JR, Shannon R, Kaldjian EP, et al: *Mod Pathol* 6:663–668, 1993.)

tween Ki-67 score and labeling index. The PCNA score and labeling index did not correlate with histologic diagnosis or clinical outcome.

Conclusion.—Immunostaining of Ki-67 with MIB 1 can aid in the distinction between benign and malignant adrenocortical tumors in routinely processed, formalin-fixed, paraffin-embedded tissue sections. In these neoplasms, Ki-67 may also be of prognostic importance. The Ki-67 score may be a more rapid and equally accurate method of estimating the proliferative index of a tumor, and it can be more readily adapted for routine diagnostic use.

▶ Any pathologist will tell you that he or she is examining increasing numbers of adrenal lesions to exclude malignancy. The incidence of adrenal incidentalomas detected by serendipity is approximately 5% in large centers, with a range of 2% to 8%. Because the distinction between benign and malignant adrenal masses less than 3 cm in diameter can be extremely difficult, any technique that facilitates making the distinction is welcome.

Does the technique described here work? A good picture is worth a thousand words. Figure 5–5 demonstrates the appearance of adrenocortical adenoma with Ki-67 monoclonal antibody. As one can see, less than 1% of the

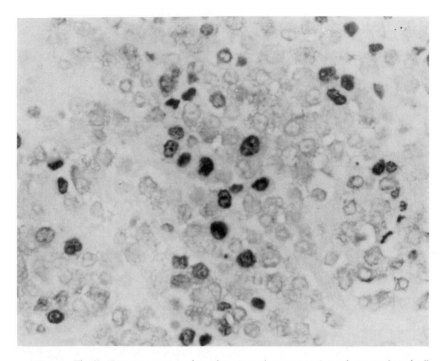

Fig 5–6.—The Ki-67 immunostaining of an adrenocortical carcinoma. A significant number of cell nuclei (19%) are strongly positive with the Ki-67 MIB 1 antibody. (Courtesy of Goldblum JR, Shannon R, Kaldjian EP, et al: *Mod Pathol* 6:663–668, 1993.)

cells are immunopositive. Figure 5–6 demonstrates Ki-67 immunopositivity in adrenocortical carcinoma, where 19% of the cells are strongly positive. The principle underlying the test takes advantage of the fact that Ki-67 monoclonal antibody recognizes nuclear proteins of 345-kd and 395-kd molecular weight only in cells that are proliferating during all non-Go phases of the cell cycle. Because carcinoma tissue contains more cells in the proliferative phase than adenoma tissue, the cells in the malignant tissue show strong immunopositivity. The authors have convincingly demonstrated that the Ki-67 score was significantly higher in malignant tumors than in adenomas. Further, the Ki-67 score correlated well with the more formal mitotic index and did have some predictive value regarding clinical outcome.

As interesting as these data are, the seasoned pathologist will tell you that the technique is still too new and has not been adequately evaluated. The top 4 parameters still used by most pathologists to determine malignancy in an adrenal lesion are nuclear volume, nuclear pleomorphism, DNA-ploidy, and loss of polarity. The importance of nuclear DNA patterns in the recognition of adrenocortical malignant lesions has been elegantly addressed by Diaz-Cano et al. (*Virchows Arch A Pathol Anat Histopathol* 423:323, 1993).

On a genetic level, considerable attention has been focused on the tumorigenesis of benign adenoma into adrenal carcinoma. The *p53* gene has been implicated in the process. Lin et al. (*J Clin Endocrinol Metab* 78:483, 1994) have demonstrated a high degree of *p53* mutation in adrenal neoplasia. Because *p53* gene protein is an important regulator of guanine nucleotide synthesis, loss of the physiologic inhibitory regulation by this mutation of the *p53* gene allows increased availability of guanosine triphosphate, resulting in increased transduction of signals essential for cell growth and hormone expression in functional adrenocortical tumors. Interesting as these molecular biological observations are, the nature and course of adrenocortical carcinoma remain unchanged, as will be seen with the next abstract.—C.R. Kannan, M.D.

Adrenal Adenocarcinoma: A Review of 53 Cases
Zografos GC, Driscoll DL, Karakousis CP, Huben RP (Roswell Park Cancer Inst, Buffalo, NY)
J Surg Oncol 55:160–164, 1994   112-95-5-13

Introduction.—Because adrenal carcinomas are relatively uncommon and may reach a considerable size without clinical evidence of disease, diagnosis is often made at an advanced stage. All patients with adrenal adenocarcinoma seen at Roswell Park Cancer Institute in Buffalo, New York, during the past 40 years were evaluated for presenting signs and symptoms; biochemical, hormonal, and radiographic changes; surgical treatment; survival; and metastatic sites.

Patients and Methods.—Thirty men and 23 women (median age, 51 years) were treated for adrenal carcinoma between 1950 and 1990. Tumors were classified as "functioning" if there was clinical evidence of endocrine disease. Staging of tumors was based upon size, nodal status, local invasion, and metastases.

Results.—The primary location of the tumor was the left adrenal gland in 32 patients and the right adrenal in 19; 2 patients had synchronous bilateral involvement. The median diameter was 14 cm for right adrenal tumors and 11 cm for left adrenal tumors. Twenty-nine patients were stage IV at diagnosis, with positive nodes and local invasion or distant metastases. Flank pain was the most common symptom. The median time between first symptoms and diagnosis was 8 months. Diagnosis was made incidentally in 16 of 32 patients for whom this information was available. Nineteen patients had endocrine manifestations from functioning tumors. Arteriography had the highest sensitivity (95%) of various radiographic localization techniques, followed by CT (94%), ultrasonography (92%), and IV pyelography (81%). Forty-three patients underwent 1 or more operations, and 21 were found to have extra-adrenal extension of the tumor. Complete surgical removal of all gross tumor was possible in 24 patients. The overall median survival time was 8 months. Only 3 of the 53 patients are alive, 1 with disease 6 years after diagnosis and 2 free of disease at 8 and 13 years after diagnosis.

Conclusion.—Adrenocortical carcinoma accounts for only .02% of all cancers. Diagnosis is often delayed until metastasis is seen. The key to cure is early and complete resection of the tumor. Factors significantly related to survival were detection at an early stage and completeness of the surgical procedure.

▶ Nothing ever changes with adrenocortical carcinoma, a diagnosis that brings in its wake dismay, disappointment with therapy, dissemination, and death. Several well-known observations are highlighted in the series described in Abstract 112-95-5-13. As we have known for years, adrenal carcinoma is usually missed in the early stages, when the odds are best to improve outcome. This study reaffirms that, first, the initial diagnosis, before establishing the diagnosis, was incorrect in 91% of cases indicating that a low index of suspicion exists for this disease. Second, as expected, a CT scan was diagnostic in all but 1 patient with adrenal carcinoma. Surprisingly, MRI was not mentioned. Third, only 36% had endocrine manifestations from functioning tumors. Fourth, 76% of patients were found to have metastases at the time of diagnosis. And, finally, the overall median survival time was 8 months. For a comparison of results of treatment in a different series dealing with large numbers of patients with adrenal carcinoma, the reader is referred to the 1994 YEAR BOOK OF ENDOCRINOLOGY, p 156. In this series, the authors measured 17-ketosteroids in the urine as a measure of androgen excess and found elevated levels in 13 of 53 patients.

A recent report focused on the mechanism of abnormal androgen production in patients with adrenocortical carcinoma. Sakai et al. (*J Clin Endocrinol Metab* 78:36, 1994) have suggested that high concentrations of adrenal androgens in these patients are mainly caused by diminished activity of 3β-hydroxysteroid dehydrogenase activity in the tumor tissue. These data should be viewed in light of another article that suggests, based on studies of a human adrenocortical carcinoma cell line, that cancer cells contain the enzyme P450C17 mRNA, which can be induced by ACTH with steroid production very similar to normal tissue (Rainey et al: *J Clin Endocrinol Metab* 77:731, 1993). So, is the adrenocortical carcinoma cell a weak producer or a brisk secretor of steroid hormones? It is difficult to tell.—C.R. Kannan, M.D.

Subclinical Hormone Secretion by Incidentally Discovered Adrenal Masses
Caplan RH, Strutt PJ, Wickus GG (Gundersen/Lutheran Med Ctr, La Crosse, Wis)
Arch Surg 129:291–296, 1994   112-95-5-14

Introduction.—Incidentally discovered adrenal masses occur in .6% to 1.4% of patients undergoing diagnostic imaging for other disorders, but this rarely occurs in patients with primary aldosteronism, Cushing's syndrome, and pheochromocytoma. These incidentalomas are often regarded as insignificant; however, they may produce serious complications. The prevalence of incidentally discovered adrenal masses and the importance of subclinical hormone secretion in them were studied.

Methods.—Eighty-nine patients with adrenal abnormalities were identified by review of 1,779 CT scans performed during a 1-year period. Patients in whom primary aldosteronism, adrenal hemorrhage, or nonadrenal malignant neoplasms was subsequently diagnosed were excluded, leaving 26 patients for study. Serum potassium levels identified patients with hypokalemia. Plasma renin activity, aldosterone levels, cortisol secretion, corticotropin levels, and urinary free catecholamine levels were measured.

Results.—Four of the 26 patients were hypokalemic; diuretic therapy caused the hypokalemia in 3, and low plasma renin activity and high plasma aldosterone levels identified aldosteronism in 1. Cortisol secretion was normal in 22 and borderline in 2 of the 24 patients tested. Four patients had low corticotropin levels; 1 of these patients also had abnormal diurnal variation of plasma cortisol concentration, and 3 had low urinary excretion of 17-ketosteroids, but all had normal cortisol secretion and excretion. Two patients had elevated urinary excretion of norepinephrine, but they had normal epinephrine and dopamine excretion. No patients had abnormal free catecholamine excretion.

Discussion.—There was a 5% prevalence of incidentally discovered adrenal masses. Excluding patients with diagnosed adrenal abnormalities, the prevalence was 1.9%. Subclinical hormone secretion of these masses is more significant than has been thought. Cortisol secretion occurred in 12% of these patients. Patients with subclinical adrenal disease may be at higher risk of hypertensive crisis or adrenal insufficiency with anesthesia, surgery, and other stressful circumstances.

▶ This article should come as good news to those endocrinologists who believe that all patients with adrenal incidentalomas should be thoroughly examined. The 5% incidence of adrenal incidentalomas in this series is similar to the experience in other large centers. In 26 patients with truly incidentally discovered adrenal masses, 12% had subclinical Cushing's syndrome, and another 12% had unrecognized causes of secondary hypertension.

This study is important for 2 reasons: First, it suggests that hormonal hypersecretion is underrecognized in incidentalomas; and second, it emphasizes the danger of perioperative problems due to contralateral adrenal suppression after removal of the incidentaloma. Unfortunately, there is no single test that routinely can identify subclinical Cushing's syndrome. Neither the overnight dexamethasone suppression test nor the urine free cortisol concentration test is consistently effective in detecting subclinical Cushing's syndrome. Two tests might help the clinician in this situation. One is the NP-59 iodocholesterol scan, which is good for outlining the functional tumor mass as well as for demonstrating lack of uptake in the suppressed contralateral gland. The second is evaluating the ACTH response to CRH, which would be blunted in patients with subclinical Cushing's syndrome. Unfortunately, neither of these tests are routinely available and hence, inevitably, subclinical

Cushing's syndrome will continue to elude us despite intensive screening. The practical approach is to be cautious and watchful in the perioperative period to detect any signs of adrenal failure, with prompt subsequent intervention—C.R. Kannan, M.D.

Hyperandrogenism

Enhanced Adrenocortical Activity as a Contributing Factor to Diabetes in Hyperandrogenic Women
Buffington CK, Givens JR, Kitabchi AE (Univ of Tennessee, Memphis)
Metabolism 43:584–590, 1994   112-95-5–15

Introduction.—Abnormally high testosterone levels in women may play a role in glucose intolerance. To investigate the role of testosterone in the development of glucose intolerance, the relationships among androgens, insulin sensitivity, and glucose tolerance were analyzed in obese diabetic and nondiabetic women with polycystic ovarian syndrome (PCO).

Methods.—Fourteen patients with normal glucose tolerance and PCO, 11 patients with PCO and mild NIDDM (PCO/D), and 14 obese control patients (OC) were studied. All patients underwent an oral glucose tolerance test, an insulin tolerance test, and a corticotropin stimulation test. Blood samples were analyzed to determine insulin binding and insulin degradation rates and the concentrations of testosterone, androstenedione, and the corticotropin-stimulated adrenal steroids—dehydroepiandrosterone (DHEA), dehydroepiandrosterone sulfate (DHEA-S), and cortisol.

Results.—After glucose challenge, the PCO/D group was hyperglycemic, but insulin levels were similar to those seen in the nondiabetic PCO group and significantly higher than those in the controls. There were no significant differences in the glucose disappearance rates in response to insulin between the 2 PCO groups; both were twice as slow as the controls. In vitro assessment of insulin binding showed similar activities in both PCO groups, but insulin degradation was significantly lower in the PCO/D group than in the PCO group. The 2 PCO groups had similar testosterone and androstenedione levels, which were significantly higher than in the controls. The PCO/D patients had significantly higher levels of cortisol, DHEA, and DHEA-S than did the PCO patients, both at baseline and during dexamethasone suppression and corticotropin stimulation.

Discussion.—Insulin resistance was not responsible for hyperglycemia in patients with PCO. In addition, there was no relationship between androgen levels and glucose intolerance. Glucose intolerance in diabetic patients with PCO was closely associated with elevated adrenocortical hormones, although the mechanism by which adrenocortical activity influences glucose metabolism in these patients is unclear. However, in vitro studies of insulin binding and degradation suggest that the defects in insulin action occur after binding.

▶ This article was selected for its "jolt value." Every once in awhile, one reads an article that challenges long-held, entrenched, and traditional beliefs. The constellation of PCO, hypertestosteronemia, hyperinsulinism, insulin resistance, and diabetes is intertwined with the belief that the central event here is elevated testosterone. An interesting observation in this study was that the hyperglycemia in the patients with diabetes did not correlate with their testosterone levels or insulin resistance but did correlate positively with adrenal hypersecretion. Also, these patients demonstrated statistically significant elevations in basal as well as ACTH-stimulated levels of cortisol, DHEA, and DHEA-S. In turn, these abnormalities correlated with the postreceptor defects in insulin action. Thus, the authors conclude that the central abnormality in patients with PCO/D is the enhanced adrenal activity. The unanswered question is whether this phenomenon is unique to patients with PCO or common in patients with NIDDM at large. Regardless, this is an excellent study by this highly respected group from the University of Tennessee. It has always been recognized that a substantial number of patients with PCO demonstrate anatomical as well as functional abnormalities in adrenocortical function. This is an exciting area that might conceivably impart a new role to adrenal androgens.

For a more conventional role of adrenal androgens, Abstract 112-95-5-16 provides a solution to a "hairy" problem.—C.R. Kannan, M.D.

Identification of Virilizing Adrenal Tumors in Hirsute Women
Derksen J, Nagesser SK, Meinders AE, Haak HR, Van De Velde CJH (Univ Hosp, Leiden, The Netherlands)
N Engl J Med 331:968–973, 1994   112-95-5-16

Background.—Hirsutism in women most often results from benign adrenal or ovarian disorders, but it also may result from adrenal carcinoma. It may, in fact, be the only sign of a virilizing adrenal tumor, but hirsutism of neoplastic origin cannot be ruled out from the history or physical findings.

Study Population.—To identify the most suitable test for determining whether hirsutism is a result of a tumor or non-neoplastic disorder, 27 women with adrenal carcinomas and 10 with adrenal adenomas were studied. Fourteen of the patients with carcinomas and 2 of those with adenomas had hirsutism as the presenting or chief symptom. Seventy-three consecutive women with hirsutism of non-neoplastic origin also were studied, as were 31 normal young women who had regular menstrual cycles.

Findings.—Serum steroid levels and urinary 17-ketosteroid excretion overlapped in the groups with neoplastic and non-neoplastic hirsutism.

The duration of hirsutism did not distinguish the 2 groups. All women with neoplasms and half of those with non-neoplastic conditions had abnormal androgen levels. None of 12 women with adrenal tumors who were given dexamethasone had suppressible serum dehydroepiandrosterone sulfate levels and urinary 17-ketosteroid excretion, but all those with non-neoplastic hirsutism did. A serum cortisol of 3.3 µg/dL also distinguished between the 2 groups.

Conclusion.—A hirsute woman with normal basal serum androgen levels is not likely to have an adrenal tumor. If the levels are elevated, dexamethasone testing is a useful way of distinguishing between a tumor and non-neoplastic hirsutism.

▶ Hirsutism affects approximately 5% of women. Although 95% of these women have benign reasons for the hirsutism, the diagnostic workup is focused to exclude the tumorous etiologies, as well as conditions such as Cushing's syndrome, late-onset congenital adrenal hyperplasia (LOCAH), and polycystic ovarian syndrome (PCOS). Because the workup for hirsutism is costly and can get out of hand, any study that provides useful information for a cost-effective workup is noteworthy. The important observation here is that normal basal testosterone and dehydroepiandrosterone-sulfate (DHEA-S) levels exclude the presence of an adrenal tumor.

What about the 40% to 60% of hirsute women with elevated androgen levels? Well, according to this study, a tumor is unlikely if the serum concentrations of DHEA-S, urine 17-ketosteroid excretion, and plasma cortisol decline to the normal basal range after the 5-day dexamethasone test. I have three comments regarding this otherwise excellent study. First, urine 17-ketosteroid measurements have largely been replaced by measurement of the plasma level of adrenal androgens and would be superfluous, cumbersome, and an added expense. Second, 17-α-hydroxyprogesterone levels were not included in the profile. Clearly, the patients with LOCAH would be suppressible to dexamethasone; hence, the diagnosis might have been missed unless tested with basal and/or corticotropin-stimulated precursor levels. Third, the testing focuses on exclusion of neoplastic causes of hirsutism but not on inclusion of other causes such as PCOS, which can, in a subset of patients, be associated with unremarkable androgen levels in the circulation. I suppose the article makes great sense if one wishes to follow the "hirsutism-nihilistic" approach, i.e., the only question that needs to be addressed would be whether an adrenal tumor underlies the hirsutism. Toward that end, measurement of basal DHEA-S and testosterone levels, coupled with a 5-day dexamethasone test when basal levels are elevated, would be admirably adequate.—C.R. Kannan, M.D.

Adrenocorticotrophin Stimulation and HLA Polymorphisms Suggest a High Frequency of Heterozygosity for Steroid 21-Hydroxylase Deficiency in Patients With Turner's Syndrome and Their Families

Larizza D, Cuccia M, Martinetti M, Maghnie M, Dondi E, Salvaneschi L,

Severi F (Univ of Pavia, Italy; IRCCS Policlinico S Matteo, Pavia, Italy)
Clin Endocrinol 40:39–45, 1994   112-95-5–17

Objective.—A 17-year-old girl with Turner's syndrome, evidenced by a 45,X karyotype, was found to have a simple virilizing form of congenital adrenal hyperplasia (CAH) characterized by 21-hydroxylase deficiency (21-OHD). The frequency of 21-OHD in 52 Italian patients with Turner's syndrome (mean age, 14.7 years) and in 26 of their relatives was determined.

Methods.—The serum level of 17-hydroxyprogesterone (17-OHP) was determined before and after intramuscular administration of .25 mg of ACTH [1–24]. Basal levels of testosterone and dehydroepiandrosterone (DHEA) were estimated in the patients with Turner's syndrome. The results of ACTH testing were examined in relation to HLA class I and class II alleles.

Results.—Eleven of the patients with Turner's syndrome (group A) had an increased 17-OHP response to ACTH, whereas 40 (group B) had a normal response. The group A patients had responses very similar to those of control subjects heterozygous for 21-OHD. Clitoromegaly was found in 54.5% of group A patients and in only 5% of group B patients, a significant difference. Nine patients with abnormal 17-OHP responses had a 45,X karyotype. Two of 10 patients with elevated baseline testosterone levels and 5 of 10 with elevated DHEA levels had increased 17-OHP responses to ACTH. No patient with an increased 17-OHP response had HLA-B8. Eight of the 26 relatives studied had biochemical findings typical of the heterozygous state. Three individuals from the same family had the cryptic form of the disorder, with 17-OHP values typical of the nonclassical form of CAH but no clinical signs of disease.

Implication.—If a patient with Turner's syndrome has an enlarged clitoris, particularly if the karyotype lacks a Y chromosome, adrenal function should be evaluated.

▶ The association between Turner's syndrome and 21-OHD comes as a complete surprise because the 2 disorders differ so greatly. It is bad enough that children with Turner's syndrome are underfeminized; with this combination, there is the extra burden of virilization. The fact that 12 of the 52 patients with Turner's syndrome had elevated basal and/or ACTH-stimulated levels of 17-α-hydroxyprogesterone progesterone in plasma is more than fortuituous. The observation that clitoromegaly was more common in this group further strengthens the link. Two additional observations provide credence to the linkage between the 2 disorders: First, the high frequency of carriers for 21-OHD in the relatives of patients with Turner's syndrome; and second, the high frequency with which HLA antigen and haplotype associated with 21-OHD were found in the Turner group with an abnormal level of precursors. These observations encountered in Italian patients need to be extended to patients with Turner's syndrome from other geoethnic backgrounds.

The clinical implication is that undetected heterozygous 21-OHD may compound the problems of sexual infantilism and growth retardation seen with Turner's syndrome. The presence of clitoromegaly in Turner's syndrome traditionally meant that the patient might have a cryptic Y chromosome and implied the development of a malignant gonadoblastoma in the dysgenetic gonad. Now, it seems, we must exclude concomitant heterozygous 21-OHD as well in these adolescents. Basta! Basta!—C.R. Kannan, M.D.

Suggested Reading

The following articles are recommended to the reader:

1. White PC, et al: Disorders of aldosterone biosynthesis and action. N Engl J Med 331:250–258, 1994.
2. Blumenfeld JD, et al: Diagnosis and treatment of primary hyperaldosteronism. Ann Intern Med 121:877–885, 1994.
3. Fallo F, et al: Abnormality of aldosterone and cortisol late pathways in glucocorticoid-remediable aldosteronism. J Clin Endocrinol Metab 79:772–774, 1994.
4. Wooten MD, King DK: Adrenal cortical carcinoma. Cancer 72:3145–3155, 1993.

6 The Sympathoadrenal System

Introduction

This year's selections have a decidedly clinical bent. As in previous editions, articles are grouped according to major topic area: the cardiovascular system, regulation of metabolism, and fundamental as well as clinical aspects of pheochromocytoma. An annotated suggested reading list appears at the end of the chapter.

Pressor crises in patients using cocaine continue to pose important clinical problems. Like pressor crises associated with monoamine oxidase inhibitors and clonidine withdrawal, cocaine-related hypertensive episodes involve widespread sympathetic stimulation. Five cases of toxicity after oral cocaine ingestion are summarized in Abstract 112-95-6-1. Catecholamine-stimulated increases in platelet aggregability have been thought to play a role in the pathogenesis of thrombotic events in patients with cardiovascular disease. In Abstract 112-95-6-2, interactions of norepinephrine and aspirin on platelet function are demonstrated. Failure of aspirin to completely reverse the norepinephrine-stimulated increases in platelet aggregation may limit the usefulness of aspirin as an antithrombotic agent. In Abstract 112-95-6-3, evidence indicates that circulating levels of catecholamines have an important genetic basis.

In the realm of metabolism, Abstract 112-95-6-4 demonstrates that epinephrine plays a role in regulating circulating triglyceride and HDL-cholesterol levels.

Many interesting articles about pheochromocytoma appeared this year. These tumors are well known to secrete a variety of biologically active compounds. Adrenomedullin (Abstract 112-95-6-5) and endothelin (Abstract 112-95-6-6) may contribute to blood pressure abnormalities in patients with pheochromocytoma. Assessment of malignant potential in pheochromocytomas has been a challenging problem; in Abstract 112-95-6-7, evidence is provided supporting the observation that nondiploid tumors are much more likely to demonstrate malignant behavior than are diploid tumors.

Diverse clinical manifestations of pheochromocytoma continue to challenge clinicians. In patients described in Abstracts 112-95-6-8 and 112-95-6-9, elevations of serum amylase erroneously suggested the diagnosis of acute pancreatitis. Both patients had pulmonary edema, and it seems likely that the increased levels of amylase originated in the lung. In

Abstract 112-95-6-10, endoscopic removal of pheochromocytoma in 5 patients is described. Although investigational at present, this technique may eventually replace conventional surgery in selected patients with this tumor.

Lewis Landsberg, M.D.

The Cardiovascular System

Adrenergic Crisis From Crack Cocaine Ingestion: Report of Five Cases

Merigian KS, Park LJ, Leeper KV, Browning RG, Giometi R (Univ of Tennessee, Memphis; The Toxicology Ctr, Memphis, Tenn)
J Emerg Med 12:485–490, 1994   112-95-6-1

Introduction.—Crack cocaine refers to a form of alkaloidal cocaine that has been converted from cocaine hydrochloride. It is believed that crack cocaine is poorly absorbed and, therefore, essentially nontoxic when swallowed. Five patients experienced severe toxicity after oral ingestion of crack cocaine.

Clinical Features.—All 5 patients, aged 16–27 years, exhibited adrenergic crisis 30–180 minutes (average, 78 minutes) after swallowing 5–28 nuggets of crack cocaine (table). In the most severe case, the patient had cardiopulmonary arrest after multiple seizures. The other patients experienced extreme agitation or a state of frenzy, hypertension, tachycardia, and hyperthermia. Electrocardiograms showed signs of cardiac ischemia and repolarization abnormalities; 2 patients had signs of myocardial infarction. However, none of the patients had increased creatinine phosphokinase enzyme MB fraction. One patient died of complications associated with subclinical status epilepticus; the other patients improved, with normal electrocardiograms on discharge.

Treatment and Discussion.—Initial treatment consists of rapid therapeutic hypnosis with benzodiazepines, followed by IV control of blood pressure and pulse with β-adrenoreceptor blockade. Moderate doses of lorazepam are effective and safe by enhancing both the presynaptic- and postsynaptic-inhibiting effects of gamma-aminobutyric acid on dopamine. The addition of haloperidol, a highly effective postsynaptic dopamine antagonist, may have had additional effects in 1 patient, but its use is controversial because of its theoretical ability to lower the seizure threshold. The hyperadrenergic states respond to the lytic effects of beta adrenoreceptor blockade. Because of its rapid onset and ultrashort half-life, esmolol is the β-blocker of choice, using a loading dose of 500 mcg/kg/min infused during 1 minute, followed by a maintenance infusion of 50–200 mcg/kg/min. Most patients will recover within 48 to 72 hours.

Presentation on Arrival in the Emergency Department

Case Number	Patient Age (Years)	Sex	Number of Crack Nuggets Ingested	Time to Signs and Symptoms (Minutes)	Mental Status on Admission	Blood Pressure (mmHg)	Pulse (Beats/ Minute)	Respirations (Breaths/ Minute)	Temperature (°C[°F])	Clinical Findings
1	22	Female	28	60	Coma	0	0	0	Unknown	Generalized seizures Full cardiac arrest
2	18	Male	13	30	Frenzy	220/90	190	30	38.6 (101.5)	Extreme agitation
3	27	Male	7	60	Agitated	190/128	132	24	37.7 (99.9)	Extreme agitation
4	24	Male	15	180	Agitated	190/120	160	32	39.9 (103.8)	Extreme agitation Generalized seizures
5	16	Male	5	60	Agitated	220/120	180	28	38.1 (100.5)	Extreme agitation

(Courtesy of Merigian KS, Park LJ, Leeper KV, et al: *J Emerg Med* 12:485–490, 1994.)

▶ Many of the untoward consequences of cocaine abuse involve cocaine-induced potentiation of adrenergic responses. This potentiation results from the blockade of catecholamine uptake into sympathetic nerve terminals, a fundamental pharmacologic property of cocaine. Because uptake into nerve terminals is a major method of inactivation, potentiation of central and peripheral actions of catecholamines results from cocaine use. The patients reported in this article suffered typical adrenergic pressor crises, with hypertension, tachycardia, fever, and agitation. Fever is a consequence of increased heat production (stimulated by catecholamines) and impaired heat dissipation (secondary to peripheral vasoconstriction). Although not present in this series of patients, rhabdomyolysis with myoglobinuric renal failure and myocardial infarction are well-described complications of cocaine. The authors recommend treatment with rapidly acting benzodiazepines and β-blockers. Alpha-receptor antagonists should also be used to control hypertension. As pointed out by the authors, severe pressor crises can occur after the *oral* ingestion of large amounts of crack cocaine.—L. Landsberg, M.D.

Norepinephrine-Induced Human Platelet Activation In Vivo Is Only Partly Counteracted by Aspirin
Larsson PT, Wallén NH, Hjemdahl P (Karolinska Hosp, Stockholm, Sweden)
Circulation 89:1951–1957, 1994   1 12-95-6–2

Introduction.—The risk of thrombus formation may be increased by circulating norepinephrine as well as epinephrine because norepinephrine is in greater concentration in blood than epinephrine. Platelet aggregation is inhibited by aspirin by obstructing thromboxane's platelet-stimulating properties. It has been shown, in vitro and in vivo, that the antiplatelet properties of aspirin are counteracted by catecholamines. The interaction of aspirin and catecholamines on platelet aggregation was studied.

Methods.—Eleven males, 25–34 years of age, volunteered to be subjects. They were nonsmokers, had not taken aspirin for 14 days before the study, and had fasted overnight and abstained from caffeine. Overnight urine specimens were collected. There were 2 experimental conditions separated by 2 weeks; 1 condition with and 1 without aspirin. After 1 hour of rest, 1 mg/mL of noradrenaline diluted in cold saline with .1 mg/mL ascorbic acid, as an antioxidant, was infused into an antecubital vein at a low (.15 nmol/kg/min) or moderately high (.75 nmol/kg/min) dose. Blood samples and platelet function was performed after the rest period and during the infusion. Heart rate was continually monitored. Platelet aggregability was measured by filtragometry. β-Thromboglobulin (urine and plasma for platelet aggregability), catecholamines, 11-dehydrothromboxane B_2 (urine, for platelet secretion) were assayed. In 1 condition, 500 mg of aspirin was ingested 12 hours before the tests.

Results.—During infusion, epinephrine remained constant, and norepinephrine rose twofold (low dose) and tenfold (high dose). Systolic blood pressure increased 11 and 28 mm Hg during the low- and high-dose infusions. Diastolic blood pressure increased 6 and 14 mm Hg during the low- and high-dose infusions. Heart rate increased by 7 beats during the high-dose infusion. Aspirin did not affect these data. Platelet aggregability was significantly enhanced according to the infusion concentration. Platelet secretion was increased during the high-dose infusion. Aspirin pretreatment reduced excretion of 11-dehydrothromboxane B_2 and attenuated resting platelet aggregability. Although resting levels and excretion of β-thromboglobulin (an index of platelet secretion) were unaffected by aspirin, its norepinephrine-induced increase was abolished.

Conclusion.—The levels of catecholamines were consistent with those seen during exercise. These levels enhance platelet aggregability and secretion in healthy males. During sympathoadrenal activation, aspirin may not be an effective antithrombotic drug.

▶ This study is interesting in 2 respects. First, it demonstrates that circulating levels of norepinephrine exert important effects on platelet aggregability similar to those exerted by epinephrine. This is not unexpected because both epinephrine and norepinephrine are potent agonists for the α-2-adrenergic receptor that mediates the effect of catecholamines on platelet aggregation. Second, the study demonstrates that norepinephrine infusion antagonizes, but does not completely reverse, the effect of aspirin on platelet aggregation; the relationship between plasma norepinephrine and platelet aggregation is shifted to the right by aspirin. The study does suggest, moreover, that platelet secretion from the marrow, also stimulated by norepinephrine, is blocked by aspirin. Thus, although the stimulatory effects of norepinephrine on platelet aggregation are not completely blocked, aspirin does exert a protective effect even when norepinephrine levels are elevated. The authors speculate that this may, in part, account for the beneficial effects of aspirin on reducing the incidence of myocardial infarction in the early morning waking hours, a time when plasma catecholamines are elevated.—L. Landsberg, M.D.

Genetic Influences on Plasma Catecholamines in Human Twins
Williams PD, Puddey IB, Beilin LJ, Vandongen R (Univ of Western Australia; Royal Perth Hosp, Western Australia)
J Clin Endocrinol Metab 77:794–799, 1993   1 12-95-6–3

Background.—Both genetic and environmental factors influence blood pressure variability. At rest and at times of stress, the sympathetic nervous system is important in the regulation of blood pressure. Both essential and borderline hypertensives can have elevated plasma catecholamines. The genetic and environmental influences can be ascertained by studying normotensive twins with the goal of determining the role of the sympathetic nervous system on normal blood pressure.

Methods.—A total of 109 pairs of monozygous (MZ) and dizygous (DZ) twins were studied. On one visit, blood samples were taken after a 20-minute rest. On a second visit, supine blood pressures were measured every 2 minutes for 20 minutes, discarding the first measurement and averaging the remaining readings. A 24-hour urine specimen was collected for measurement of sodium excretion. The 2 sessions were designed to separate possible anxiety effects on blood pressure from the venipuncture. Catecholamines and dopamine were analyzed by enzymatic techniques.

Results.—There were 31 DZ females, 44 MZ females, 9 DZ males, 14 MZ males, and 11 DZ opposite-sex pairs. Body mass index was not related to norepinephrine or dopamine in either males or females. There was a weak negative correlation between body mass index and epinephrine in each sex. The overall epinephrine levels were lower in females and norepinephrine increased with age. There was no relationship between blood pressure and epinephrine in either sex or between norepinephrine and blood pressure in females. There was a positive relationship between norepinephrine and diastolic blood pressure in males. Dopamine was negatively correlated with both systolic and diastolic blood pressure in females. The relationship disappeared when age, body mass index, and sex were controlled. Genetic effects accounted for 57% of the variability in norepinephrine, whereas environment accounted for 27% and age accounted for 16% of the variability. Genetics explained 64% (females) and 74% (males) of the variability in epinephrine. Genetics explained 72% and environment explained 28% of the variability in dopamine levels.

Conclusion.—Genetics can account for 60% to 70% of the variability in catecholamines, suggesting considerable genetic control. A consistent relationship between blood pressure and catecholamines was not demonstrated. This genetic influence on circulating catecholamines adds understanding of the role of the sympathetic nervous system in early stages of essential hypertension.

▶ This study provides evidence that heredity accounts for a substantial portion of the variance in plasma catecholamine levels. Because plasma norepinephrine provides an index of sympathetic nervous system activity, the finding that 57% of the variance in plasma norepinephrine was accounted for by heredity supports an important effect of genetic background on sympathetic outflow. Poor correlation of plasma norepinephrine with blood pressure was noted in this study; better correlation is frequently observed in hypertensive, as compared with normotensive subjects, such as the cohort examined here. Also of note is the inverse correlation between plasma epinephrine and body mass index. This is in agreement with other evidence that epinephrine is diminished in obesity (Troisi et al: *Hypertension* 17:669, 1991) and suggests, along with other evidence, that diminished epinephrine may contribute to the development of obesity (Leigh et al: *Int J Obes* 16:597, 1992).—L. Landsberg, M.D.

Regulation of Metabolism

The Relationship of Epinephrine Excretion to Serum Lipid Levels: The Normative Aging Study

Ward KD, Sparrow D, Landsberg L, Young JB, Vokonas PS, Weiss ST (Brigham and Women's Hosp, Boston; Harvard Med School, Boston; Charles A Dana Research Inst, Boston; et al)

Metabolism 43:509–513, 1994   112-95-6–4

Objective.—Lipid metabolism is influenced in several ways by catecholamines and by adrenergic activity. Increases in HDL cholesterol and decreases in triglyceride levels appear to result from β-adrenergic receptor stimulation. Obesity has been associated with increased urinary norepinephrine excretion and decreased epinephrine excretion, which are markers of sympathetic nervous system and adrenal medullary activity, respectively. Thus, catecholamines may play a role in the lipid abnormalities of obesity. The associations between urinary catecholamine excretion and serum lipid and lipoprotein levels in men were assessed.

Methods.—The Normative Aging Study is a continuing, longitudinal study of the effects of aging, begun in 1961. The current analysis included 615 community-dwelling men from this study (age range, 43–85 years). Each subject underwent high-performance liquid chromatographic measurement of urinary catecholamine levels in 24-hour urine samples. The relationship between urinary catecholamine excretion and lipids and other variables were assessed.

Results.—Epinephrine excretion was positively correlated with HDL cholesterol and with the HDL/LDL ratio, inversely correlated with triglycerides, and unrelated to total or LDL cholesterol levels. Norepinephrine and dopamine excretion were unrelated to any of the lipid levels. After adjustment for age, smoking, physical activity, alcohol intake, body mass index, abdomen/hip ratio, and postcarbohydrate insulin level,

Adjusted Mean (SE) HDL Cholesterol (HDL-C) Levels,
HDL/LDL Cholesterol Ratio, and Triglyceride Levels by
Tertiles of Urinary Epinephrine Excretion ($n = 615$)

Textile of Ephinephrine Excretion (µg/24h)	HDL-C (mmol/L)	HDL/LDL Ratio	Triglycerides (mmol/L)
I (0.9-4.9)	1.24 (0.03)	0.32 (0.01)	1.61 (0.06)
II (5.0-7.5)	1.29 (0.03)	0.34 (0.01)	1.56 (0.06)
III (7.6-30.0)	1.34 (0.03)	0.35 (0.01)	1.47 (0.06)
P for linear trend	<.0001	.01	.05

Note: Values are adjusted for age, smoking status and amount, ln physical activity level, ln alcohol intake, body mass index, abdomen-to-hip ratio, and ln postcarbohydrate insulin level.

(Courtesy of Ward KD, Sparrow D, Landsberg L, et al: *Metabolism* 43:509–513, 1994.)

HDL cholesterol levels increased from 1.24 to 1.34 mmol/L across tertiles of epinephrine excretion (table). These relationships persisted after multiple linear regression analyses with adjustment for selected covariates.

Conclusion.—Epinephrine appears to play a key role in the regulation of lipid and lipoprotein metabolism in human beings. In obese individuals, the commonly observed dyslipidemia—with increased triglyceride and decreased HDL cholesterol levels—may be influenced by decreased adrenal medullary activity. Thus, the increases in cardiovascular risk associated with the insulin resistance syndrome may involve the sympathoadrenal system in addition to hyperinsulinemia.

▶ Obesity is associated with a characteristic dyslipidemia consisting of high triglyceride and low HDL cholesterol levels. The hyperinsulinemia that accompanies obesity is known to play a role in this lipid abnormality, which is thought to convey considerable cardiovascular risk (Ward et al: *Int J Obes* 18:137, 1994). The major finding reported in this article is that epinephrine also contributes to this dyslipidemia. Even after adjustment for obesity, body fat distribution, and insulin levels, epinephrine remained directly correlated with HDL cholesterol and inversely with triglycerides. Low levels of epinephrine, therefore, may contribute to the dyslipidemia of obesity because, as noted above in the comments pertaining to Abstract 112-95-6-3, epinephrine levels may be low in the obese. Interestingly, high triglyceride and low HDL cholesterol is the pattern of dyslipidemia that accompanies β-adrenergic blockade. Antagonism of the effects of epinephrine on lipid metabolism may underlie this undesirable effect of β-receptor blockers.—L. Landsberg, M.D.

Pheochromocytoma

Synthetic Human Adrenomedullin and Adrenomedullin 15–52 Have Potent Short-Lived Vasodilator Activity in the Hindlimb Vascular Bed of the Cat

Santiago JA, Garrison EA, Ventura VL, Coy DH, Bitar K, Murphy WA, McNamara DB, Kadowitz PJ (Tulane Univ, New Orleans, La)
Life Sci 55:PL85–PL90, 1994   112-95-6-5

Purpose.—The newly discovered hypotensive peptide adrenomedullin, isolated from human pheochromocytoma cells, is distributed in several different organ tissues but not in the CNS. It is found in the plasma of normal and hypertensive subjects and may act as a circulating hormone. Studies in rats have shown that adrenomedullin has potent, long-lasting hypotensive activity in systemic and isolated mesenteric vascular beds and increases platelet levels of cyclic adenosine monophosphate (cAMP). The vascular responses to adrenomedullin in the hindlimb vascular bed of the cat were studied under constant flow conditions.

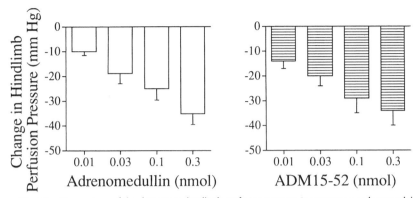

Fig 6–1.—Comparison of the decrease in hindlimb perfusion pressure in response to adrenomedullin (**left**) and the carboxy terminal 15-52 fragment of adrenomedullin (**right**) in doses of .01-.3 nmol in the hindlimb vascular bed of the cat. Responses to adrenomedullin and ADM15-52 were investigated in 9 cats with the exception of the .01-nmol dose of ADM15-52, which was studied in 7 animals. (Courtesy of Santiago JA, Garrison EA, Ventura VL, et al: *Life Sci* 55:PL85-PL90, 1994.)

Methods.—Responses to synthetic human adrenomedullin were assessed in the perfused and denervated hindlimb vascular beds of 18 anesthetized cats and compared with the responses to bradykinin and acetylcholine. Further experiments compared the vasodilator responses to the carboxy terminal 15-52 fragment of adrenomedullin (ADM15-52) with the vasodilator responses to adrenomedullin.

Results.—Dose-related decreases in hindlimb perfusion pressure occurred when .01 to .30 nmol of adrenomedullin and ADM15-52 was injected into the hindlimb perfusion circuit (Fig 6-1). This response peaked within 20-30 seconds of injection; depending on the injected dose, hindlimb perfusion pressure returned to baseline within 100-200 seconds. On comparison of identical nmol doses, vasodilator activity was similar for adrenomedullin, ADM15-52, and bradykinin; acetylcholine was approximately 10 times more potent. At the doses studied, the half-life of the vasodilator responses ranged from 55 to 80 seconds for adrenomedullin and ADM15-52 and from 20 to 45 seconds for bradykinin and acetylcholine.

Conclusion.—Synthetic human adrenomedullin and ADM15-52 both cause significant dose-related decreases in perfusion pressure in the hindlimb vascular bed of the cat. Because blood flow was constant, the observed decreases directly reflect hindlimb vascular resistance; because the adrenergic nerves to the vascular bed were sectioned, the responses are not dependent on changes in sympathetic vasomotor tone. Adrenomedullin-induced dilation of vascular smooth muscle may occur via increasing cAMP levels.

▶ It is well recognized that pheochromocytomas synthesize and secrete a variety of biologically active compounds, some of which have important clinical manifestations. Neuropeptide-Y, ACTH, PTH-related protein, erythropoietin, and a variety of opioids have all been associated with this tumor. Cushing's syndrome, hypercalcemia, and polycythemia (Jacobs and Wood: *Am J Med* 97:307, 1994) have all been documented as ectopic hormone syndromes in patients with pheochromocytoma. Neuropeptide-Y and endogenous opioids, in addition, have been postulated to play a role in some of the blood pressure abnormalities that occur in patients with this disease.

One of the puzzling and least well understood manifestations of pheochromocytoma is hypotension. Volume depletion and blunted adrenergic reflexes, the traditional explanations for the associated orthostatic hypotension, probably contribute to the profound cardiovascular collapse that sometimes occurs in patients with these tumors. It has also been suggested that a hypotensive compound secreted by the tumor may be responsible for these depressor episodes. Epinephrine and dopamine have both been candidate hypotensive agents, but these catecholamines seem unlikely choices because they both raise the blood pressure except in very small doses. Adrenomedullin, a hypotensive peptide isolated originally from human pheochromocytoma cells, appears to be an excellent candidate depressor substance. As shown in Figure 6–1, this peptide and its carboxy terminal fragment cause a dose-related decrease in isolated hindlimb perfusion pressure consistent with a direct vasodilator effect. The potency of this peptide is similar to that of bradykinin. It seems likely that pheochromocytomas associated with depressor crises may produce this or related hypotensive peptides. Interestingly, adrenomedullin seems to be related structurally to another hypotensive peptide, calcitonin gene–related peptide.—L. Landsberg, M.D.

Elevated Immunoreactive Endothelin Levels in Patients With Pheochromocytoma
Oishi S, Sasaki M, Sato T (Kumamoto Univ, Japan)
Am J Hypertens 7:717–722, 1994   112-95-6-6

Introduction.—The potent vasoconstrictor peptide endothelin-1 (ET-1) produces sustained pressor responses when given by IV injection to rats. Blood pressure elevations have also been reported with ET-1 infusion for as long as 1 week. The possible role of ET-1 in blood pressure regulation raises the question of whether the elevated blood pressure observed in patients with pheochromocytoma results from the tumor-produced catecholamine alone or from additive ET-1 changes. Plasma and tissue ET-1 levels were assessed in patients with pheochromocytoma.

Methods.—The subjects were 44 patients with pheochromocytoma, 31 patients with essential hypertension, and 20 healthy controls. Of the pheochromocytoma patients, 24 were hypertensive and 20 were normotensive. All subjects underwent measurement of plasma ET-1 by radioimmunoassay. Seventeen of the pheochromocytoma group underwent measurement of plasma ET-1 before and after surgery. Tissue ET-1 levels were measured in 26 tumors obtained at operation and in 7 normal adrenal medullas obtained at autopsy.

Results.—The mean plasma ET-1 concentration in the pheochromocytoma group was 18 fmol/mL, significantly greater than the level in the control and hypertensive groups, which is about 7 fmol/mL. Within the pheochromocytoma group, plasma ET-1 concentrations were nonsignificantly higher in the hypertensive patients than in the normotensive patients, 23 vs. 12 fmol/L. The hypertensive pheochromocytoma patients also had slightly higher plasma norepinephrine levels than did their normotensive counterparts.

Plasma ET-1 was significantly correlated with blood pressure in the pheochromocytoma group but not in the control or essential hypertension groups. However, blood pressure was more strongly correlated with plasma norepinephrine than with ET-1. In the 17 patients studied postoperatively, the mean plasma ET-1 levels declined from 17 to 8 fmol/L within 2 weeks after surgery. The mean tumor tissue ET-1 concentration was 1.4 pmol/g of wet tissue, significantly higher than in the normal adrenal medullas.

Conclusion.—Patients with pheochromocytoma have significantly elevated plasma ET-1 concentrations. The evidence suggests that excessive amounts of this peptide are produced and secreted by pheochromocytomas. Plasma ET-1 levels normalize after adrenalectomy; any role of ET-1 in this tumor is eliminated when the tumor is removed. In patients with pheochromocytoma, plasma norepinephrine appears to contribute directly to blood pressure maintenance.

▶ This study provides convincing evidence that the potent vasoconstrictive peptide ET-1 is secreted by pheochromocytomas. Previous studies (including one in last year's selections) had demonstrated that pheochromocytomas contain endothelin messenger RNA; in this study, plasma levels of ET-1 before and after pheochromocytomas were resected support secretion of this peptide by the tumor. Although in this particular study blood pressure correlated better with norepinephrine levels than with ET-1 levels, it seems likely that endothelin contributes to hypertension in some patients with pheochromocytoma, because carefully measured sequential changes in circulating catecholamine levels have not always correlated well with alterations in blood pressure. Many diverse manifestations of pheochromocytoma may reflect the complex interplay of biologically active compounds produced and secreted by these tumors.—L. Landsberg, M.D.

Flow Cytometric DNA Analysis for the Determination of Malignant Potential in Adrenal and Extra-Adrenal Pheochromocytomas or Paragangliomas

Pang L-C, Tsao K-C (Chang Gung Mem Hosp, Taipei, Taiwan, China; Chang Gung Med College, Taipei, Taiwan, China)
Arch Pathol Lab Med 117:1142–1147, 1993   112-95-6-7

Background.—Only about 10% of adrenal and extra-adrenal pheochromocytomas or paragangliomas are malignant. However, these malignancies cannot be identified on the basis of their histologic features alone; a rigorous definition of malignancy would be the presence of metastases or direct invasion in a site where there should be no embryologic remnant of paraganglionic tissue. Flow cytometry is widely used to determine the nuclear DNA content and ploidy pattern of many common human tumors. Pheochromocytoma or paraganglioma cells obtained from paraffin-embedded tissues were evaluated for malignant behavior.

Methods.—Extracted nuclei from 53 adrenal, 13 carotid body, 14 retroperitoneal, 2 intrathoracic, 2 urinary bladder, and 1 cauda equina pheochromocytomas or paragangliomas were subjected to DNA ploidy

DNA Ploidy Pattern by Flow Cytometry in 79 Patients With
Adrenal and Extra-Adrenal Pheochromocytomas
or Paragangliomas

DNA Histogram Pattern	Site	No. of Patients		
		Benign	Malignant	Total
Diploid	Adrenal	36	0	36
	Extra-adrenal	20	0	20
Subtotal		**56**	**0**	**56**
Tetraploid	Adrenal	2	3	5
	Extra-adrenal	5	2	7
Subtotal		**7**	**5**	**12***
Aneuploid	Adrenal	5	1	6
	Extra-adrenal	4	1	5
Abnormal DNA content (including tetraploid and aneuploid)		16	7	23†
Subtotal		**9**	**2**	**11‡**
Total		**72**	**7**	**79**

* $P = .0037$.
† $P = .0003$.
‡ $P = .0248$.
(Courtesy of Pang L-C, Tsao K-C: *Arch Pathol Lab Med* 117:1142–1147, 1993.)

studies by flow cytometry. Nine percent of the tumors were classified as clinically malignant based on the finding of regional or distant metastases, extensive local invasion, or local recurrence with extensive invasion of adjacent organs.

Results.—The DNA histograms resembled those of normal adrenal tissue, and thus were considered normal DNA diploid patterns, in 71% of the tumors. Another 15% had tetraploid peaks, with DNA indexes ranging from 1.91 to 2.11, and 14% had aneuploid histograms, with DNA indexes ranging from 1.14 to 1.51. Five of the 12 patients whose tumors showed a tetraploid pattern had direct invasion of the adjacent organs or distant metastases; 3 of these tumors originated in the adrenal gland, 1 from the carotid body, and 1 from the retroperitoneal area. Two of the 11 tumors with an aneuploid pattern showed extensive invasion of the adjacent organs, including 1 adrenal and 1 retroperitoneal tumor. Malignancies were significantly more frequent in these 2 groups than in the normal DNA diploid group (table).

Conclusion.—Flow cytometric analysis suggests that nondiploid pheochromocytomas or paragangliomas are more prone to aggressive behavior than diploid tumors. Aneuploidy is not a definite diagnostic indicator of malignancy, but it may suggest that the tumor is a potentially persistent and/or invasive one. Thus, patients with nondiploid pheochromocytomas or paragangliomas should be monitored carefully.

▶ Determination of the malignant potential of pheochromocytomas is difficult, if not impossible, using conventional histologic techniques. Metastatic deposits, vascular invasion, and local recurrence have been the clinical features associated with malignancy. After surgical resection, follow-up is required to assess the possibility of residual or recurrent disease. The usual recommendations are an annual clinical assessment and a 24-hour urinary collection for catecholamines and metanephrines. It is generally recommended that yearly screening continue for at least 5, and preferably 10, years because late recurrences or metastases are a distinct possibility. Flow cytometric DNA analysis, as described in this article, may allow identification of a subgroup that requires especially close follow-up. As shown in the table, no diploid tumor displayed malignant activity in comparison to those tumors displaying tetraploidy or aneuploidy. Even those patients with diploid tumors, however, need long-term follow-up because benign tumors may recur if incompletely resected.—L. Landsberg, M.D.

Phaeochromocytoma Presenting as Acute Hyperamylasaemia and Multiple Organ Failure

Gan TJ, Miller RF, Webb AR, Russell RCG (Duke Univ, Durham, NC; The Middlesex Hosp, London)
Can J Anaesth 41:244–247, 1994   112-95-6-8

Introduction.—The bizarre signs and symptoms from a pheochromocytoma are accounted for because the tumor secretes catecholamines. The most common sign is sustained or paroxysmal hypertension, although fewer than 1% of patients who are hypertensive have the tumor. A case is reported in which the tumor caused hyperamylasemia and multiple organ failure.

Case Report.—Male, 58, received a diagnosis of acute relapsing pancreatitis and was referred for analysis of a mass on the tail of the pancreas. Before this admission, he had a history of sudden abdominal pain and fever. A similar pattern occurred 9 years earlier. His blood pressure was 110/75 mm Hg with diffuse abdominal pain. Blood test results included hemoglobin of 15.5 g/dL, hematocrit of 45%, and platelet count of 185,000/μL with a marginally elevated creatinine. Serum amylase was 4,308 units/L. The patient received a diagnosis of acute pancreatitis. Hyperglycemia and hypoxemia developed suddenly. A chest radiograph showed diffuse lung infiltration. Wedge pressure was consistent with adult respiratory distress syndrome. The patient was mechanically ventilated for 11 days. On day 3 of ventilation, disseminated intravascular coagulopathy developed, hemoglobin fell to under 10 g/dL, white cell count rose to 18,000/μL, platelets rose to 35,000/μL, and prothrombin and partial thromboplastin times were increased with ensuing acute renal failure. Blood pressure varied between 80/65 mm Hg and 170/100 mm Hg. Colloid administration controlled the hypotensive episodes. Although abdominal ultrasound showed no biliary tract or gallbladder stones and a normal pancreatic head and body, a 7 × 7 cm mass was detected at the pancreatic tail. He was discharged, but returned again 2 weeks later with similar clinical signs followed by acute respiratory failure. Amylase was 4,235 units/L. The same mass was detected on ultrasound. A pancreatic tumor was suspected. During a percutaneous biopsy of the mass, his blood pressure ranged from 40/20 mm Hg to 230/130 mm Hg with excess sweating and vasoconstriction, and he was transferred to the ICU. The T waves on the ECG were inverted in the lateral chest leads. A pheochromocytoma was suspected. Urinary vanillylmandelic acid was elevated by a factor of 10. The patient's blood pressure continued to fluctuate. Surgery was scheduled for the third day, during which a 9 × 8 cm adrenal mass above the left kidney was removed.

Comment.—The 2 episodes of respiratory failure were thought to be the result of the excess catecholamines producing a toxic effect on pulmonary capillaries. Hyperamylasemia is an unusual occurrence in pheochromocytoma. The widely changing blood pressure and headache are not common in the aspiration of a pancreatic mass. Biopsies of the tumor are not regularly attempted because of the chance of a hypertensive crisis, although only half of patients with pheochromocytoma have hypertensive episodes. Although this pattern of symptoms is unusual, the differential diagnosis of a suspected peripancreatic mass should include consideration of a pheochromocytoma before biopsy or surgical exploration.

▶ Adult respiratory distress syndrome is a rare but recognized consequence of pheochromocytoma. Catecholamine-induced damage to the pulmonary capillary endothelium may be responsible. Aggressive supportive care and appropriate use of adrenergic blocking agents will frequently permit recovery. Two additional features of the patient reported here are noteworthy. First, the untoward response to needle aspiration of an unsuspected pheochromocytoma is well documented. Large swings in blood pressure may occur, as were noted here, and the induced pressor crisis may be fatal. Pheochromocytoma should be excluded before percutaneous biopsy or other manipulation of a mass in the region of the adrenals. Second, the elevated serum amylase suggested the diagnosis of acute pancreatitis. What is the origin of the amylase? Read on.—L. Landsberg, M.D.

Malignant Pheochromocytoma Masquerading as Acute Pancreatitis: A Rare But Potentially Lethal Occurrence

Dugal Perrier NA, Van Heerden JA, Wilson DJ, Warner M (Mayo Clinic and Found, Rochester, Minn)
Mayo Clin Proc 69:366–370, 1994   112-95-6-9

Background.—Pheochromocytoma can express itself in a confusing array of symptoms and lead to an emergency. A patient with acute abdominal pain and hyperamylasemia, which are indicative of pancreatitis, is discussed.

Case Report.—Healthy male, 68, came to the emergency room with acute midabdominal pain and vomiting that awoke him from sleep. Severe cervical pain and cardiac palpitations were also noted. Blood tests included hemoglobin of 14.7 mg/dL, hematocrit of 53.3%, leukocyte count of 22.9 × 10⁹/L and platelet count of 346 × 10⁹/L. Serum amylase was 2,526 units/L (salivary-type was 2,278 U/L) and lipase was normal. Serum calcium and phosphorus were 8.6 and 5.4 mg/dL, respectively. The chest x-ray film showed a normal cardiac silhouette and clear lungs. The initial diagnosis was acute pancreatitis because of the elevated amylase, and rehydration and analgesics were begun. During the next 5 hours, his normal blood pressure rose to 180/100 mm Hg and heart rate increased to 180 beats/min. Bibasilar rales and hypoactive bowels were detected. An echocardiogram showed a dilated left ventricle, global hypokinesia, and an ejection fraction of 11%. During 10- to 20-minute intervals, systolic blood pressure would fluctuate from 65 to 260 mm Hg. He was admitted to the ICU. Abdominal ultrasound showed a normal liver, gallbladder, and kidneys and a 6-cm mass in the area of the right adrenal gland. Computed tomography confirmed the mass and showed a normal pancreas. Urinary and plasma catecholamines and creatine kinase were increased. After 8 hours in the ICU his blood pressure varied, at 2- to 4-minute intervals, between 30 and 320 mm Hg, and his heart rate varied from 120 to 220 beats/min. Pulmonary edema and large amounts of frothy fluid forced intubation to maintain an airway. An emergency adrenalectomy was performed. A large mass, dissected from the vena cava, was found in the right suprarenal region. After ligation from the right adrenal vein, the fluctuations in blood pressure diminished, and the tumor was successfully removed. The 100-g malignant tumor extended into the blood vessels. The amylase concentration within the tumor was 1,520 units/L. During the following week, the ejection fraction improved to 45%, and amylase and catecholamine levels decreased to normal levels.

Comment.—Although the initial diagnosis suggested pancreatitis, the hemodynamic instability and elevation of the S-fraction of amylase lead to alternative diagnoses. Two reasons for the elevated amylase might include ischemic injury to amylase-containing tissues, particularly lung tissue, or amylase produced by the tumor itself. Because amylase levels in the tumor were similar to the serum, the source of the enzyme was likely the lungs. Although rare, the possibility of a pheochromocytoma masquerading as pancreatitis should be considered, especially in conjunction with hemodynamic instability and elevated S-type amylase. When ultrasound shows a normal pancreas, examination of the adrenal glands is needed. Overlooking a pheochromocytoma can lead to a fatal outcome.

▶ This patient was similar to the patient described in Abstract 112-95-6–8 with prominent abdominal pain, elevated serum amylase, and pulmonary edema. In this patient, unlike the previous one, the pulmonary edema was cardiogenic as judged by evidence of depressed cardiac function. The latter is a well-recognized complication of both hypertension and catecholamine-induced cardiomyopathy. In this case, fractionation of the amylase revealed that it was of the S-type, the isotype present in salivary glands and lung. The lipase level was normal. The authors conclude that the lung is the source of the increased amylase in patients with pheochromocytoma who have pulmonary edema. The constellation of pulmonary edema, abdominal pain, and high amylase should raise the suspicion of pheochromocytoma, especially in the face of elevated or fluctuating blood pressure. A normal lipase is helpful in excluding acute pancreatitis, although infarction of the pancreas in association with pheochromocytoma has also been described (Al-Dawoud et al: *Dig Dis Sci* 38:1338, 1993).—L. Landsberg, M.D.

Early Experience With Laparoscopic Approach for Adrenalectomy
Gagner M, Lacroix A, Prinz RA, Bolté E, Albala D, Potvin C, Hamet P, Kuchel O, Quérin S, Pomp A (Hôtel-Dieu de Montréal; Univ of Montreal; Loyola Univ, Maywood, Ill)
Surgery 114-1120–1125, 1993   112-95-6–10

Background.—Among the several approaches to adrenalectomy, the posterior or transabdominal approaches result in considerable postoperative pain because the incisions are close to the intercostal nerves. Experience with a laparoscopic approach to adrenal disease is presented.

·

Methods.—During a 1-year period, 25 laparoscopic adrenalectomies were performed on 22 patients with a variety of adrenal disorders (5 had pheochromocytoma). For operations on the left side, the patients were placed in a decubitus position, the abdomen was inflated with CO_2 to 15 mm Hg, and an 11-mm trocar was inserted in the anterior axillary line. Under direct visualization, 3 more trocars were inserted in the flank, under the 12th rib. A similar procedure was performed on the right side, taking care to avoid insufflation in the liver parenchyma. This was checked before with a syringe. The third trocar was inserted dorsally after avoiding the kidney.

Results.—The average age of the patients was 42 years, and the study included 15 women and 7 men. Nine operations were performed on the right gland, 10 were done on the left, and 6 were bilateral. The operations took an average of 2.3 hours, with the left approach taking slightly less than 2 hours and the right just more than 2.5 hours. Bilateral surgeries took 5.3 hours. Hospital stays averaged 4 days. The tumors averaged 4.1 cm, and the operation was successful in all but 1 patient who required laparotomy because of ineffective exposure. Complications were few (perioperative bleeding controlled by suturing, partial pancreatic dissection, hypertension during bag extraction), and there were only 5 narcotic injections. There were no deaths.

Comment.—In spite of preoperative adrenergic blockade, hypertension developed in 2 patients with pheochromocytoma. Laparoscopy can be a safe procedure. Less postoperative pain and rapid return to normal activity may make this the preferred method for surgical removal of most adrenal gland lesions.

▶ The revolution in endoscopic and minimally invasive surgery has progressed so rapidly that it should not be surprising to find adventurous surgeons operating on pheochromocytomas by the laparoscopic approach. In this series of 25 patients with different adrenal lesions, 5 pheochromocytomas were successfully removed via laparoscope. Despite adrenergic blockade (details not given), 2 patients experienced hypertension during the procedure. The feasibility of endoscopic removal of pheochromocytomas is enhanced by the excellent localization techniques now available (CT or MRI).

Although this technique is potentially attractive in terms of simplicity and shortened convalescence, further experience is required before it can be considered for routine treatment of patients with pheochromocytoma. The incidence of perioperative complications and long-term results (including recurrence rates) will have to be established in large series of patients. Careful preoperative preparation with adrenergic blocking agents will, of course, be required. Within the next few years, in centers with extensive laparoscopic experience, the use of laparoscopic techniques may begin to replace conventional surgery for removal of pheochromocytomas in selected patients.—L. Landsberg, M.D.

Suggested Reading

The following articles are recommended to the reader:

Noshiro T, Shimizu K, Way D, et al: Angiotensin II enhances norepinephrine spillover during sympathetic activation in conscious rabbits. *Am J Physiol* H1864–H1871, 1994.
▶ This study provides additional evidence of a physiologically significant prejunctional facilitory effect of angiotensin II on norepinephrine release in response to sympathetic neuronal impulse traffic. Activation of the renin-angiotensin system enhances noradrenergic responses by increasing norepinephrine release at sympathetic neuroeffector junctions.

Lembo G, Capaldo B, Rendina V, et al: Acute noradrenergic activation induces insulin resistance in human skeletal muscle. *Am J Physiol* E242–E247, 1994.
▶ This interesting study demonstrates that under physiologic activation of the sympathetic nervous system, sensitivity to insulin is diminished. Other evidence indicates that insulin stimulates the sympathetic nervous system via central neurons related to the ventral medial hypothalamus. These and other observations indicate that the sympathetic nervous system may be involved in the relationship between insulin and hypertension.

Kurpad AV, Khan K, Calder AG, et al: Muscle and whole body metabolism after norepinephrine. *Am J Physiol* E877–E884, 1994.
▶ Improved precision in the determination of oxygen consumption has resolved the long-standing debate over whether norepinephrine increases oxygen consumption (metabolic rate) in humans and has shown that norepinephrine infusions do in fact increase metabolic rate by up to 10%, as was the case in this study. Substantial debate remains, however, on the site of origin and the metabolic processes involved in this increased energy expenditure. This carefully performed study finds no evidence for skeletal muscle as a site of norepinephrine-induced thermogenesis. It indicates that substrate cycling of fatty acids in and out of triglycerides is quantitatively significant.

Bornstein SR, Gonzalez-Hernandez JA, Ehrhart-Bornstein M, et al: Intimate contact of chromaffin and cortical cells within the human adrenal gland forms the cellular basis for important intra-adrenal interactions. *J Clin Endocrinol Metab* 78:225–232, 1994.
▶ The close anatomical association between the adrenal cortex and medulla has engendered continuing speculation about an underlying teleologic basis for the morphologic proximity. The high corticosteroid content of blood draining the cortex into the medulla via a portal venous system appears to have a role in inducing the epinephrine-forming enzyme, phenolethanolamine-N-methyl transferase. In this article, close anatomical connection between cortical cells throughout the adrenal medulla and chromaffin cells throughout the adrenal cortex provide an anatomical basis for intra-adrenal paracrine mechanisms that might operate in both directions.

Granneman JG, Lahners KN: Analysis of human and rodent β_3-adrenergic receptor messenger ribonucleic acids. *Endocrinology* 135:1025–1031, 1994.
▶ Regular readers of these pages will recall last year's selections on the β_3-adrenergic receptor. This study provides further evidence of important species differences in receptor structure and function. The data here indicate heterogeneity of human and rat β_3-receptor messenger RNA. This is potentially important because β_3-adrenergic receptor agonists are being investigated as therapeutic agents for the treatment of obesity. The rodent is clearly not a good model for testing activity of these compounds for possible use in humans.

Jönsson A, Hallengren B, Manhem P, et al: Cardiac pheochromocytoma. *J Intern Med* 236:93–96, 1994.

▶ Pheochromocytomas can be located almost anywhere. This large tumor (4 × 5 cm) was located in the right atrium. Scanning with contrast-enhanced CT, ECG-gated MRI, and metaiodobenzylguanidine identified the tumor.

Aprill BS, Drake AJ III, Lasseter DH, et al: Silent adrenal nodules in von Hippel-Lindau disease suggest pheochromocytoma. *Ann Intern Med* 120:485–487, 1994.

▶ Pheochromocytoma occurs commonly in patients with von Hippel-Lindau disease. The incidence seems to vary in different kindreds, and in some affected families, 60% to 70% of patients have pheochromocytomas. As noted here, clinically silent adrenal nodules in patients with von Hippel-Lindau disease should be assumed to be pheochromocytomas.

Tanaka K, Noguchi S, Shuin T, et al: Spontaneous rupture of adrenal pheochromocytoma: A case report. *J Urol* 151:120–121, 1994.

▶ Severe pressor crises in patients with pheochromocytoma are frequently thought to represent areas of hemorrhagic infarction with subsequent release of stored catecholamines. In this case, hemorrhage in the pheochromocytoma dissected out of the adrenal and caused substantial retroperitoneal hematoma.

Freier DT, Thompson NW: Pheochromocytoma and pregnancy: The epitome of high risk. *Surgery* 114:1148–1152, 1993.

▶ Pheochromocytoma in pregnant women continues to carry a high risk for the fetus. Spontaneous vaginal delivery is disastrous for both mother and child. Alpha- and beta-adrenergic blockade instituted after diagnosis have markedly improved the prognosis for the mother. Surgical removal during the mid-trimester or cesarean section followed by tumor extirpation when the fetus is of sufficient size is usually recommended for patients diagnosed in the third trimester. Despite modern techniques, fetal wastage remains high—about 15% in large series. In this study, the 2 fetal deaths were planned terminations.

Munden R, Adams DB, Curry N: Cystic pheochromocytoma: Radiologic diagnosis. *South Med J* 86:1301–1305, 1993.

▶ Pheochromocytomas are usually solid tumors. As pointed out here, however, resorption of hemorrhagic areas may leave large cysts that may confuse the radiologic diagnosis.

Orchard T, Grant CS, van Heerden JA, et al: Pheochromocytoma: Continuing evolution of surgical therapy. *Surgery* 114:1153–1159, 1993.

▶ An interesting and comprehensive update of the Mayo Clinic experience.

7 Islet Cell Tumors, Paraneoplastic Syndromes, and Multiple Endocrine Neoplasia

Introduction

The year 1994 will be remembered as the year when octreotide scintigraphy became commercially available for diagnostic use in the United States. Readers of the YEAR BOOK OF ENDOCRINOLOGY will recall that the lead articles for this section in the past 4 years have involved somatostatin-receptor imaging in one way or another. Ever since the original description of the procedure by Lamberts' group in Rotterdam, considerable improvements have been made in refining this important imaging technique. The result is indium-labeled pentetreotide (Octreoscan) for imaging tumors of neuroendocrine origin as well as their metastases. The procedure will undoubtedly receive much scrutiny with regard to its potential in one particular area: Will octreotide scintigraphy score well in localizing primary tumors of neuroendocrine origin that have eluded detection by conventional thin-slice CT or MRI? The 2 other areas that will benefit by somatostatin-receptor imaging are the ability to predict responsiveness to octreotide therapy and the ability to predict the neuroendocrine origin of a tumor in cases in which metastatic lesions manifest in the absence of a known primary lesion. Several articles chosen for this year's section have to do with octreotide scintigraphy in the diagnosis and treatment of gastroenteropancreatic tumors of endocrine origin.

The second major area of interest that saw a breakthrough in 1994 is the MEN-IIA gene. Two separate groups identified a unique mutation in the *RET* gene in affected family members with this syndrome. (Hofstra et al: *Nature* 367:375, 1994; Eng et al: *Hum Mol Genet* 3:237, 1994). This important localization, which consists of mutations in exon 10 or 11 of the *RET* proto-oncogene, will be of enormous help in identifying family members who are carriers of the gene. More importantly, it will afford substantial peace of mind to those family members who are not carriers and could, by such unambiguous validation, obviate the need for expensive hormonal testing.

In addition to these 2 discoveries, there were significant additions to our knowledge. We learned that endoscopic ultrasonography has lived up to its original expectations in its ability to localize small islet cell tumors that defy localization by high-resolution CT/MRI (Abstract 112-95-7-2). Treatment for amine precursor uptake decarboxylation cell malignancies using radioactive metaiodobenzylguanidine became an exciting, although slightly disappointing, reality(Abstract 112-95-7-3). We also learned that somatostatin scintigraphy can be added to that ever-enlarging diagnostic armamentarium of tests used for localization of the occult ectopic ACTH-producing bronchial carcinoid tumor (Abstract 112-95-7-11). A great deal was learned about the hypoglycemia caused by non–islet cell tumors (Abstract 112-95-7-15). And, finally, the first report on a head-to-head comparison between DNA testing and hormonal testing for the detection of MEN-IIA has been published (Abstract 112-95-7-18). All this, and more, made the past year interesting, if not riveting.

C.R. Kannan, M.D.

Neuroendocrine Tumors—Localization and Treatment

Preoperative Localization of Gastrointestinal Endocrine Tumors Using Somatostatin-Receptor Scintigraphy
Weinel RJ, Neuhaus C, Stapp J, Klotter H-J, Trautmann ME, Joseph K, Arnold R, Rothmund M (Phillips-Univ Marburg, Germany)
Ann Surg 218:640–645, 1993   112-95-7-1

Background.—High-affinity somatostatin receptors are found in most endocrine tumors. With pentatreotid, a stable, ^{111}In-labeled somatostatin analogue that binds to these receptors, somatostatin-receptor positive tumors can be detected scintigraphically. The value of somatostatin-receptor scintigraphy (SRS) in the preoperative localization of gastrointestinal endocrine tumors was investigated.

Methods.—Nine patients with various gastrointestinal endocrine tumors underwent SRS, CT, and ultrasonography before surgery. The results of preoperative imaging studies and intraoperative ultrasound were compared with surgical findings.

Findings.—At surgical exploration, 12 primary tumors were found in 8 patients. These tumors were identified correctly by SRS in 5 patients, ultrasonography in 4, and CT in 3. In 1 patient with Zollinger-Ellison syndrome, scintigraphic findings suggested a tumor in the hepatoduodenal ligament region. The results of CT and ultrasonography in this case were negative. In 4 patients with metastases, scintigraphy, CT, and ultrasonography were comparable.

Conclusion.—This new technique appears to be useful in preoperatively localizing gastrointestinal endocrine tumors. However, SRS has some disadvantages. It seems unlikely to reach a sensitivity and specificity high enough to replace conventional imaging methods. Rather, SRS can serve as a complement to such methods.

▶ The year 1994 will be remembered as the year when somatostatin-receptor imaging with the indium-tagged pentetreotide, "Octreoscan," was approved for use by the Food and Drug Administration in the United States. Octreoscan imaging should (1) provide information regarding localization of the primary tumor undetected by conventional methods, (2) validate the neuroendocrine source of lesions demonstrated by other imaging techniques, and (3) serve as a predictor of benefits with therapy using octreotide. The authors give octreotide imaging a slight edge over CT and ultrasonography in detecting primary tumors, whereas all 3 were equally good for detecting metastases. The catch here is that for a tumor outside the liver to visualize with pentetreotide, the tumor must contain a significant number of somatostatin receptors. Obviously, not all tumors (carcinoids, gastrinoma, and insulinoma included) are receptor-rich for somatostatin. In the 1 patient with gastrinoma in whom the scintigraphy suggested a tumor in the hepatoduodenal ligament (and the CT and ultrasound studies were negative), extensive exploration failed to reveal a tumor in that location. This raises the question of false positive results. The authors' conclusion that octreotide scintigraphy is not sensitive enough to stand alone is well worth noting. Hence, ultrasonography, CT, and even invasive procedures continue to play a role in localization of gastrointestinal endocrine tumors.

For a slightly different view on the same subject, Scherubl et al. (*Gastroenterology* 105:1705, 1993) compared indium pentetreotide scintigraphy in 40 patients with neuroendocrine gastroenteropancreatic tumors and was able to visualize 11 of 17 foregut tumors, 14 of 16 midgut tumors, and 7 of 7 metastatic neuroendocrine tumors with unknown primary. These are among the best results that tout the sensitivity of octreotide scintigraphy. In 16 patients, tumor tissue that had escaped conventional imaging techniques was detected by indium pentetreotide imaging. Thus, these authors concluded that indium pentetreotide was a "safe and sensitive procedure for in vivo imaging of gastroenteropancreatic neuroendocrine tumors." New somatostatin analogues are also under investigation; Breeman et al. (*Eur J Nucl Med* 20:1089, 1993) evaluated the potential usefulness of the radioiodinated octapeptide RC-160. The search goes on. For a comparison between scintigraphy and endoscopic ultrasonography, Abstract 112-95-7–2 will provide the answer.—C.R. Kannan, M.D.

Localisation of Neuroendocrine Tumours of the Upper Gastrointestinal Tract
Zimmer T, Ziegler K, Bäder M, Fett U, Hamm B, Riecken E-O, Wiedenmann B (Free Univ, Berlin)
Gut 35:471–475, 1994   112-95-7–2

Sensitivities of Various Imaging Procedures in Detecting Primary Lesions of
Neuroendocrine Tumors Depending on Functional State

	Endoscopic US	US	CT	NMR	SRS
Sensitivity total	22/25 (88)	8/25 (32)	9/25 (36)	6/25 (24)	13/25 (52)
Sensitivity gastrinomas	4/5 (80)	3/5 (60)	3/5 (60)	3/5 (60)	5/5 (100)
Sensitivity insulinomas	7/8 (87)	0/8 (0)	1/8 (12)	0/8 (0)	1/8 (12)
Sensitivity carcinoid	1/1 (100)	1/1 (100)	1/1 (100)	1/1 (100)	1/1 (100)
Sensitivity non-functional tumours	10/11(91)	4/11 (36)	4/11 (36)	2/11 (18)	6/11 (54)

Abbreviations: US, ultrasonography; *NMR,* nuclear magnetic resonance imaging; *SRS,*
somatostatin-receptor scintigraphy.
Note: Numbers in parentheses are percentages.
(Courtesy of Zimmer T, Ziegler K, Bäder M, et al: *Gut* 35:471-475, 1994.)

Background.—Neuroendocrine tumors of the foregut type comprise a
subgroup of tumors located primarily in the pancreas, stomach, and duodenum. Depending on their size, functional neuroendocrine tumors
can be diagnosed before operation by various imaging procedures. The
value of endoscopic ultrasound, somatostatin-receptor scintigraphy
(SRS), ultrasonography, CT, and MRI in diagnosing primary tumors and
local spread was investigated.

Methods.—Eighteen patients with a total of 25 primary tumors were
studied. All had been verified histologically in tissue obtained at surgery
or by ultrasonography or endoscopy-guided biopsy. Tumors were located in the pancreas in 17 patients, in the duodenum in 6, in the stomach in 1, and the liver in 1.

Findings.—Endoscopic ultrasonography showed the highest sensitivity
(88%) for detecting tumor, followed by SRS, CT, transabdominal ultrasonography, and MRI, with sensitivities of 52%, 36%, 32%, and 24%,
respectively (table). Endoscopic ultrasonography was especially sensitive
in tumors smaller than 2 cm in diameter. Among the pancreatic tumors,
endoscopic ultrasonography showed a sensitivity of 94%. Six of the 8
extrapancreatic tumors were identified by endoscopic ultrasonography, 5
by SRS, and only 1 each by CT, transabdominal ultrasonography, and
MRI. One neuroendocrine tumor not identified by endoscopic ultrasonography was identified correctly by SRS. Endoscopic ultrasonography enabled correct determination of tumor size and spread into the
parapancreatic structures, especially in the large vessels, in all 14 patients
undergoing surgery. The lymph node stage was identified correctly in 10
of these patients.

Conclusion.—Endoscopic ultrasonography and SRS were the most
sensitive imaging modalities for localizing neuroendocrine tumors of the
foregut. These modalities should be used early to accurately stage neuroendocrine tumors of this type.

▶ YEAR BOOK readers will remember that endoscopic ultrasonography literally exploded into the diagnostic arena in 1992 (1993 YEAR BOOK OF ENDO-

CRINOLOGY, p 226). Lightdale et al. (*N Engl J Med* 326:1721, 1992) were among the first to report that this procedure had a sensitivity of 82% in localizing endocrine pancreatic tumors in patients with negative CT and ultrasonography, whereas angiography was diagnostic in only 27% of patients. Thus, endoscopic ultrasonography was superior to any of the invasive procedures. Here we have a head-to-head comparison between the various modalities. There were 3 unique situations where endoscopic ultrasonography was clearly superior: small tumors (less than 2 cm in diameter), nonfunctional tumors, and detection of tumor that had spread into the parapancreatic structures. Notably, even the extrapancreatic tumors visualized surprisingly well by endoscopic ultrasonography. The message from this study is that the combination of endoscopic ultrasonography and octreotide scintigraphy have such a high accuracy in localization and therefore obviate wasting effort and resources with CT, MR, and transabdominal ultrasonography. The limitation here is that these techniques are not generally available in the United States.—C.R. Kannan, M.D.

Treatment of Malignant Phaeochromocytoma, Paraganglioma and Carcinoid Tumours With ^{131}I-Metaiodobenzylguanidine
Bomanji J, Britton KE, Ur E, Hawkins L, Grossman AB, Besser GM (St Bartholomew's Hosp, London)
Nucl Med Commun 14:856–861, 1993   112-95-7-3

Introduction.—Radioiodinated metaiodobenzylguanidine (MIBG) is known to concentrate in malignant pheochromocytoma, paraganglioma, and carcinoid tumors, and it has been used to treat tumors of neural crest origin. Treatment of these neoplasms with external beam radiation and chemotherapy has generally been unrewarding.

Series.—Four patients with metastatic carcinoid tumors, 3 with paraganglioma, and 2 with malignant pheochromocytoma were treated with ^{131}I-MIBG. In all cases pretreatment scans made with ^{123}I-MIBG had demonstrated metastases in soft tissue and, in 2 instances, in bone as well. The patients were followed up for 8 months to 9 years after receiving ^{131}I-MIBG in cumulative doses of 4.8–40.1 GBq.

Results.—None of the patients had a complete response, but 3 had a partial response lasting 40, 50, and 108 months, respectively, and have remained in remission. Three patients had progressive disease. In all, 47 lesions were detected on baseline diagnostic and treatment images, whereas only 20 were detected after treatment. Five of the 9 patients had a complete symptomatic response to treatment and 3 others had a partial response. The one serious adverse effect was mild liver failure in a patient with extensive hepatic metastases.

Conclusion.—Treatment with ^{131}I-MIBG, although not curative, does provide temporary palliation for some patients with metastatic pheochromocytoma, paraganglioma, and carcinoid tumors.

▶ One of the visionary prophecies in the treatment of those neuroendocrine tumors that visualize by octreotide scintigraphy is the potential for delivering radiolabeled octreotide as a form of radiation therapy. The analogy here between pheochromocytoma and MIBG is inevitable. When MIBG scintigraphy was first used to localize pheochromocytoma almost 2 decades ago, it was suggested that in the future it could be used to deliver radiation to malignant pheochromocytomas, exploiting the affinity of these neural crest tumors for MIBG. This study indicates that this approach also works in carcinoid tumors that also can concentrate MIBG. Unfortunately, complete responses did not occur with this therapy. Thus, at best, it is palliative. It won't be too long before radioactive octreotide could be tried in a similar fashion to treat malignant or metastatic endocrine pancreatic tumors. Who would have thought that radioactive iodine therapy for metastatic differentiated thyroid cancer would have had such far-reaching analogies 40 years later?—C.R. Kannan, M.D.

Insulinoma

Islet Amyloid Polypeptide in Human Insulinomas: Evidence for Intracellular Amyloidogenesis

O'Brien TD, Butler AE, Roche PC, Johnson KH, Butler PC (Mayo Clinic and Found, Rochester, Minn; Univ of Minnesota, St Paul)
Diabetes 43:329–336, 1994   112-95-7-4

Background.—Amyloid deposits are the characteristic lesions in the pancreatic islets in NIDDM and in insulinomas. These deposits are derived from islet amyloid polypeptide (IAPP), which is produced primarily by pancreatic β-cells and is co-packaged and co-secreted with insulin. IAPP-derived deposits could aggregate in β-cells and then be released into the extracellular space. Such a question could be addressed by careful study of insulinoma specimens.

Objectives.—Twenty human insulinomas were studied by immunohistochemistry and electron microscopy to determine the frequency of IAPP-derived amyloid deposits in human insulinomas and the potential importance of intracellular IAPP aggregation and fibrillogenesis in the degeneration and destruction of β-cells.

Results.—The tumors consisted of solid cords or palisading ribbons of insulin-immunoreactive tumor cells (Fig 7–1), which were often separated by dense collagenous stroma or cavernous vascular sinuses. Sixteen of the 20 tumors had detectable cellular IAPP immunoreactivity (Fig 7–2). Tumor sections showed small, globular or irregular amyloid deposits within the cytoplasm of many tumor cells in 10 of 13 (77%) amyloid-containing insulinomas, and these deposits corresponded to the

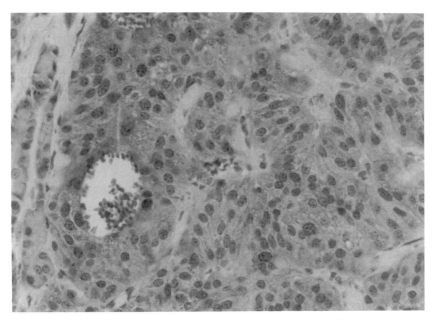

Fig 7–1.—Photomicrograph of an insulinoma showing immunoreactivity (red-brown stain) in most of the tumor cells. Insulin-immunoperoxidase/Schmitt's hematoxylin stain; original magnification, ×100. (Courtesy of O'Brien TD, Butler AE, Roche PC, et al: *Diabetes* 43:329–336, 1994.)

dense, punctate, intracellular foci of IAPP immunoreactivity within tumor cells. Ubiquitin immunoreactivity supported the intracellular origin for these deposits. The appearance of pathologic IAPP aggregates by electron microscopy varied with 3 tumors showing intracellular aggregates of IAPP-immunoreactive amyloid fibrils often were free in the cytoplasmic matrix adjacent to the nucleus and mitochondria and lacked delimiting membranes. In β-cells that were surrounded by hemorrhage and isolated from surrounding tumor cells and connective tissues, large (up to 10 μm in greatest dimension) amyloid deposits were completely surrounded by β-cell cytoplasm and often displaced normal cellular organelles.

Discussion.—These observations suggest the intracellular formation of IAPP-derived amyloid deposits that are subsequently released to the extracellular space by exocytosis of the membrane-bound structures or after necrosis of the tumor cells, or both. It is also possible that IAPP-derived islet amyloid deposits may be initially formed within the cytoplasm of β-cells, thus leading to β-cell necrosis and a reduction of the β-cell mass, as seen in NIDDM.

▶ That there can be a common link between NIDDM that results in hyperglycemia and insulinoma that causes hypoglycemia is curious. The insulinoma cell may indeed hold the key for the β-cell damage seen in patients with

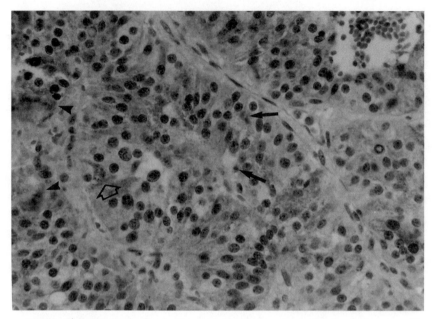

Fig 7–2.—Photomicrograph of an insulinoma showing dense, punctate (*filled arrows*) or more diffuse (*open arrow*) cytoplasmic islet amyloid polypeptide (IAPP) immunoreactivity in many tumor cells. Extracellular amyloid deposits (*arrowheads*) also have a strong IAPP immunoreactivity. IAPP-immunoperoxidase/Schmitt's hematoxylin stain; original magnification, × 100. (Courtesy of O'Brien TD, Butler AE, Roche PC, et al: *Diabetes* 43:329–336, 1994.)

NIDDM, whose pancreases also show IAPP. Abnormal amyloidogenesis might be responsible for cytolysis during its transit from intracellular to extracellular locations. Obviously, the large mass of insulinoma cells overrides this effect in islet cell tumors but may result in β-cytolytic effects in the pancreas of patients with NIDDM. As Alice would have said, things are getting curiouser!—C.R. Kannan, M.D.

Zollinger-Ellison Syndrome

A Prospective Study of Intraoperative Methods to Diagnose and Resect Duodenal Gastrinomas

Sugg SL, Norton JA, Fraker DL, Metz DC, Pisegna JR, Fishbeyn V, Benya RV, Shawker TH, Doppman JL, Jensen RT (Natl Cancer Inst, Bethesda, Md; Natl Inst of Arthritis, Diabetes, Digestive and Kidney Diseases, Bethesda, Md)
Ann Surg 218:138–144, 1993   112-95-7-5

Background.—Duodenal gastrinomas are an increasingly common finding in patients with Zollinger-Ellison syndrome (ZES). Some authors advocate intraoperative endoscopy with transillumination (IOE) at surgery to detect these tumors; others recommend routine duodenotomy (DX).

Methods.—To determine whether DX should be done routinely in patients with ZES, 35 such patients were studied prospectively. The ability of DX to detect gastrinomas was compared with that of palpation, intraoperative ultrasound, and IOE.

Findings.—Thirty-three patients (94%) had tumors detected and excised. Twenty-seven (77%) had duodenal gastrinomas excised. The mean duodenal tumor size was .8 cm, which was significantly smaller than the pancreatic and lymph node tumors found in this series. Standard palpation after a Kocher maneuver identified 61% of the duodenal tumors, and intraoperative ultrasound showed only 26% and no new lesions. With IOE, 64% of duodenal gastrinomas and 6 new lesions were identified. All of the duodenal tumors and 5 additional lesions were identified with DX. Morbidity occurred in 17%. One patient had a duodenal fistula after surgery but later recovered. None of the patients died.

Conclusion.—The duodenum is the most common location for gastrinomas in patients with ZES. These gastrinomas occur in 77%. Duodenotomy should be performed routinely in patients with ZES to detect and remove duodenal gastrinomas.

▶ This confirms what has been suspected all along: that most ZES patients with gastrinoma have tumors in the duodenum and not in the pancreas. I have not previously seen the high frequency of duodenal gastrinomas in patients with ZES. Duodenal gastrinomas are easy to miss because they are notoriously difficult to find. Because of their small size, it is not surprising that conventional ultrasonography, CT, and MR were poor at localizing them. Even intraoperative ultrasound provided localization in only 26% of cases. The 2 most helpful localization procedures were intraoperative endoscopic ultrasound (see Abstract 112-95-7-2) and standard palpation by the surgeon, which gave a diagnostic sensitivity of 64% and 61%, respectively. In many instances, the only procedure that documented the gastrinoma was duodenectomy, with careful dissection of the removed tissue. The fact that the duodenal gastrinoma tends to be more malignant than does pancreatic gastrinoma underscores the need for early removal of the tumor within the duodenum. Apparently, duodenectomy is not associated with undue morbidity. The inescapable conclusion of this study is that when all else fails and you can't locate the gastrinoma, do a diagnostic duodenectomy! Clearly, this article adds a new focus to our understanding of ZES.—C.R. Kannan, M.D.

Long-Term Prognosis of Zollinger-Ellison Syndrome in Multiple Endocrine Neoplasia

Melvin WS, Johnson JA, Sparks J, Innes JT, Ellison EC (Ohio State Univ, Columbus)
Surgery 114:1183–1188, 1993   112-95-7-6

Introduction.—The Zollinger-Ellison syndrome (ZES), first described in 1955, is now recognized as a distinct clinical entity caused by a gastrin-secreting tumor. It occurs either sporadically or as a part of the familial MEN syndrome, and these 2 forms follow a different course. The long-term prognosis of patients with ZES and MEN was reviewed.

Methods.—The records of 76 patients with a diagnosis of ZES were reviewed. Patients were classified as having MEN when ZES occurred in conjunction with pituitary adenomas, hyperparathyroidism, or pheochromocytoma. All patients were routinely screened on a regular basis for determination of levels of serum calcium, PTH, and PRL.

Results.—Nineteen patients were given a diagnosis of gastrinoma as a manifestation of MEN. In 10 cases, the patients were thought to have MEN when ZES was first diagnosed. A total of 28 abdominal operations were performed on 17 patients, resulting in 12 total gastrectomies and 11 pancreatic resections or tumor enucleations. Only 1 patient achieved a biochemical cure after surgical resection of gastrinoma. Hyperparathyroidism was present in 20% of all patients with ZES and in 79% of those with MEN. In 6 patients, hyperparathyroidism was diagnosed before ZES (average, 7.7 years). The diagnosis was made synchronous with ZES in 3 patients and after that of ZES (average 11.5 years) in 6 patients. Surgical excision of the parathyroid glands was required in all 15 cases. Three patients were given a diagnosis of pheochromocytoma, a rare development, and 3 of pituitary adenoma. Sixteen patients were followed for at least 10 years and 12 for more than 20 years. The actual survival rates at 5, 10, 15, and 20 years after the diagnosis of ZES were 94%, 75%, 61%, and 58%, respectively. In contrast, patients with sporadic ZES had 5-, 10-, 15-, and 20-year survival rates of 62%, 50%, 37%, and 31%, respectively.

Discussion.—In this group of patients with ZES and MEN, endocrinopathies were diagnosed as early as 17 years before and as late as 39 years after diagnosis of ZES, indicating a need for lifelong surveillance. Most patients had an indolent course, although some did exhibit severe, progressive multiple endocrine dysfunction. Medical therapy can now be used in place of surgery to achieve symptomatic relief. Surgical cure of ZES is uncommon in patients with MEN. The prolonged survival of patients with ZES and MEN vs. sporadic ZES is probably the result of the indolent behavior of multiple endocrine tumors. Metastases were associated with decreased survival.

▶ The gastrinomas seen in association with MEN-1 differ in 6 important ways from the sporadic variety. They (1) are much smaller (less than .5 cm) "microgastrinomas"; (2) show immunopositivity to either pancreatic polypeptide, insulin, or glucagon and are usually gastrin-negative (larger gastrinomas may demonstrate gastrin immunopositivity); (3) are found more frequently in the duodenum, where they may be too small to detect even by palpation, and yet may already have metastasized to a regional lymph node; (5) are likely to be more malignant than their sporadic counterpart; and (6) may have a slightly higher incidence of enterochromaffin-like cell hyperplasia of the stomach. This paper indicates that the 10-year survival in patients with ZES without metastases associated with MEN-1 (100%) is longer than in sporadic ZES (70%). With hepatic metastases, however, for unclear reasons the 10-year survival rate decreased to 40% for patients with MEN and to 25% for patients with sporadic gastrinoma. This paper is among the few that bode well for patients with ZES and MEN. It does come as a surprise.

In a related area, Fraker et al. (*Ann Surg* 220:320, 1994) studied the effect of surgery on the natural history of ZES. Their data indicate that for the patient with ZES without metastases, curative gastrinoma resection alters the natural history of the disease in the following manner: hepatic metastases developed in only 3% of patients who had gastrinoma resection, whereas 23% of patients in the medically treated group had hepatic metastases develop. This, too, comes as a surprise.—C.R. Kannan, M.D.

Carcinoid Syndrome

Metastatic Carcinoid Disease Presenting Solely as High-Output Heart Failure

Yun D, Heywood JT (Loma Linda Jerry L Pettis Memorial Veterans Hosp, Calif; Loma Linda Univ, Calif)
Ann Intern Med 120:45–46, 1994   112-95-7–7

Introduction.—Typically, congestive heart failure in metastatic carcinoid disease is caused by progressive endocardial fibrosis of right-sided chambers and valves. An unusual case of metastatic carcinoid disease with high-output congestive heart failure without the typical features of cutaneous flushing and valvular lesions was described.

Case Report.—Man, 54, had signs and symptoms of congestive heart failure. Echocardiogram showed a hyperdynamic left ventricle with an ejection fraction of .75 and 4-chamber dilatation. There was no evidence of clinically significant tricuspid regurgitation or pulmonary stenosis; the valves were not thickened. Thermodilution cardiac output was 15.4 L/min, and systemic vascular resistance was calculated at 389 dynes/sec/cm^{-5}. Liver biopsy revealed a carcinoid tumor, but urinary level of 5-hydroxyindole acetic acid (5-HIAA) was relatively low at 36.1 µmol/24 hours. However, substance P, another important tumor marker in the diagnosis of carcinoid syndrome, was markedly elevated at 283 pmol/L.

Summary.—Carcinoid heart disease may present only as high-output failure without the typical right-sided fibrotic lesions when substance P is the primary neurohormone produced. The markedly elevated cardiac output with low systemic vascular resistance is consistent with the potent vasodilating effect of high substance P values.

▶ Now we can add one more facet to the spectrum of carcinoid heart disease. The similarities between this and thyrotoxic high-output cardiac failure are striking. The cardiac output of 15.4 L seen in this case is probably a record! In addition to the magnitude of the high output, this case is unique in that the patient had no demonstrable valvular disease, no significant dilatation of cardiac chambers, only mild elevation in the urinary 5-HIAA levels, and markedly elevated substance P levels in the plasma. Substance P is now believed to be the humoral mediator of the carcinoid flush, and yet in this patient the flushing was conspicuous by its absence. The vasodilatation caused by substance P can be profound, leading to the eventual development of high-output failure. It is also interesting that this patient did not have orthostatic changes either. The concept that substance P can cause such profound vasodilatation to result in cardiac failure, and yet not cause flushing or orthostatic hypotension, is difficult to reconcile. Regardless, all patients with high-output congestive heart failure need to be screened for thyrotoxicosis and carcinoid heart disease . . . and Paget's disease and beriberi and arteriovenous fistulae, and so on, and so on.—C.R. Kannan, M.D.

Serotonin, Catecholamines, Histamine, and Their Metabolites in Urine, Platelets, and Tumor Tissue of Patients With Carcinoid Tumors
Kema IP, de Vries EGE, Slooff MJH, Biesma B, Muskiet FAJ (Univ and Univ Hosp of Groningen, The Netherlands)
Clin Chem 40:86–95, 1994   112-95-7–8

Introduction.—Depending on their site of origin, carcinoid tumors can give rise to excessive synthesis, storage, and release of biogenic amines and polypeptides. In addition, production of catecholamines and histamine by carcinoid tumors is also conceivable given their confinement to the amine precursor uptake and decarboxylation (APUD) system. The long-term concentrations of platelet serotonin and urinary serotonin, 5-hydroxyindoleacetic acid, and 7 catecholamine metabolites were monitored in patients with carcinoid tumors.

Methods.—Forty-four patients with carcinoid tumors of foregut, midgut, and hindgut origin were studied during a median follow-up of 11 months (range, 1 day to 5 years). Tumor serotonin and catecholamine contents were measured in 11 patients and urinary concentrations of histamine and N-methylhistamine in 15.

Results.—The platelet serotonin content was the most sensitive and consistently increased marker during long-term monitoring, being present in 96% and 43% of patients with midgut and foregut carcinoids, respectively. None of the patients with hindgut tumors showed consistently increased platelet serotonin content. The urinary catecholamine metabolites were also frequently increased, particularly in patients with midgut carcinoids. The urinary dopamine metabolites were more frequently increased than norepinephrine and epinephrine metabolites, and urinary 3-O-methylated catecholamines had the highest sensitivity and consistency of all catecholamine metabolites. Tissue samples from midgut carcinoid tumors had the highest serotonin content, whereas catecholamine concentrations were independent of tumor location. Neither tumor serotonin nor catecholamine contents consistently correlated with platelet serotonin content for urinary excretion of catecholamine metabolites. Occurrence of the carcinoid syndrome was related to increased serotonin production. Increased histamine production was not an important feature in patients with lung carcinoids or liver-metastasized ileum carcinoids.

Discussion.—The platelet serotonin content is the most sensitive and consistently increased marker during long-term monitoring of patients with carcinoid tumors, notably in patients with midgut and foregut carcinoids. Urinary concentrations of catecholamines are also increased, but their origin in carcinoid tumors remains unclear. The lack of a relationship between tumor amine content and urinary metabolite concentrations may be caused by differences in tumor amine storage capacity, catabolizing activity, and the frequency of release.

▶ Will the new replace the old in the diagnostic testing for the carcinoid syndrome? According to this article, the answer is "yes," and the new marker will be increased platelet serotonin concentrations. What's new and exciting in this article is the revelation that carcinoid tumors possess an impressive capacity to synthesize, store, and release catecholamines and their metabolites. About one third of patients in this study with midgut carcinoids also showed increased excretion of urinary normetanephrine and metanephrine levels. Even more impressive is the observation that urinary dopamine metabolites were consistently increased in 38% of patients with carcinoid tumors of midgut origin. This should not be terribly surprising, because the carcinoid and the adrenal medullary cell lines both have APUD cell origins. Both carcinoids and pheochromocytomas are versatile secretors, capable of causing dramatic hormonal events; both secrete chromogranin A and related peptides; concentrate metaiodobenzylguanidine, albeit not to the same extent; and possess somatostatin receptors. Now comes additional evidence that carcinoid tumors are impressive secretors of catecholamines. Whether this phenomenon represents de novo secretion, the result of malignancy-related stress, or concomitant activation of the sympathetic system is not clear. Regardless, this pulls these 2 tumors closer than ever before.

For an excellent review on the management of patients with advanced carcinoid tumors, the reader is referred to the article by Moertel et al. (*Ann Intern Med* 120:302, 1994). Also, McDermott et al. (*Br J Surg* 81:1007, 1994) have analyzed the prognostic variables and outcome measures in 188 patients with gastrointestinal carcinoid tumors. Finally, the clinical efficacy of octreotide scintigraphy in patients with midgut carcinoid tumors and evaluation of intraoperative scintillation detection is discussed in an interesting article from Sweden (Ahlman et al: *Br J Surg* 81:1144, 1994).—C.R. Kannan, M.D.

Glucagonoma

The Long-Acting Somatostatin Analogue Octreotide Alleviates Symptoms by Reducing Posttranslational Conversion of Prepro-Glucagon to Glucagon in a Patient With Malignant Glucagonoma, But Does Not Prevent Tumor Growth

Jockenhövel F, Lederbogen S, Olbricht T, Schmidt-Gayk H, Krenning EP, Lamberts SWJ, Reinwein D (Universität, Essen, Germany; Laborärztliche Gemeinschaftspraxis, Heidelberg, Germany; Erasmus Univ, Rotterdam, The Netherlands)
Clin Investig 72:127–133, 1994   112-95-7–9

Introduction.—Glucagonoma is a rare tumor of the pancreatic alpha cells that may lead to necrolytic migratory erythema, hyperglycemia, loss of body weight, and anemia. The symptoms tend to be nonspecific, however, and the correct diagnosis may not be made until the tumor has invaded locally or spread to the liver. Octreotide, a long-acting somatostatin analogue, has proven clinically effective in a small number of patients despite the fact that plasma levels of glucagon remained elevated.

Case Report.—Woman, 51, was seen with epigastric pain and was found to have a tumor in the pancreatic head and metastases in the liver. She lost weight, became hyperglycemic, and had a skin rash. A pancreatic alpha-cell tumor that stained positive for glucagon and chromogranin A (CGA) was discovered. The plasma level of glucagon was extremely high. The patient became anemic and deteriorated gradually. A skin biopsy specimen confirmed necrolytic migratory erythema. The patient refused laparotomy to reduce the tumor mass and instead was given octreotide in increasing doses up to a maintenance level of 200 μg 3 times daily. The treatment did not inhibit the growth of the tumor, but it did reduce the plasma level of glucagon from more than 8 to as low as 2.2 μg/L. The level of CGA also declined. Her weight loss ceased for a time and the eruption resolved. The plasma level of glucagon rose to above pretreatment levels after 3 months, and the level of CGA rose after 14 months. The erythema recurred after a year of treatment and the patient died after 2 years in a cachectic state. Doses of octreotide as high as 600 μg 4 times daily had been given without producing serious side effects. The estimates of immunoreactive glucagon showed a treatment-related reduction in the ratio of glucagon to preproglucagon from 1.8 to .6.

Discussion.—The biochemical studies indicated that octreotide inhibited post-translational processing of preproglucagon in this patient, thereby lowering the circulating level of bioactive glucagon. The treatment reduced the symptoms, but it did not control the growth of the tumor.

▶ This is among the first reports of treating malignant glucagonoma with the somatostatin analogue octreotide. It is probably the only report that evaluates the long-term effect of octreotide as the single agent used in treatment of this rare malignancy. The results are as one would have anticipated. Octreotide caused a prompt reduction in glucagon levels, induced an impressive remission of clinical symptoms, i.e., the vanishing of the disabling necrolytic migratory erythema, and necessitated progressively increasing doses of the drug with protracted therapy. The latter is very reminiscent of the effects of octreotide in malignant carcinoid syndrome. As with other islet cell malignancies, the drug had no effect on tumor growth. The authors have also demonstrated a novel action of octreotide in this instance. For the first time, octreotide was shown here to block the post-translational conversion of preproglucagon to glucagon, thereby reducing circulating levels of bioactive glucagon. It is also noteworthy that the tumor "lit up" with octreotide scintigraphy, indicating presence of somatostatin receptors in the tumor, and hence predicting a favorable response to therapy with octreotide.—C.R. Kannan, M.D.

Somatostatinoma

Clinical Features of Duodenal Somatostatinomas

O'Brien TD, Cheijfec G, Prinz RA (Loyola Univ, Maywood, Ill; VA Hosp, Hines, Ill)
Surgery 114:1144–1147, 1993 112-95-7–10

Introduction.—Somatostatin-producing tumors rarely occur in the duodenum. Their clinical characteristics are different from those of pancreatic somatostatinomas, generally displaying local symptomatology rather than the effects of hyperproduction of somatostatin. Four patients with duodenal somatostatinomas were studied to characterize the clinical and pathologic profile of these tumors.

Methods.—The records were reviewed of 4 patients; 3 men and 1 woman, aged 54 to 71 years, who were treated for duodenal somatostatinoma between 1988 and 1992. The patients were followed for 1 to 4 years.

Results.—Three patients complained of dyspepsia and early satiety at presentation. Biopsies obtained from submucosal masses during upper gastrointestinal endoscopy in those 3 patients supplied the diagnosis of neuroendocrine tumor. In the fourth patient, the tumor was found incidentally. The tumors were excised in all cases. Immunohistochemical analysis of the excised tumors revealed a strong presence of somatostatin. The patient with the incidentally discovered tumor died of cardiac disease 2 years after resection. The other 3 patients were surviving without recurrence 1, 2, and 4 years after the tumor resection.

Discussion.—Although patients with pancreatic somatostatinomas generally have diabetes mellitus, steatorrhea, and cholelithiasis, patients with duodenal somatostatinomas generally have only local symptoms or no symptoms at all. It appears that local resection of small tumors and pancreaticoduodenectomy and resection of metastatic lesions provides definitive therapy, but long-term follow-up study is needed.

▶ Since the first description of the somatostatin-producing tumor of the duodenum in 1979, interest has been focused on distinguishing duodenal and pancreatic somatostatinomas. Given the rarity of duodenal somatostatinoma, the authors here have an impressive series. Duodenal somatostatinomas do not produce the "syndrome" (i.e., the triad of diabetes mellitus, cholelithiasis, and steatorrhea) associated with pancreatic somatostatinomas, are often asymptomatic, and are detected because of local pressure effects. The 2 new pieces of information from this article are that psammoma bodies are a distinct histologic feature of duodenal (but not pancreatic) somatostatinoma, and that intra-arterial methylene blue injection may help localize small tumors during operation. Incidentally, none of the 4 patients in this series had neurofibromatosis.

Richnel et al. (*J Comput Assist Tomogr* 18:427, 1994) studied the imaging characteristics of somatostatinoma with MR, CT, ultrasonography, and angiography in 4 patients. Surprisingly enough, in contrast to glucagonoma or insulinoma, the pancreatic somatostatinoma visualized well with CT and MRI. The tumor was of low signal intensity on the T1-weighted image and showed high signal intensity in the T2-weighted image, very much like a pheochromocytoma. As expected, MR failed to detect the duodenal somatostatinoma. Incidentally, for those taking the Boards, here is an item of trivia: von Recklinghausen's type of neurofibromata is associated with duodenal (but not pancreatic) somatostatinoma.—C.R. Kannan, M.D.

Ectopic ACTH Secretion

Somatostatin Analogs for the Localization and Preoperative Treatment of an Adrenocorticotropin-Secreting Bronchial Carcinoid Tumor
Phlipponneau M, Nocaudie M, Epelbaum J, De Keyzer Y, Lalau JD, Marchandise X, Bertagna X (Centre Hospitalier Régional Universitaire, Amiens, France; Centre Hospitalier Régional Universitaire, Lille, France; INSERM U-159, Paris)
J Clin Endocrinol Metab 78:20–24, 1994   112-95-7-11

Introduction.—A bronchial carcinoid tumor may be difficult to detect by CT or MRI. Because neuroendocrine cells frequently express somatostatin receptors, the somatostatin analogue octreotide might prove helpful in locating a nonpituitary tumor in patients with ectopic ACTH syndrome.

Case Report.—Woman, 45, had symptomatic hypokalemia of 3.1 mmol/L and hypercortisolism. Her appearance was typical for moderate Cushing's syndrome. Bone mineral density in the spine was markedly reduced. The serum cortisol was 1,448 nmol/L, and the plasma ACTH was 21.4 pmol/L. Urinary free cortisol excretion was unchanged during a high-dose dexamethasone suppression test, and plasma ACTH did not respond to stimulation with ovine corticotropin-re-leasing factor. Abdominal CT scans showed moderate enlargement of the adre-nal glands and the head of the pancreas. Thoracic CT scans revealed a possible 7-mm nodule in the left upper lobe. A 3-day course of octreotide led to marked clinical improvement and a substantial decline in plasma and urinary cortisol lev-els. Scintigraphy with ^{111}In-pentetreotide (Octreoscan) revealed a focus of abnor-mal uptake in the upper left lung at the exact site of the suspected nodule. Ex-ploration, done after a month of octreotide therapy, revealed a small tumor at the expected site that was associated with a plasma ACTH gradient. The lesion proved to be a carcinoid tumor that contained immunoreactive ACTH in a con-centration of 198 pmol per mg of wet tissue weight.

Conclusion.—Radioanalogue scintigraphy with somatostatin is an ac-curate and noninvasive means of localizing occult neuroendocrine tu-mors. It may provide an alternative to inferior petrosal sinus sampling in patients suspected of having ectopic ACTH secretion whose pituitary is normal on MRI.

▶ The distinction between the CT/MR-negative pituitary-dependent hyper-cortisolism and the occult ectopic ACTH-producing tumor can be vexing. Although selective inferior petrosal sinus sampling can provide reasonable assurance that the hypercortisolism is of nonpituitary origin, localization, which is often problematic, was achieved here with indium-labeled pentet-reotide. Four points are noteworthy: First, the octreotide scintigraphy worked with laser-like precision in locating the tumor, which was found dur-ing surgery in the predicted location. Second, octreotide therapy dramati-cally lowered the free cortisol level from 1,738 to 441 nmol/day after 3 days of administration. This is an important phenomenon that may soon be-come a test for distinguishing pituitary-dependent ACTH excess from ec-topic ACTH excess.

In fact, Woodhouse et al. (*Am J Med* 95:305, 1993) used this test (50 to 500 μcg every 8 hours for 24 hours to 72 hours) to distinguish pituitary from ectopic ACTH hypersecretion. These workers recommend a short trial of octreotide in patients with Cushing's syndrome with no demonstrable pitu-itary tumor, and a reduction in cortisol levels should alert the physician to the possibility of an ectopic ACTH source, as happened in this case. Third, the excised nodule showed strong immunopositivity to ACTH and contained the messenger RNA for proopiomelanocortin by Northern blot. Finally, the tumor contained appreciable amounts of somatostatin receptors, which accounts for its capacity to be localized as well as its therapeutic response to octreo-tide.

Will somatostatin-receptor scintigraphy find a firm place in the investiga-tion of hypercortisolism? I think the door is wide open. To wit, let us look at a report by de Herder et al. (*Am J Med* 96:305, 1994) on the feasibility of this test in patients with ectopic ACTH syndrome. These workers studied 10 pa-tients with Cushing's syndrome, 9 with ectopic ACTH production, and 1 with ectopic CRH production and were able to successfully identify the primary tumors or their metastases in 8 of 10 patients. In contrast, all 8 patients with pituitary-dependent hypercortisolism, used as contols, had normal scans. These authors concluded that somatostatin analogue scintigraphy can be included as a diagnostic step when one suspects an ectopic ACTH- or CRH-secreting tumor. The inescapable question is whether octreotide scintigraphy could obviate the need for the invasive inferior petrosal sinus sampling. This question cannot be answered without a larger database. Debate will be generated concerning the best method to localize the "occult" ectopic ACTH-secreting tumor. It is widely held that properly performed CT and MR will routinely detect bronchial carcinoids 1 cm or larger. However, cross-sectional state-of-the-art imaging with CT/MR is at the limits of its resolution and cannot provide a definite answer when the occult tumor is smaller than 1 cm. The advantage of the scintigraphy with octreotide is that it focuses on the functional rather than the anatomical nature of the tumor. Therefore, the procedure will work when the tumor has sufficient numbers of somatostatin receptors and will fail when it does not. I believe octreotide scintigraphy will be evaluated at great length and depth in the years to come. Until then, one can only wait, watch, and read.—C.R. Kannan, M.D.

Adrenocorticotropic Hormone-Secreting Islet Cell Tumors: Are They Always Malignant?

Doppman JL, Nieman LK, Cutler GB Jr, Chrousos GP, Fraker DL, Norton JA, Jensen RT (Warren G Magnuson Clinical Ctr, Bethesda, Md; Natl Inst of Child Health and Human Development, Bethesda, Md; Natl Cancer Inst, Bethesda; et al)

Radiology 190:59–64, 1994   112-95-7-12

Introduction.—In cases of ACTH-dependent Cushing's syndrome of extrapituitary origin, the need to exclude small ACTH-producing pancreatic islet cell tumors by using more invasive studies has remained questionable. To define more clearly the nature of islet cell tumors and the frequency of malignant, readily imaged versus benign occult (less than 2 cm) islet cell tumors responsible for the ectopic ACTH syndrome, experience and previously reported cases were reviewed.

Results.—Ten patients with Cushing's syndrome caused by the production of ACTH by a pancreatic islet cell tumor were seen in an 8-year period. All had malignant islet cell tumors, ranging from 2.5 to 6.0 cm in diameter. All patients had metastases to the liver at presentation. Five are dead, 4 are alive with liver metastases, and 1 is alive without clinical evidence of residual tumor 8 months after distal pancreatectomy and right hepatectomy. In addition to ACTH, 8 tumors produced gastrin.

Fifty-three cases of ACTH-secreting islet cell tumor have been reported in the English literature. There was only 1 benign adenoma with a prolonged follow-up. Twenty-six percent of these tumors secreted gastrin.

Discussion.—An islet cell tumor that causes ectopic ACTH production is large and malignant and has usually metastasized to the liver by the time the Cushing's syndrome is diagnosed. To date, a small, radiographically occult islet cell tumor producing ectopic ACTH has not been detected. These findings suggest that if careful imaging fails to detect a pancreatic mass or liver metastases in a patient with ectopic ACTH syndrome, an islet cell tumor can be ruled out for all practical purposes.

▶ This group from the National Institutes of Health probably has the most experience in the multidisciplinary diagnostic approach to Cushing's syndrome. And we learn 3 significant facts regarding ectopic ACTH production caused by islet cell tumors. First, there is no such thing as an "occult" ACTH-producing pancreatic islet cell carcinoid. When Cushing's syndrome occurs, these malignant tumors have become large, are readily visualized by conventional imaging procedures, and are usually metastatic. This obviates the need for invasive diagnostic testing when thin-slice CT is negative. This contrasts with ectopic ACTH production by bronchial carcinoids, which are usually very small, difficult to detect, and of low-grade malignancy. Second, we learn that concomitant gastrin hypersecretion is very common in ectopic ACTH-producing islet cell tumors. And finally, the prognosis is usually poor in those patients with ectopic ACTH production.—C.R. Kannan, M.D.

Ectopic GHRH Secretion

Somatotroph Hyperplasia Without Pituitary Adenoma Associated With a Long Standing Growth Hormone-Releasing Hormone-Producing Bronchial Carcinoid

Ezzat S, Asa SL, Stefaneanu L, Whittom R, Smyth HS, Horvath E, Kovacs K, Frohman LA (Univ of Toronto; Univ of Illinois, Chicago)
J Clin Endocrinol Metab 78:555–560, 1994   112-95-7-13

Introduction.—The hypersecretion of GH seen in patients with acromegaly usually comes from a pituitary somatotroph adenoma. However, rare cases of acromegaly caused by ectopic GH-releasing hormone (GHRH) hypersecretion have been reported, mainly involving pancreatic, pulmonary, or gastrointestinal tumors. These patients have exhibited varying pituitary morphologic features. Pituitary function and morphologic features were studied in a patient who had a disseminated bronchial carcinoid producing GHRH for 10 years.

Case Report.—Woman, 28, had a long history of headaches and soft tissue swelling. Her pituitary gland was diffusely enlarged on MRI. An endobronchial carcinoid tumor had been excised 10 years earlier, but she had breast, chest wall, and ovarian metastases. She had elevated serum GH levels, which were not inhibited after glucose ingestion but were further stimulated by TRH. Administration of GHRH and GnRH did not affect GH levels. Octreotide therapy improved symptoms but did not reduce the pituitary size or reduce GH levels. A nonselective transsphenoidal anterior hypophysectomy completely resolved her headaches and swelling and reduced serum GH levels. Light microscopic examination of the resected pituitary gland identified somatotroph hyperplasia with enlarged acini and preserved reticulin fibers. Immunocytochemical analysis revealed marked cellular GH immunopositivity. Electron microscopic examination revealed that most cells were somatotrophs but that other cell types were intermingled. There was an abundance of GH mRNA identified in in situ hybridization. Histologic examination identified well-differentiated carcinoid tumor, and most of the tumor cells immunostained strongly for GHRH. In in vitro studies of pituitary tissue cultures, GH was stimulated by GHRH, TRH stimulated GH release inconsistently, and octreotide and somatostatin inhibited GH release.

Discussion.—The pituitary in this patient exhibited somatotroph hyperplasia but no adenoma. The paradoxical response of GH to TRH administration is more typical of ectopic GHRH than of GH-producing pituitary adenomas. The differing GH responses to GHRH seen in vivo and in vitro suggest that nontumorous somatotrophs downregulate the response to continuous GHRH exposure.

▶ This report is a reminder that ectopic GHRH secretion is rare but does occur. It also illustrates the indolent nature of malignant bronchial carcinoid tumors. This case is reminiscent of a similar case that was reviewed in these pages a few years ago (1993 YEAR BOOK OF ENDOCRINOLOGY, p 243). The remarkable aspect of this case was the development of somatotroph hyperplasia without pituitary adenoma. In this regard, the situation is analogous to that of pituitary-dependent Cushing's disease developing from ectopic CRH production. The pituitary response to these releasing hormones is apparently generalized, resulting in enlargement of the whole pituitary. Perhaps the large volume of the population of the somatotrophs is the reason for the poor therapeutic response to octreotide, necessitating total hypophysectomy for cure of acromegaly. The message for the clinician is that ectopic GHRH secretion should be considered as a cause of acromegaly when exogenous GHRH administration fails to evoke a robust release of GH. For yet another unusual example of ectopic GHRH secretion, proceed to Abstract 112-95-7–14.—C.R. Kannan, M.D.

Demonstration of Biological Activity of a Growth Hormone–Releasing Hormone–Like Substance Produced by a Pheochromocytoma
Saito H, Sano T, Yamasaki R, Mitsuhashi S, Hosoi E, Saito S (Saito Hosp, Tokushima, Japan; Univ of Tokushima, Japan)
Acta Endocrinol 129:246–250, 1993   112-95-7–14

Background.—Pheochromocytomas may produce a large number of peptides, including a growth hormone–releasing hormone (GHRH)-like substance. Some pheochromocytomas have been associated with acromegaly, but it is not clear whether this association is causative or fortuitous. More than 30 definitively diagnosed extracranial GHRH-producing tumors associated with acromegaly have been reported.

Case Report.—Woman, 62, had been hypertensive for 13 years and had occasionally noted palpitations and sweating. Blood pressures ranged from 140/90 mm Hg to as high as 212/128 mm Hg. Plasma epinephrine and norepinephrine levels were as high as 341 and 9,130 ng/L, respectively. A left suprarenal mass was found, and 51 g of tumor tissue were removed and confirmed as classic pheochromocytoma. Immunohistochemical study demonstrated immunoreactive GHRH-positive cells within the tumor, which contained 29.8 μg/kg wet weight of GHRH. Inferior caval catheterization confirmed that the tumor released GHRH into the blood.

Hormonal Studies.—Gel filtration chromatography using distinct GHRH antisera recognizing the N- and C-termini of true GHRH(1-44)NH$_2$ showed the tumor hormone to be molecularly heterogeneous, but a component corresponding to the authentic hormone predominated. Studies of dispersed rat anterior pituitary cells demonstrated a dose-related increase in GH release at levels of .125–2 nmol/L. This increase was comparable to what occurred using synthetic GHRH(1-44)NH$_2$.

Conclusion.—Patients with a GHRH-producing pheochromocytoma may have acromegaly as a result.

▶ Despite the fact that the tumor was immunopositive for GHRH that was biologically active in vitro, the patient did not have acromegaly and her plasma GH, IGF-I, and immunoreactive GHRH levels were all normal. This implies that even though the adrenal tumor secreted immunoreactive and bioactive GHRH, it had no clinical consequences. Flash back to 1986, when Roth et al. (*J Clin Endocrinol Metab* 63:1421, 1986) described a patient with pheochromocytoma, acromegaly, and somatotroph hyperplasia secondary to ectopic GHRH secretion by the adrenal tumor. The secretory versatility of the pheochromocytoma continues to unfold.—C.R. Kannan, M.D.

Ectopic IGF-II Secretion

A Case of Hepatoma Associated With Hypoglycaemia and Overproduction of IGF-II (E-21): Beneficial Effects of Treatment With Growth Hormone and Intrahepatic Adriamycin
Hunter SJ, Daughaday WH, Callender ME, McKnight JA, McIlrath EM, Teale JD, Atkinson AB (Royal Victoria Hosp, Belfast, Northern Ireland; Washington Univ, St Louis, Mo; St Luke's Hosp, Guildford, England)
Clin Endocrinol 41:397–401, 1994   112-95-7-15

Background.—Hypoglycemia associated with some non–islet cell tumors has been frequently reported. The mechanism is thought to be associated with the production of peptides with insulin-like activity, in particular insulin-like growth factor II (IGF-II). A recent advance in this area has been the development of a radioimmunoassay directed against the first 21 amino acids of the E-domain of pro-IGF-II that allows direct plasma estimation of larger molecular forms of IGF-II without interference from normal IGF-II. Recurrent hypoglycemia associated with hepatoma was described.

Case Report.—Man, 64, was admitted unconscious and found to be hypoglycemic. Physical examination showed that the liver edge extended 7 cm below the costal margin, although there were no stigmata of chronic liver disease or signs of hepatic decompensation. Hepatitis B surface antigen was negative. On CT and isotope scan, a mass was seen to occupy most of the right lobe and extend into the left. Histology revealed a well-differentiated hepatoma. Plasma was obtained for measurement of serum IGF-II, pro-IGF-II and IGF-I, and a diagnosis of IGF-II-producing hepatoma was made. During a fast, the man became hypoglycemic. Serum insulin was undetectable. Plasma IGF-II was not elevated, although 71% of plasma IGF-II was seen as big IGF-II, which could represent a nonglycated form of pro-IGF-II. The GH response to hypoglycemia was reduced and plasma levels of both IGF-I and the GH-dependent IGF-binding protein (IGFBP-3) were low. Treatment with GH led to an increase in mean plasma glucose and a reduction in hypoglycemic attacks. A rise in IGFBP-3 and a small increase in insulin-like growth factors was also seen. Subsequent treatment with the octreotide did not result in a significant change in plasma glucose levels or insulin-like growth factors. Levels of E-21 were restored to normal by 2 courses of intrahepatic Adriamycin. Total IGF-II remained normal, and IGF-I increased. Growth hormone treatment was stopped with no effect on plasma glucose or growth factor levels and the patient remained free of hypoglycemia. Two years later, he developed malignant ascites, but there was still no recurrence of hypoglycemia, and E-21 and insulin-like growth factor concentrations were normal. After an initial response to intravenous chemotherapy with mithozantrone, he deteriorated and died 26 months after presentation.

Conclusion.—This case report demonstrates that E-21 is useful in the diagnosis of non-islet tumor hypoglycemia. It also shows that GH was beneficial in the initial treatment. However, the most effective therapy was intrahepatic Adriamycin, which significantly influenced plasma E-21 concentration. Hypoglycemia was successfully eliminated. The decrease in circulating growth factors may have had a beneficial effect on tumor growth, as shown by the patient's prolonged remission and excellent quality of life before the eventual development of malignant ascites.

▶ The continuing saga of tumor hypoglycemia seems to get more complex each year. Readers may remember the unique case abstracted in last year's volume (1994 YEAR BOOK OF ENDOCRINOLOGY, p 187). Interestingly enough, well-studied case reports have made major contributions to our understanding of the subject. For example, back in 1966, Unger first suspected that hypoglycemia in patients with non–islet cell tumors was not mediated by insulin

(*Am J Med* 40:325, 1966). Two decades later, Daughaday et al. showed that hypoglycemia associated with a leiomyosarcoma resulted from ectopic IGF-II secretion (*N Engl J Med* 319:1434, 1988). The riddle was in trying to explain why total IGF-II immunoreactivity was normal in these patients. The concept of "big" IGF-II was introduced and fully explored by Zapf et al. (*J Intern Med* 234:543, 1993) and is further delineated here. What then is the mechanism of hypoglycemia in these cases? Back to physiology. Growth hormone and 2 specific IGF binding proteins (150 and 50 kDA) circulate in the plasma and mutually control each other. Increased production of IGF-II suppresses GH and results in a shift in the 2 IGF-binding complexes. As a consequence, the 150-kDA complex formation decreases, whereas the 50-kDA complex increases and it now carries IGF II, changing its half-life and increasing its bioavailability to tissues.

In this case, the authors have demonstrated that even though the total serum IGF-II levels were in the normal range, a specific assay directed against the first 21 amino acids of the E-domain, i.e., the pro IGF-II fraction, was greatly elevated. This assay is not subjected to interference by normal IGF binding proteins. In addition to providing us with a novel diagnostic method, in using GH therapeutically the authors add a new facet to the treatment of this rare disorder. The question is, did GH therapy reduce the frequency and severity of the hypoglycemic attacks by causing a shift in the IGF-II binding proteins that altered the bioavailability of IGF-II, or was it the result of reduced tissue sensitivity to "big" IGF-II at the insulin-receptor level? Regardless, GH therapy appears to work, at least initially. Of course, intrahepatic Adriamycin therapy directed at the primary neoplasm provided longer-lasting relief in this palliative setting.

We have come a long way since 1966, when Dr. Unger referred to this syndrome as "the most baffling of the unsolved para-endocrine puzzles." —C.R. Kannan, M.D.

Multiple Endocrine Neoplasia-I

A Family Pedigree Exhibiting Features of Both Multiple Endocrine Neoplasia Type 1 and McCune-Albright Syndromes

O'Halloran DJ, Shalet SM (Christie Hosp, Manchester, England)
J Clin Endocrinol Metab 78:523–525, 1994   112-95-7–16

Objective.—This report documents for the first time the occurrence of McCune-Albright and MEN type I syndromes in the same kindred.

Case Report.—The index patient was a member of a large family with MEN-I syndrome. At age 7 years, she had vaginal bleeding and clinical evidence of early puberty, but no other abnormalities. She had regular menses at age 11 years and underwent a right oophorectomy for painful ovarian cyst at age 15 years. Further investigations showed persistently elevated serum PRL levels, but imaging of the hypothalamic-pituitary region was normal. She subsequently experienced a painful right hip, and subsequent radiologic examinations were consistent with polyostotic fibrous dysplasia. A diagnosis of McCune-Albright syndrome was made.

Discussion.—McCune-Albright and MEN-I share many clinical and biochemical characteristics, although their mode of inheritance differs: MEN-I shows an autosomal pattern, and McCune-Albright syndrome is apparently sporadic as a result of postzygotic mutation. McCune-Albright syndrome is associated with tissue-specific expression of activating mutations in the gene encoding the α-subunit of the stimulatory G-protein, resulting in the formation of the putative *gsp* oncogene. Because there may be a functional link between MEN-I and McCune-Albright syndromes, a search for G-protein gene mutations as a mechanism of disease in MEN-I is mandatory.

▶ This is an exciting paper, not merely because of the possible expansion of the MEN-I syndrome to include the McCune-Albright phenotype, but because it suggests that a G-protein mutation may play a role in the tumorigenesis of MEN-I. It is now well accepted that McCune-Albright is caused by a genetic mutation, resulting in the formation of the putative *gsp* oncogene responsible for the increased cell growth and hyperfunction present in this syndrome. The striking family history of MEN-I in this case can hardly be ignored, even though the mode of inheritance for both diseases is believed to be quite different. Yet, the possibility that a *gsp* oncogene underlies both is not far-out. Even though it is accepted that MEN-I is caused by a deletion of a recessive oncogene on chromosome 11q13, how this deletion affects glandular hyperfunction is not clear. The ubiquity of the G-protein holds the key for the diverse features of McCune-Albright syndrome. Would it take a huge leap of faith to implicate G-protein abnormalities in MEN-I? I am not so sure.—C.R. Kannan, M.D.

Multiple Endocrine Neoplasia-II

Prevalence of Pheochromocytoma and Hyperparathyroidism in Multiple Endocrine Neoplasia Type 2A: Results of Long-Term Follow-Up
Howe JR, Norton JA, Wells SA (Washington Univ, St Louis, Mo)
Surgery 114:1070–1077, 1993   112-95-7–17

Introduction.—Multiple endocrine neoplasia type IIA is an autosomal dominant condition in which nearly all gene carriers will express medullary thyroid carcinoma (MTC), whereas the penetrance of pheochromocytoma and hyperparathyroidism is variable. The prevalence of pheochromocytoma ranges from 5% to 95%, and the prevalence of hyperparathyroidism ranges from 0% to 70%. Members of MEN-IIA kindreds with more than 10 years of follow-up were studied to more accurately estimate the prevalence and age at diagnosis of pheochromocytoma and hyperparathyroidism in affected members.

Subjects.—A total of 86 patients from 12 separate kindred were studied. The diagnosis of pheochromocytoma was based on histologic examination, and hyperparathyroidism was defined as preoperative serum calcium levels at or above 10.5 mg/dL and histologic diagnosis of parathyroid hyperplasia. The mean follow-up was 15.8 years for 85 patients with MTC, 12.9 years for 79 patients with pheochromocytoma, and 15.0 years for 78 patients with hyperparathyroidism. All but 1 patient had MTC, including 44 (51.2%) with MTC only, 15 (17.4%) with MTC and pheochromocytoma, 9 (10.5%) with MTC and hyperparathyroidism, and 18 (20.9%) with MTC, pheochromocytoma, and hyperparathyroidism.

Results.—The overall prevalence of pheochromocytoma was 42%, and the prevalence by kindred ranged from 5.5% to 100%. Pheochromocytoma was diagnosed at the same time or before MTC in 30% of patients, whereas the mean interval until diagnosis of pheochromocytoma was 11.8 years in 70%. If the 9 patients who underwent thyroidectomy before 1968 were excluded and therefore not screened for urinary catecholamines, then 42% of individuals who developed pheochromocytoma did so after being diagnosed with MTC. The overall prevalence of hyperparathyroidism was 35%, and the prevalence by kindred ranged from 0% to 53%. In 63% of patients, hyperparathyroidism was diagnosed at the same time or before MTC and at a mean interval of 17.3 years from the diagnosis of MTC in the remaining 37%. Mean age was 29 years at diagnosis of MTC, 37 years for pheochromocytoma, and 36 years for hyperparathyroidism.

Conclusion.—In MEN-IIA the penetrance of pheochromocytoma and hyperparathyroidism is incomplete relative to MTC, and the degree of penetrance varies widely among kindreds. Including all other previous reports of MEN-IIA the overall prevalence of pheochromocytoma is 38.3% and that for hyperparathyroidism is 23.8%. There is no genetic test yet for determining which individuals will have pheochromocytoma or hyperparathyroidism.

▶ In a patient with MEN-II with only 1 expression of the syndrome, the pertinent question, naturally, is when will the other shoe drop? To answer that question, it is essential to learn the natural history of this rare syndrome provided by this study. The answer is that it seems highly variable. The remarkable finding in this study was that of the 33 patients with pheochromocytoma, only 3 patients had the adrenal tumor before the MTC. This contrasts with the European experience relating to MEN-II, where pheochromocytoma was the first sign of MEN-II in nearly half the cases.

Although a similar situation was noted for hyperparathyroidism, the percentage of patients with primary hyperparathyroidism occurring contemporaneously with MTC was twice as high in comparison to the pheochromocytoma-MCT combination occurring simultaneously. The other remarkable aspect of this study is that pheochromocytoma and primary hyperparathyroidism were detected as late as 12 to 17 years after the MTC was discovered. This underscores careful follow-up beyond 10 years. As we all know, hormonal testing to detect the pheochromocytoma of MEN-II can be frustrating. This extends even to the hormonal diagnosis of MTC. This extends even to the hormonal diagnosis of MTC when the thyroid tumor is small or in the C-cell hyperplasia stage. Can we do better with modern gene technology? Abstract 112-95-7–18 addresses this issue.—C.R. Kannan, M.D.

Clinical Screening as Compared With DNA Analysis in Families With Multiple Endocrine Neoplasia Type 2A
Lips CJM, Landsvater RM, Höppener JWM, Geerdink RA, Blijham G, Van Veen JMJ-S, Van Gils APG, De Wit MJ, Zewald RA, Berends MJH, Beemer FA, Brouwers-Smalbraak J, Jansen RPM, Van Amstel HKP, Van Vroonhoven TJMV, Vroom TM (Univ Hosp Utrecht, The Netherlands; Westeinde Hosp, The Hague, The Netherlands; Clinical Genetics Ctr, Utrecht, The Netherlands)

N Engl J Med 331:828–835, 1994   112-95-7–18

Introduction.—Multiple endocrine neoplasia type IIA (MEN-IIA), an inherited disease with an autosomal dominant pattern, is characterized by medullary thyroid carcinoma (MTC) together with pheochromocytoma and sometimes parathyroid adenoma. Screening for the biochemical signs of MTC has allowed early surgical treatment and improved survival. It is also possible to identify carriers of the MEN-IIA gene by DNA analysis. Four large families with MEN-IIA were screened to compare the reliability of biochemical tests with that of DNA analysis.

Methods.—Three hundred members of the families have been repeatedly studied since 1974. Screening was carried out annually starting between the ages of 5 and 10 years; after age 35 years, the examinations were performed every 3 years. Studies involved measurements of basal and stimulated plasma calcitonin concentrations, urinary excretion of catecholamines and catecholamine metabolites, and serum calcium concentrations. Carrier status was assessed by linked genetic markers until 1993 and more recently by analysis of mutations in the *RET* gene.

Results.—Biochemical and radiologic tests, pathologic examinations, and DNA analysis identified 80 MEN-IIA gene carriers. Sixty-six had abnormal plasma calcitonin values and MTC. Eight of 14 young carriers with normal plasma calcitonin had small foci of MTC detected at thyroidectomy; the other 6 carriers have not undergone operations. Sixty-eight of the remaining 220 family members were found by DNA analysis not to carry the MEN-IIA gene. Six of these 68 individuals had elevated plasma calcitonin concentrations and underwent thyroidectomy but had only C-cell hyperplasia. None of the 68 had MTC or pheochromocytoma.

Conclusion.—Analysis of DNA is more accurate than biochemical tests in identifying MEN-IIA gene carriers. There have been no false positive or false negative results in the families studied, thereby allowing unaffected family members to discontinue screening for the disease. In addition, total thyroidectomy can be postponed until results of the stimulation test become positive or have remained negative annually to age 12 or 13 years.

▶ This is the first large-scale study to compare hormonal screening and DNA analysis to detect gene carriers for the MEN-II syndrome. In the process, these workers from the Netherlands have provided us with a first-class study. The truth, it seems, will be unmasked by DNA testing and not by pentagastrin-stimulated calcitonin and catecholamine studies. The remarkable finding here is that DNA analysis revealed the carrier state even when pentagastrin-stimulated calcitonin levels were normal, thus justifying preventive surgical intervention. When the DNA linkage is normal, the implication here is that the patient is not at risk of MTC or pheochromocytoma developing. The fiscal implication of such unambiguous validation of being a noncarrier for the gene is that expensive hormonal testing can be abandoned. The MEN-IIA gene carrier state was identified in this study with a high degree of reliability by linkage analysis with no false positives—so far. The study also confirms our long-held suspicion regarding the sensitivity and limitation of the plasma calcitonin stimulation test. Several questions come to mind. Assuming that one has access to reliable DNA analysis, if the DNA test is normal and fails to reveal the specific *RET* mutations of MEN-IIA, can we safely assume that all is well, reassure the patient that there is no risk, and forever abandon clinical, hormonal, and radiologic surveillance? If the DNA linkage studies reveal the specific *RET* mutations, should the patient undergo thyroidectomy even if calcitonin stimulation tests are normal? Would one also recommend prophylactic bilateral adrenalectomy as well to prevent pheochromocytoma, or would one pursue only hormonal surveillance? Can the results of this European study be extended to other geoethnic patients? The answers to these and other questions relating to the *RET* proto-oncogene and its specific mutations will be eagerly sought in the years to come.—C.R. Kannan, M.D.

▶ As noted in the editorial accompanying this article (Utiger: *N Engl J Med* 331:870, 1994), all patients with MTC should be tested for *RET* mutations. Using an immunoradiometric assay for calcitonin after pentagastrin stimulation, Barbot et al. (*J Clin Endocrinol Metab* 78:114, 1994) suggested that those with peak values above 100 ng/L should undergo surgery, whereas surgery may be postponed when values between 30 and 100 ng/L are obtained if the probability of being gene carriers is low. The availability of genetic screening will certainly resolve this issue. Patients with persistent elevated serum calcitonin levels after surgery for medullary cancer have residual disease that is often difficult to detect. Technetium-99m dimercaptosuccinic acid is a sensitive, safe, and useful localization technique for detecting occult disease by single-photon emission computed tomography (Udelsmann et al: *Surgery* 114:1083, 1993). Moley et al. have carried out reoperation in the neck for persistent medullary cancer, resulting in normalization of the serum calcitonin levels in 28% and a decrease by 40% or more in another 42% of patients (*Surgery* 114:1090, 1993). Treatment of advanced MTC with a combination of cyclophosphamide, vincristine, and dacarbazine offered some improvement, but further studies are warranted (Wu et al: *Cancer* 73:432, 1994). Three patients with coexistent papillary and medullary cancers of the thyroid have been reported (Lax et al: *Virchows Arch* 424:441, 1994).—L.E. Braverman, M.D.

Suggested Reading

The following articles are recommended to the reader:

Lamberts SW, et al: A role of somatostatin analogs in the differential diagnosis and treatment of Cushing's syndrome. *J Clin Endocrinol Metab* 78:17–24, 1994.
Jensen RT, Fraker DL: Zollinger Ellison syndrome. *JAMA* 272:1429–1435, 1994.
Zapf: Non-islet-cell tumor hypoglycemia. *Clin Endocrinol* 41:402, 1994.
Moertel CG, et al: The management of patients with advanced carcinoid tumors and islet cell carcinomas. *Ann Intern Med* 120:302–309, 1994.

8 Obesity, Metabolism, Exercise, and Energy

Introduction

The bad news is that the American population is still gaining body weight at an alarming rate (Abstract 112-95-8-1). Approximately one third of the American population is considered overweight, and the prevalence is even higher in specific minority groups. The public health and economic repercussions of this trend are of significant concern. My suspicion is that the increase in body weight is related to the decline in physical activity, although I have not seen epidemiologic data on this issue. We presently have several National Institutes of Health–funded Obesity and Nutrition Research Centers scattered around the country that are carefully examining the causes of obesity from a behavioral, physiologic, and molecular approach. A call to increase federal funding in the obesity and nutrition areas would seem to be justified, given the increased prevalence of obesity. On the other end of the energy balance spectrum, it appears that a body fat level constituting 5% to 6% of our total body weight is considered to be the lower limit of acceptable body fatness in human beings (Abstract 112-95-8-2).

We found several interesting papers that support metabolic differences in multiple subtypes of individuals. Specifically, restrained eaters (Abstract 112-95-8-5) and postobese individuals (Abstract 112-95-8-4) were shown to have a reduced ability to oxidize fat in response to a fat-containing meal. This metabolic problem would favor an accelerated pattern of fat storage. The observation that human beings are not "calorie blind" has been the subject of considerable research interest and has prompted numerous investigations on the impact of fat intake (independent of total energy intake) on obesity.

Body fatness has emerged as a significant predictor of the increased sympathetic nervous system activity in some individuals. In 1994, Scherrer et al. (Abstract 112-95-8-6) found that high levels of body fat are directly related to increased firing of sympathetic outflow in the muscle, and in 1993, Khort et al. (Abstract 112-95-8-9) showed an inverse relation between body fatness and the increase in catecholamines during submaximal exercise. The central role of the sympathetic nervous system as a mediator of thermogenesis, blood pressure, and insulin resistance continues to attract a great deal of interest.

Resistance training is the exercise of choice these days. In the elderly, "pumping iron" shows promise as a clinical intervention to increase muscular strength, to improve daily function, and to enhance daily energy requirements. These concepts are derived from 2 interesting studies (Abstracts 112-95-8-10 and 112-95-8-11) that found that resistance-trained elderly individuals demonstrated increased muscular strength, spontaneous physical activity, and resting metabolic rate.

In the Energy Expenditure section, a study performed in female athletes showed they do indeed consume a large quantity of calories, which is consistent with their high levels of energy expenditure (Abstract 112-95-8-13). Although many investigators may find these findings self-evident, there were previous suggestions that highly trained women were able to maintain body weight on miniscule quantities of calories. Small sex-related differences in resting metabolic rate were revealed in a study by our laboratory, which showed that on average, women burned approximately 50 kcal less per day compared with men after data were normalized for differences in body composition (Abstract 112-95-8-14). Can the lower levels of energy expenditure in women possibly contribute to their higher levels of body fat?

Finally, I was encouraged to read that long-term runners were having fewer problems with their knees than are long-term couch potatoes. We hope you enjoy the reading.

Eric T. Poehlman, Ph.D.

Edward S. Horton, M.D.

Body Fatness

Increasing Prevalence of Overweight Among US Adults: The National Health and Nutrition Examination Surveys, 1960 to 1991
Kuczmarski RJ, Flegal KM, Campbell SM, Johnson CL (Ctrs for Disease Control and Prevention, Hyattsville, Md)
JAMA 272:205–211, 1994   112-95-8–1

Background.—The economic cost of disease associated with overweight is high. Trends in the prevalence of excess weight and body mass index (BMI) in the United States adult population were reported.

Methods.—Nationally representative cross-sectional surveys with personal interviews and a medical assessment were performed. A total of 6,000 to 13,000 adults, aged 20–74 years, were examined at 4 times—1960–1962, 1971–1974, 1976–1980, and 1988–1991—in 4 different surveys.

Findings.—From 1988 to 1991, 33.4% of the sample were estimated to be overweight. Dramatic increases in prevalences occurred over time in all racial groups and for both sexes. Overweight prevalence increased 8% between the 1976–1980 and 1988–1991 surveys. The mean BMI in-

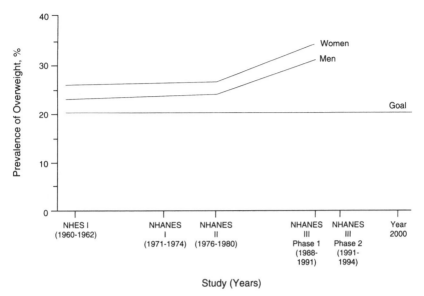

Fig 8–1.—Trends in age-adjusted prevalence of overweight for the United States population 20–74 years of age, compared with the year 2000 health objective for overweight. *Abbreviations: NHES*, National Health Examination Survey; *NHANES*, National Health and Nutrition Examination Survey. (Courtesy of Kuczmarski RJ, Flegal KM, Campbell SM, et al: *JAMA* 272:205–211, 1994.)

creased from 25.3 to 26.3 during this time, and mean body weight rose by 3.6 kg.

Conclusion.—Notable increases in overweight have occurred in the past decade. The objective of reducing the prevalence of overweight among adults in the United States to 20% or below by the year 2000 may not be achieved (Fig 8-1).

▶ The "fattening of America" continues to be an alarming problem. One third of the United States population is estimated to be overweight, and this figure has increased within the past 10 years, despite the plethora of exercise videos, low-calorie products, etc. An even more striking finding was the estimated 50% prevalence of obesity in black women. This striking increase in fatness may have important implications for our health care system. The prevalence of metabolic and functional problems that accompany an overweight status (e.g., IDDM, gout, osteoarthritis, etc.) may increase as a result of these trends. Public health strategies aimed at the prevention of obesity by urging individuals to decrease food intake and increase physical activity, although seemingly simple and straightforward, have proven difficult to implement.—E.T. Poehlman, Ph.D.

Lower Limit of Body Fat in Healthy Active Men

Friedl KE, Moore RJ, Martinez-Lopez LE, Vogel JA, Askew EW, Marchitelli LJ, Hoyt RW, Gordon CC (US Army Research Inst of Environmental Medicine, Natick, Mass; Martin Army Community Hosp, Fort Benning, Ga)
J Appl Physiol 77:933–940, 1994   112-95-8-2

Background.—Quantifying minimum body fat (BF) in human beings has been difficult. Anthropometric assessments of BF, established in comparison with hydrodensitometry, consistently overestimate lean individuals. Dual-energy x-ray absorptiometry (DEXA), a new technology, provides another opportunity to evaluate extremes of body composition.

Methods.—Body composition changes were assessed in 55 healthy young men during an 8-week Army combat leadership training course. The course involved strenuous exercise and low-energy intake, with an estimated energy deficit of 5 MJ/day and a result of 15.7% loss of weight.

Findings.—Percent BF, determined by DEXA, averaged 14.3% at the beginning of the course and 5.8% at the end. Men achieving a minimum percent BF—4% to 6%—by week 6 had only small additional total and subcutaneous fat losses in the final 2 weeks, sacrificing increasingly greater proportions of fat-free mass. Percent BF estimated from skinfold thicknesses reflected relative changes in fat mass. However, actual percent BF was overestimated. After fat stores were substantially depleted, abdominal, hip, and thigh girths continued to decrease with body weight loss rather than reaching a plateau.

Conclusion.—A 4% to 6% BF, or 4 skinfolds under 20 mm, appears to be the minimum BF achievable in healthy men. In healthy young men with a mean 15% BF, the rapid loss of 16% of body weight results in a virtual depletion of fat stores, which is excessive.

▶ At the other end of the energy balance spectrum, a rigorous Army training course was used as a model to estimate the lower limit of BF in healthy men. The lower limit of 4% to 6% BF was suggested, which corresponds to the low levels of BF observed in the Minnesota study on human starvation. Such low levels of BF are rarely observed in humans, with the exception of high-caliber endurance-trained athletes. After cessation of the Army training course, levels of BF in the majority of recruits rebounded to their pretraining level, which suggests a set point for the maintenance of body fatness in younger males.—E.T. Poehlman, Ph.D.

Substrate Oxidation

Effect of Alcohol on Postmeal Fat Storage

Sonko BJ, Prentice AM, Murgatroyd PR, Goldberg GR, van de Ven MLHM,

Coward WA (MRC Dunn Clinical Nutrition Centre, Cambridge, England)
Am J Clin Nutr 59:619–625, 1994   112-95-8-3

Background.—The role of alcohol consumption in the etiology of obesity remains a question. Past studies have explored the effects of alcohol on fat, protein, and carbohydrate oxidation but have not investigated macronutrient balance further downstream in the process. These effects were studied within the context of a normal pattern of eating.

Methods.—Thermogenesis and whole-body indirect calorimetry were used to study macronutrient balances after meals with and without alcohol. Studies were done 20.5 hours after ingestion. Five healthy men with a mean age of 35 years were studied. Each subject was studied 3 times, acting as his own control using a within-subject analysis. Three meal treatments were randomly given to the subjects: the control (C), alcohol substitution (S), and alcohol addition (A). The fat:carbohydrate:protein:ethanol composition of the test meals expressed as a percent of energy were: meal C = 40:46:14:0; meal S = 40:23:14:23; and meal A = 34:36:12:18. Meals were labeled with ^{13}C. Stable isotope procedures were used to track ^{13}C and distinguish between endogenous and exogenous fat oxidation. The results were analyzed by within-subject paired t-test.

Findings.—The thermogenic effect of alcohol was similar to carbohydrate. There was no evidence of heat dissipation as an explanation for the lack of weight gain when excess energy was consumed as alcohol. Alcohol suppressed the oxidation of carbohydrate and fat. The data show a hierarchy in which alcohol dominates oxidative pathways because of a lack of storage capacity in the body and because the imperative is for oxidative detoxification. A net increase in fat storage from alcohol occurred only when it was added to the control meal. Alcohol was seen to behave like a carbohydrate; however, its high reactivity caused a temporal displacement in fat balance. This is believed to be caused by alcohol's domination of oxidative pathways.

Conclusion.—In this small study, alcohol appears to cause weight gain only when consumed in excess of normal energy needs. Alcohol has a fat-sparing effect that is similar to carbohydrate. Long-term studies of macronutrient balance are needed for further investigation of the adipogenic potential of alcohol.

▶ The strengths of this study lie in the simulation of a real-life condition in which there is a slight overconsumption of energy in the form of alcohol. Thereafter, substrate oxidation patterns were monitored for an extended period in a room calorimeter. This meticulously performed study shows that alcohol calories are only fattening when consumed in excess of daily energy needs. In fact, the thermogenic potential of alcohol was similar to that of ingested carbohydrates. This is possibly because alcohol suppresses oxidation of carbohydrate and fat. Although there have been previous reports regarding the absence of weight gain when excess calories are consumed in the form of alcohol, this study supports the notion that alcohol calories "behave" metabolically in a fashion similar to carbohydrate calories.—E.T. Poehlman, Ph.D.

Failure to Increase Lipid Oxidation in Response to Increasing Dietary Fat Content in Formerly Obese Women
Astrup A, Buemann B, Christensen NJ, Toubro S (Royal Veterinary and Agricultural Univ, Frederiksberg, Denmark; Univ of Copenhagen)
Am J Physiol 266:E592–E599, 1994   112-95-8-4

Background.—Obesity is a prevalent disease in the Western world, and those with excess body fat are at increased risk for many diseases. Whether the fat-to-carbohydrate oxidation ratio adjusts appropriately to the fat-to-carbohydrate intake ratio after a few days of consuming diets with realistic differences in dietary fat content was investigated. Also examined was whether formerly obese women would respond differently than normal-weight women would to the dietary changes.

Methods.—In a case-control study, 9 formerly obese, currently weight-stable women were matched with 9 normal-weight women for height, weight, age, and body composition. Initially, all women were started on a diet with 30% of energy from fat, 55% from carbohydrates, and 15% from protein. They were then randomly assigned after a 1- to 2-month washout period) to either a low-fat diet (20% of energy from fat) or a high-fat diet (50% of energy from fat). The experimental diets were consumed for 3 days immediately before the subjects were placed in a respiratory chamber for a 24-hour period. Two open-circuited respiratory chambers were used to measure 24-hour energy expenditure and substrate oxidation rates.

Results.—The 24-hour fat balance was increased significantly when the dietary fat content was increased, after adjustment for 24-hour energy intake equal to 24-hour energy expenditure. When the low- and medium-fat diets were compared, no differences in macronutrient balances were found between groups, but on the high-fat diet the postobese women failed to increase the ratio of fat to carbohydrate oxidation appropriately, resulting in a positive adjusted fat balance and a negative carbohydrate balance. The 24-hour energy expenditure of the normal-weight women was unaffected by the low-fat diet, but the 24-hour energy expenditure of the postobese women increased significantly while on the low-fat diet.

Conclusion.—An increase in dietary fat content to 50% of energy results in preferential fat storage, impaired suppression of carbohydrate oxidation, and a reduction of 24-hour energy expenditure in postobese women, independent of energy balance. Therefore, an increase in dietary carbohydrate content at the expense of fat is the appropriate dietary part of a therapeutic strategy to treat obesity.

▶ This study was chosen because it clearly shows that metabolic abnormalities may persist in the postobese state that may promote a regain of body fat. Postobese individuals were unable to increase their level of fat oxidation when presented with a challenge of a high-fat meal. This would favor a metabolic pathway of preferential fat storage. To our knowledge, this study also presented the first evidence that high-fat diets may also suppress daily energy expenditure in postobese individuals. Evidence has accumulated that suggests that the obese state is a reflection of both an energy and substrate imbalance.—E.T. Poehlman, Ph.D.

Substrate Utilization in Man: Effects of Dietary Fat and Carbohydrate
Verboeket-van de Venne WPHG, Westerterp KR, ten Hoor F (Univ of Limburg, Maastricht, The Netherlands)
Metabolism 43:152–156, 1994   112-95-8-5

Background.—To maintain a stable body weight over time, the energy intake should equal the energy expenditure and intakes of protein, fat, and carbohydrate should equal the oxidation of each substrate. A high-fat intake is often associated with an increasing prevalence of obesity, and metabolic differences between persons in handling dietary fat may be related to obesity. The effect of an isoenergetic exchange of fat and carbohydrate on substrate metabolism was investigated, and metabolic responses to dietary fat and carbohydrate among persons who were more or less susceptible to becoming obese were determined.

Study Design.—Fourteen young healthy female subjects were fed a low-fat, mixed, and high-fat diet over 3-day intervals. The relationship between substrate intake and substrate oxidation with each diet was studied by comparing the 24-hour respiratory quotient (RQ) with the food quotient (FQ). By means of their scores on the psychometric questionnaires, the subjects were classified as "restrained" or "unrestrained" eaters.

Results.—For all 3 diets, the subjects remained in energy balance, with the difference between energy intake and energy expenditure averaging 86 kJ/day. The composition of the diet strongly affected the RQ. On a low-fat or mixed diet, the RQ was significantly lower than the FQ, whereas the RQ did not differ from the FQ on a high-fat diet. The RQ and nonprotein RQ were significantly higher in restrained-eating subjects on a high-fat diet, suggesting a relatively lower oxidation ratio of fat to carbohydrate for restrained eaters. Fat and carbohydrate oxidation significantly increased with increasing fat and carbohydrate content of the diet for both restrained and unrestrained eaters. On a high-fat diet, restrained eaters showed a decreased fat oxidation, compared with unrestrained-eating subjects, resulting in a positive fat balance for restrained-eating subjects. On a low-fat diet, the fat balance was negative for both restrained- and unrestrained-eating subjects, indicating a net endogenous fat oxidation.

Conclusion.—Restrained-eating subjects have more difficulty in handling a high-fat diet, possibly explaining their higher susceptibility to becoming obese. Because there is a greater net endogenous fat oxidation on a low-fat than on a high-fat diet, a low-fat diet appears to be a useful tool in the treatment of obesity.

▶ This study supports the notion that a restrained eating pattern is associated with a lower fat oxidation pattern in response to a high-fat meal than is an unrestrained eating pattern. We have previously shown that restrained eaters also have a lower resting metabolic rate and higher levels of body fat than unrestrained eaters (Poehlman et al: *Can J Physiol Pharmacol* 69:320, 1991). Collectively, these results add to a growing body of literature reflecting that restrained eating patterns are associated with metabolic disturbances that may facilitate weight gain. It is unclear, however, whether the restrained eating pattern was a primary or secondary event that leads to alterations in postmeal substrate oxidation and alterations of energy expenditure.—E.T. Poehlman, Ph.D.

Sympathetic Nervous System Activity

Body Fat and Sympathetic Nerve Activity in Healthy Subjects
Scherrer U, Randin D, Tappy L, Vollenweider P, Jéquier E, Nicod P (CHUV, Lausanne, Switzerland; Univ of Lausanne, Switzerland)
Circulation 89:2634–2640, 1994   112-95-8-6

Introduction.—Although obesity is known to be associated with an increased incidence of cardiovascular complications, the mechanism of this association is unknown. Animal models have demonstrated a link between overfeeding and sympathetic activation, and adrenergic mechanisms appear to contribute to cardiovascular complications. Sympathetic nerve activity and the functional consequences of sympathetic nerve discharge were examined in a group of human subjects across a broad range of percent body fat.

Methods.—The study sample comprised 37 healthy volunteers (mean age, 31 years) with percent body fat ranging from 8% to 41%. All underwent measurement of resting postganglionic sympathetic nerve discharge to skeletal muscle using intraneural microelectrodes. Simultaneous measurements of calf vascular resistance, arterial pressure, and energy expenditure were obtained to evaluate the possible functional consequences of sympathetic nerve discharge. Further studies were performed to determine whether acute elevation of plasma insulin in 5 lean subjects to the levels seen in fasting overweight subjects stimulated sympathetic nerve activity.

Results.—There was a direct correlation between resting rate of sympathetic nerve discharge to skeletal muscle and body mass index and percent body fat, $r = .67$ and $.64$, respectively (Fig 8–2). Sympathetic nerve activity was also correlated with age, plasma insulin concentration,

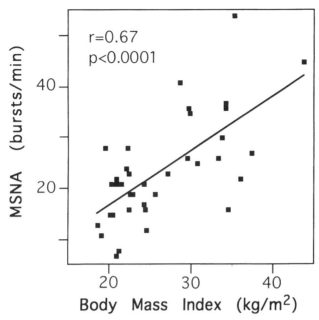

Fig 8–2.—Plot of relation between body mass index and rate of sympathetic nerve discharge to skeletal muscle vasculature. *Abbreviation:* MSNA, muscle sympathetic nerve activity. (Courtesy of Scherrer U, Randin D, Tappy L, et al: *Circulation* 89:2634–2640, 1994.)

and plasma lactate concentration. The combination of these 3 variables with body fat explained 58% of the observed variance in muscle sympathetic nerve activity. Although sympathetic nerve discharge to calf blood vessels was directly correlated with calf vascular resistance, it did not predict energy expenditure. Insulin infusion studies in lean subjects showed that increasing plasma insulin concentrations evoked marked sympathetic activation.

Conclusion.—Sympathetic nerve activity bears a close and direct relation to percent body fat and body mass index in healthy subjects. The sympathetic activation associated with overweight might be 1 mechanism of the increased incidence of cardiovascular complications in overweight individuals. This mechanism could operate by triggering acute events or by contributing to the sustained elevation of arterial pressure.

▶ The use of microneurography, a technique that permits a direct assessment of sympathetic outflow in muscle, has recently provided some unique insights into the relationships between obesity and sympathetic nervous system activity. The results of this study support the notion that higher levels of body fatness are positively related to higher firing rates of sympathetic discharge in the muscle and to increased vascular resistance. The functional consequences of this relationship at this time are unclear, but the heightened sympathetic outflow in individuals with higher levels of body fat may trigger a number of metabolic and cardiovascular events, such as a sustained elevation of arterial blood pressure, increased peripheral vascular resistance, and increased insulin resistance.—E.T. Poehlman, Ph.D.

Impaired Insulin-Induced Sympathetic Neural Activation and Vasodilation in Skeletal Muscle in Obese Humans

Vollenweider P, Randin D, Tappy L, Jéquier E, Nicod P, Scherrer U (Centre Hospitalier Universitaire Vaudois, Lausanne, Switzerland; Univ of Lausanne, Switzerland)
J Clin Invest 93:2365–2371, 1994   112-95-8-7

Background.—The responses of the sympathetic nervous system, an important regulator of metabolic and cardiovascular function, may be altered in obesity. In experimental animals, there is considerable evidence that obesity may alter the sympathetic nerve response to acute hyperinsulinemia. The sympathetic nerve discharge to skeletal muscle of obese, insulin-resistant and lean, healthy subjects was compared.

Patients and Methods.—Eight obese but otherwise healthy volunteers were age and sex matched with 8 lean, healthy volunteers. All were on a weight-maintaining diet for 3 days before testing and fasted the night before testing. By using standardized instruments, muscle sympathetic nerve activity and calf blood flow were measured simultaneously in each subject at baseline and during a 2-hour period of hyperinsulinemia induced with continuous IV infusion of crystalline insulin at a rate of 1 mU/kg/min. Throughout the testing, euglycemia was maintained and hypokalemia was avoided by monitoring and adjusting the flow of IV fluids.

Results.—In both groups, plasma concentrations of glucose during the basal period were comparable, whereas plasma concentrations of insulin were significantly higher in the obese group. The obese subjects had a significantly higher rate of sympathetic nerve firing than lean subjects at baseline, but during hyperinsulinemic testing a markedly smaller increase in burst frequency occurred, and there was no detectable effect on calf blood flow and calf vascular resistance. During the testing period, variations in plasma concentrations of glucose were comparable in both groups, whereas plasma concentrations of insulin increased to significantly higher levels in obese than in lean subjects. Plasma concentrations of norepinephrine increased significantly by the end of the 2-hour period, but concentrations of potassium remained within normal limits in both groups. The heart rate increased significantly in both groups during the testing. Blood pressure rose in both groups, but the increase was significantly greater in the obese group. Markedly less stimulation of total glucose uptake, carbohydrate oxidation, and nonoxidative glucose disposal occurred in the obese subjects.

Conclusion.—Obesity is associated with profound alterations in sympathetic nerve activity characterized by increased fasting activity and a specific attenuation of sympathetic responsiveness to hyperinsulinemia.

▶ This study provides further evidence that increases in body fat are associated with high levels of muscle sympathetic nervous system activity. The new finding, however, relates to the blunted vasodilatory and sympathoexcitatory responses of obese individuals to physiologic hyperinsulinemia. These findings add to a growing body of literature that relates to an impairment in insulin-induced stimulation of muscle blood flow as one important mechanism contributing to insulin resistance in obese humans.—E.T. Poehlman, Ph.D.

Effect of β-Adrenoceptor Blockade on Post-Exercise Oxygen Consumption

Børsheim E, Bahr R, Hansson P, Gullestad L, Hallén J, Sejersted OM (Univ of Oslo, Norway; Central Hosp, Kristianstad, Sweden)
Metabolism 43:565–571, 1994   112-95-8–8

Objective.—A sustained increase in resting oxygen uptake after strenuous exercise—termed the excess postexercise oxygen consumption (EPOC)—has recently been documented. The underlying mechanisms of the prolonged component of EPOC are unclear, although catecholamines may play a role. The effects of β-adrenoreceptor blockade on EPOC were examined in a randomized study.

Methods.—The EPOC study included 6 healthy young men who took part in 1 control experiment and 2 exercise experiments, 1 with and 1 without nonselective β-adrenoreceptor blockade. The exercise experiments included 60 minutes of cycle ergometry at 78% of maximal oxygen uptake, followed by $6\frac{1}{2}$ hours of bed rest. β-Adrenoreceptor blockade was achieved with IV propranolol, .1 mg/kg^{-1}, given immediately after exercise and again $3\frac{1}{2}$ hours later. In the control condition, the men neither exercised nor received propranolol. The difference in oxygen uptake between the exercise and control experiments was used to calculate EPOC. A supplementary study examined the effects of β-adrenoreceptor blockade on resting oxygen uptake in 15 healthy men and women.

Results.—During the recovery period after exercise, a significant increase in oxygen uptake was noted in the absence of β-adrenoreceptor blockade. The subjects showed a mean 19 mL/min^{-1} increase in oxygen uptake after bed rest. When propranolol was given during the recovery period, oxygen uptake was significantly increased for only the first 2 hours after exercise. β-Adrenoreceptor blockade yielded about a one third decrease in total EPOC, from 14.4 to 9.5 L, mainly in the prolonged EPOC component. In the supplementary study, resting oxygen uptake was unaffected by propranolol.

Conclusion.—Intravenous administration of propranolol significantly reduces the duration and magnitude of EPOC, mainly through an effect on the prolonged EPOC phenomenon. Thus, β-adrenergic stimulation appears to play a major role in the mechanisms underlying the prolonged component of EPOC, possibly through increased triglyceride-fatty acid cycling.

▶ The prolonged effects of exercise on postexercise energy expenditure continue to be a research area of continued interest. This group has made significant contributions to our understanding of the regulation of postexercise metabolism. When young subjects were administered a nonselective β-adrenoceptor blockade, the magnitude and duration of the postexercise energy expenditure was reduced by approximately 50%. These findings imply that the prolonged component of the postexercise energy expenditure (i.e., at least 1 hour after exercise cessation) is at least partially influenced by sympathetic factors. It must be kept in mind, however, that the energetic contribution of the postexercise period was 14–15 L of oxygen consumed or just 60–75 kcal, which is small in comparison to the direct energy cost of the exercise session.—E.T. Poehlman, Ph.D.

Effects of Age, Adiposity, and Fitness Level on Plasma Catecholamine Responses to Standing and Exercise

Kohrt WM, Spina RJ, Ehsani AA, Cryer PE, Holloszy JO (Washington Univ, St Louis, Mo)
J Appl Physiol 75:1828–1835, 1993   112-95-8-9

Background.—Age, adiposity, and exercise training status all affect the plasma norepinephrine (NE) and epinephrine (E) responses to various stressors, including posture change and exercise. However, the independent and interactive effects of these factors on plasma catecholamine responses remain to be determined. The interactive effects of age, adiposity, and maximal oxygen uptake on plasma catecholamines were assessed in healthy young and older subjects.

Methods.—The study subjects were 25 healthy young men and women with a mean age of 25 years and 106 older men and women with a mean age of 64 years. The basal levels of NE and E and of posture- and exercise-induced changes in these concentrations were measured in all patients. The association of these responses with adiposity and maximal oxygen uptake was examined as well. In addition, the NE and E responses were reanalyzed after 9 months of endurance exercise training in 48 of the older subjects.

Results.—There were no significant differences between the 2 groups in basal levels of NE and E. However, the older subjects showed an exaggerated NE response to standing, a mean of 696 vs. a mean of 512 pg/mL. They also had attenuated NE and E responses to exercise at 78% of maximal oxygen uptake, a mean of 1,444 vs. a mean of 1,983 pg/mL for NE and a mean of 109 vs. a mean of 228 pg/mL for E. The exercise-induced changes in NE and E were more closely related to age and maximal oxygen uptake than to adiposity. In the older subjects who completed the 9-month endurance exercise training protocol, the increase in NE was 39% lower and the increase in E was 57% lower during exercise at the same absolute intensity. The differences were correlated with the smaller exercise-induced increases in heart rate and the degree of improvement in maximal oxygen uptake.

Conclusion.—During exercise at the same relative intensity, older persons have a blunted catecholamine response, compared to that of young persons. Endurance exercise training in those who are older markedly reduces the metabolic and hemodynamic stress during exercise at a given absolute intensity. The changes in catecholamine responses after training are significantly related to the reduction in the relative intensity of the exercise as well as to the training-related decrease in plasma accumulation of lactate during exercise.

▶ In this study, the authors found no significant age-related differences in basal levels of norepinephrine between younger and older men; significant differences, however, were observed in their catecholamine responses to the stressors of standing and acute exercise. The level of body fatness was also a significant determinant of the catecholamine response to exercise, in which increments in catecholamines were negatively associated with percent body fat during submaximal exercise. Collectively, the level of body fat appears to influence sympathetic nervous system activity both at rest (Abstract 112-95-8–6) and in response to exercise.—E.T. Poehlman, Ph.D.

Resistance Training

Exercise Training and Nutritional Supplementation for Physical Frailty in Very Elderly People
Fiatarone MA, O'Neill EF, Ryan ND, Clements KM, Solares GR, Nelson ME, Roberts SB, Kehayias JJ, Lipsitz LA, Evans WJ (Hebrew Rehabilitation Ctr for Aged, Roslindale, Mass; Tufts Univ, Boston; New England Med Ctr, Boston)
N Engl J Med 330:1769–1775, 1994   112-95-8–10

Background.—Both inadequate nutrition and a lack of muscular exercise are often given as reasons elderly persons are frail, but the value of appropriate interventions has not been established. Whether training in progressive resistance exercises and supplementation with multiple nutrients lead to significant improvement in frail nursing home residents was investigated in a randomized, placebo-controlled study.

Study Plan.—One hundred nursing home residents older than age 70 years (mean age, 87 years) who were able to walk 6 meters participated in a 10-week study, during which they were randomly assigned to supervised high-intensity progressive resistance exercises of the hip and knee extensors 3 days per week or to activities of their choice. The participants also received a nutritional supplement providing 360 kcal daily, intended to increase caloric intake by about 20% and to provide one third of the daily allowances of vitamins and minerals, or a placebo supplement.

Results.—Initially, 83% of the participants required assistance to get around, and 66% had fallen in the past year. Their general level of physical activity was about one fourth that of sedentary young adults. Exercise training significantly improved muscle strength and increased muscle cross-sectional area. Gait velocity and stair-climbing ability improved, as did the overall level of physical activity. Body weight increased significantly with supplementation, but the whole body fat-free mass did not change significantly. The decline in energy intake after completion of the trial was less marked in subjects who exercised than in those given only the supplement.

Conclusion.--Ten weeks of training in resistance exercises enhance muscle strength in frail elderly subjects, make them more mobile, and augment their spontaneous level of physical activity.

▶ This interesting study combined resistance exercise and nutritional supplementation in an attempt to improve physical functioning in elderly individuals. The results add to a growing body of literature that supports exercise as a useful clinical intervention to restore age-related deficits in daily function, even in very old individuals. Of particular interest are the findings that exercise appeared to stimulate appetite and spontaneous daily physical activity.—E.T. Poehlman, Ph.D.

Increased Energy Requirements and Changes in Body Composition With Resistance Training in Older Adults
Campbell WW, Crim MC, Young VR, Evans WJ (Tufts Univ, Boston; Massachusetts Inst of Technology, Cambridge; Pennsylvania State Univ, University Park)
Am J Clin Nutr 60:167–175, 1994   112-95-8–11

Background.—Energy requirements generally decrease with age, and obesity may develop in the elderly when decreased energy expenditure is not matched by decreased energy intake. In some elderly adults, reduced energy and nutrient intakes may contribute to the development of nutritional deficiency. In the metabolic study the effects of resistance training, promoted as a means of increasing muscle strength in the elderly, were examined in 12 previously untrained men and women aged 56–80 years.

Methods.—The study participants were 8 men and 4 postmenopausal women. The 14-week study consisted of a 2-week baseline period during which participants remained sedentary and a 12-week period of progressive resistance training. During the baseline period and at the end of the study, the men and women were assessed for muscular strength, body

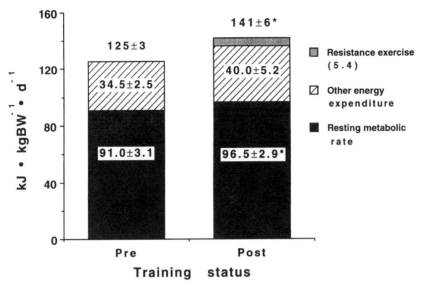

Fig 8–3.—Increased total energy intake and expenditure in 10 older individuals during resistance training. The values at the top of the stacked bars represent the total energy intake necessary to maintain body weight (BW) before and after 12 weeks of resistance training. The resting metabolic rates (RMRs) were measured in each subject by indirect calorimetry. The energy expenditure during resistance exercise was measured by indirect calorimetry in 5 men during a pilot study and assumed to be similar in all 10 study subjects. The other energy expenditure represents the portion of the energy expenditure that was not the result of RMR or resistance exercise and includes the additional thermic effect of feeding and the energy cost of nonresistance exercise daily activity. It was calculated by subtracting the daily energy expenditure because of RMR and resistance exercise from the total energy intake. *Significant increase with resistance training, $P < .05$. (Courtesy of Campbell WW, Crim MC, Young VR, et al: *Am J Clin Nutr* 60:167–175, 1994.)

composition, and energy metabolism. The participants were randomly assigned to either a lower-protein or a higher-protein diet to be followed throughout the 14-week period.

Results.—The lower- and higher-protein diet groups had similar baseline body composition, muscular strength, fasting glucose and hormone concentrations, energy intake, and resting metabolic rate (RMR). Because the effect of resistance training on these variables was not influenced by diet or gender, data for the 12 study participants were combined. Resistance training increased maximum dynamic muscular strength from 24% to 92% for all trained lower- and upper-body muscle groups. Body weight remained stable throughout the study period, fat mass and percent of body fat decreased, and fat-free mass (FFM) increased with training. The resistance training-induced changes in FFM (mean, 1.4 kg) showed a high correlation with increases in total body water (mean, 1.6 kg). The study participants required approximately 15% more energy intake to maintain body weight during the resistance-training period than during baseline. The balance between energy intake and energy expenditure during baseline and week 12 of resistance training is shown in Figure 8–3 for the 10 subjects for whom complete data sets were available.

Conclusion.—Healthy older subjects may benefit from resistance training as an adjunct to weight control programs. The 3-day-per-week resistance-exercise sessions increased energy requirements, lowered body-fat mass, and maintained metabolically active tissue mass.

▶ The use of resistance training to restore physical functioning in elderly patients has gained widespread research interest in recent years. This paper argues persuasively in favor of the use of resistance training as a means to enhance daily energy needs, preserve fat-free mass, and blunt the decline in resting metabolic rate in older individuals. It is possible that if a general level of cardiorespiratory fitness is obtained in older individuals, the exercise prescription should focus more on resistance training activities as a means to preserve function and to maintain healthy body composition.—E.T. Poehlman, Ph.D.

Dietary Supplements Affect the Anabolic Hormones After Weight-Training Exercise
Chandler RM, Byrne HK, Patterson JG, Ivy JL (Univ of Texas, Austin)
J Appl Physiol 76:839–845, 1994   112-95-8-12

Background.—It remains unclear how resistance exercise causes muscle hypertrophy. Activation of amino acid uptake by muscle contraction may promote protein synthesis, but the postexercise hormonal environment significantly influences the synthesis of contractile proteins. Carbohydrate loading and, to a lesser extent, protein consumption increase the plasma insulin level, and ingestion of both carbohydrate and protein produces a rise in insulin beyond that produced by carbohydrate alone.

Objective.—The effects of various dietary supplements, after weight-training exercise, on protein synthesis were examined in 9 experienced male weight-lifters whose mean age was 25 years. They had a mean body weight of 79 kg and a mean percent body fat of 11.8%.

Methods.—The subjects received either water or an isocaloric carbohydrate (1.5 g/kg), protein (1.38 g/kg), or carbohydrate-protein (1.06 g/kg carbohydrate and .41 g/kg protein) supplement immediately and again 2 hours after a weight-training workout. Venous blood was sampled during an 8-hour postexercise recovery period.

Findings.—Plasma glucose and insulin levels both increased after exercise. The greatest rise in insulin was associated with the carbohydrate and mixed supplements. Exercise also increased the levels of lactate, testosterone, and GH. The GH response was most marked after the mixed carbohydrate/protein supplement. The supplements did not alter levels of IGF-I, but they did lead to a significant decline in testosterone levels. Luteinizing hormone levels, however, did not decrease.

Interpretation.—It is likely that postexercise increases in muscle mass are influenced not only by the amount and intensity of exercise during training, but also by the hormonal milieu of the trained muscles. A number of anabolic hormones may influence maximum muscle growth. Supplemental nutrients taken after exercise can alter the anabolic hormonal environment. Carbohydrate, alone or combined with protein, can promote muscle growth throughout the body by increasing postexercise circulating concentrations of insulin and GH.

▶ This study was selected for inclusion in this year's volume because it examined the interaction between nutritional supplementation and the postexercise hormonal milieu (insulin, GH, testosterone, and IGF-I) as an environment that may stimulate protein synthesis and muscle hypertrophy. Of special note was that carbohydrate supplements that caused the greatest rise in insulin also caused the greatest rise in GH (but not IGF-I) 6 hours after exercise. A randomized, controlled study now needs to be undertaken to determine whether nutritional supplementation will actually increase muscle mass in response to resistance training when compared with a nonsupplemented group. The results of this study raise interesting questions regarding the interaction of nutritional supplements and resistance exercise that will potentially enhance muscle growth.—E.T. Poehlman, Ph.D.

Energy Expenditure

Energy Balance in Endurance-Trained Female Cyclists and Untrained Controls

Horton TJ, Drougas HJ, Sharp TA, Martinez LR, Reed GW, Hill JO (Vanderbilt Univ, Nashville, Tenn)
J Appl Physiol 76:1937–1945, 1994   112-95-8-13

Background.—Whether there are sex-specific differences in the response to exercise training because of the increased participation of women in endurance sports must be determined. The differences in energy balance in trained female cyclists and noncyclists were investigated.

Methods.—In a case-control study, 5 trained female cyclists and 5 noncyclists were matched for age, body weight, and height. All were healthy nonsmokers. The women completed initial assessments of maximal oxygen uptake, body composition, and determination of menstrual status and were then scheduled for 2 separate measurements of daily energy expenditure in a whole room indirect calorimeter, once on a cycling day and once on a noncycling day. The normal activity of both groups of women was measured by using a Caltrac accelerometer worn for 2 separate 7-day periods. All subjects were fed a fixed composition diet (30% energy from fat, 55% from carbohydrates, 15% from protein) for 5 days before each measurement.

Results.—Cyclists achieved energy balance on the cycling day while consuming 2,900–3,000 calories (their usual condition), and noncyclists achieved energy balance on the noncycling day while consuming 2,100–2,200 calories (their usual condition). On the cycling day, the daily energy expenditure was significantly higher in the cyclists, whereas the energy expenditure was not different in the noncyclists on the 2 days. The resting metabolic rate and thermic effect of food and activity (noncycling), the components of daily energy expenditure, were not significantly different between the groups.

Conclusion.—Trained female cyclists demonstrated no evidence of increased energetic efficiency, compared with nontrained women. These results suggest that there is no evidence of a large increase in energy efficiency in female athletes.

▶ Previous reports have suggested that endurance-trained female athletes were able to maintain body weight despite only marginal levels of food intake. The "mysterious" energetic efficiency of female athletes appears to be largely unfounded as a result of recent advances in the measurement of daily energy expenditure with the use of room calorimeters and the doubly labeled water technique. It appears that female endurance athletes consume a substantial and appropriate number of calories to meet the energetic demands of their vigorous training schedules.—E.T. Poehlman, Ph.D.

Resting Metabolic Rate Is Lower in Women Than in Men
Arciero PJ, Goran MI, Poehlman ET (Univ of Maryland, Baltimore; Univ of Vermont, Burlington)
J Appl Physiol 75:2514–2520, 1993   112-95-8-14

Introduction.—Because it accounts for up to 75% of the total daily energy expenditure, the resting metabolic rate (RMR) plays an important role in the regulation of energy balance. The absolute RMR is generally higher in men than in women because men have greater amounts of fat-free mass; however, it is unknown whether RMR differs between the sexes independently of their differences in body composition. To address this question, sex differences in RMR were examined in a large cohort of healthy volunteers across a broad spectrum of age, body mass, aerobic fitness, and adiposity.

Methods.—The retrospective study included 328 men and 194 women aged 17–81 years. All underwent measurement of RMR by indirect calorimetry using the ventilated hood technique in a clinical research center. Body composition, physical activity, peak oxygen consumption, anthropometric indices, and energy intake were also assessed. Sex differences in RMR were analyzed with adjustment for composition and aerobic fitness. Additional RMR comparisons were made in premenopausal and postmenopausal women vs. men of a similar age.

Results.—Men had an mean RMR of 1,740 kcal/day vs. 1,348 kcal/day in women, a difference of 23%. On multiple regression analysis, the

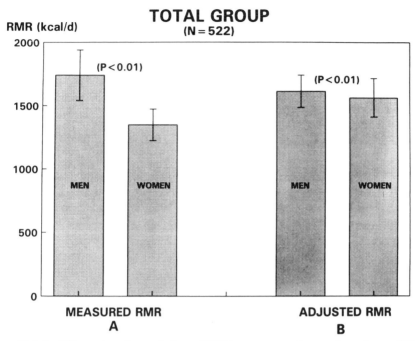

Fig 8–4.—Difference in resting metabolic rate (RMR) between men and women for total group (522 subjects). **A,** measured mean RMR for men (mean of 1,740 kcal/day) vs. women (mean of 1,348 kcal/ day). **B,** adjusted RMR values after controlling for fat-free mass, fat mass, and peak oxygen consumption for men (mean of 1,613 kcal/day) and women (mean of 1,563 kcal/day). (Courtesy of Arciero PJ, Goran MI, Poehlman ET: *J Appl Physiol* 75:2514–2520, 1993.)

variables of fat-free mass, fat mass, peak oxygen consumption, and sex accounted for 84% of the individual variation in measured RMR. After adjustment for the first 3 of these variables, the mean RMR remained 3% higher in men than in women (1,613 vs. 1,563 kcal/day (Fig 8-4). The adjusted RMR was also significantly lower in premenopausal women and postmenopausal women than in men of similar age.

Conclusion.—The RMR is lower in women than in men, independent of sex-related differences in body composition, aerobic fitness, age, and menopausal status. Given the large role of RMR in total daily energy expenditure, a small sex difference in RMR may have a significant long-term effect on the regulation of body weight and composition.

▶ The results of this study in a large population of healthy men and women spanning a broad age range support the notion that women burn calories at a slightly slower rate at rest than men. It was speculated that the lower resting metabolic rate in women (approximately 50 kcal per day) may partially contribute to their higher levels of body fat. It is likely, however, that sex-related differences in body composition cannot fully account for the lower resting metabolic rate in women. Thus, other metabolic processes may "burn at a slower rate" in women compared with men.—E.T. Poehlman, Ph.D.

Miscellaneous

Relation of Leisure-Time Physical Activity and Cardiorespiratory Fitness to the Risk of Acute Myocardial Infarction in Men

Lakka TA, Venäläinen JM, Rauramaa R, Salonen R, Tuomilehto J, Salonen JT (Univ of Kuopio, Finland; Kuopio Research Inst of Exercise Medicine, Kuopio, Finland; Natl Public Health Inst, Helsinki)
N Engl J Med 330:1549–1554, 1994   112-95-8-15

Background.—The risk of coronary heart disease is reduced in individuals with higher levels of regular physical activity and cardiorespiratory fitness. However, most studies of this issue have failed to use truly quantitative assessments of physical activity or direct measurements of maximal oxygen uptake, the most accurate method of assessing cardiorespiratory fitness.

Methods.—A detailed questionnaire was used to measure physical activity during leisure time, and exercise testing was used to determine maximal oxygen uptake in 1,453 men. The men, aged 42 to 60 years at baseline examination, had no reported cardiovascular disease or cancer. A total of 1,166 of the subjects were followed for an average of 4.9 years, during which 42 of those with initially normal ECGs had a first acute myocardial infarction. Independent associations between physical activity, maximal oxygen uptake, and the risk of acute myocardial infarction were sought.

Results.—The relative risk of myocardial infarction was .31 in men with the highest level of physical activity—more than 2.2 hr/wk—compared with the risk in those with the lowest level, after adjustment for age and year of examination. After adjustment for age, year and season of examination, weight, height, and type of respiratory gas analyzer used, the relative hazard in patients with the highest maximal oxygen uptake—more than 2.7 L/min—was .26. Even after adjustment for up to 17 confounding variables, the third of the men with the highest level of physical activity and maximal oxygen uptake continued to have relative hazards significantly less than 1 compared with men in the lowest third of each category.

Conclusion.—A strong, graded, inverse association was found between high levels of leisure-time physical activity and cardiorespiratory fitness, and risk of acute myocardial infarction in men. These findings support the notion that low levels of physical activity and cardiorespiratory fitness are independent risk factors for coronary heart disease. Physical activity of moderate-to-high intensity may be needed to decrease coronary risk.

▶ The authors' unique contribution here is that they simultaneously investigated both physical activity and cardiorespiratory fitness as predictors of cardiovascular disease. The type, duration, and frequency of physical activity that is needed to protect against coronary heart disease is presently unknown. The major point of this paper is that low levels of leisure time physical activity are associated with decreased risk of acute myocardial infarction in men. This finding is encouraging from a public health perspective because most people will only engage in low levels of physical activity.—E.T. Poehlman, Ph.D.

Growth Hormone Treatment of Obese Women for 5 Wk: Effect on Body Composition and Adipose Tissue LPL Activity
Richelsen B, Pedersen SB, Bφrglum JD, Mφller-Pedersen T, Jφrgensen J, Jφrgensen JO (Aarhus Amtssygehus, Denmark; Skejby Sygehus, Aarhus; Aarhus Kommunehospital, Denmark)
Am J Physiol 266:E211–E216, 1994   112-95-8-16

Purpose.—Obese subjects have relatively low plasma levels of GH and a diminished GH response to various stimuli. Although the reason for these conditions is unclear, they are normalized after successful weight reduction. Previous studies have shown that GH treatment in GH-deficient adults can reduce total adipose tissue mass while increasing lean body mass. The effects of GH treatment on body composition and adipose tissue lipoprotein lipase (LPL) activity of obese women were examined in a double-blind, placebo-controlled crossover study.

Methods.—The study included 9 obese women referred for weight reduction. Their mean age was 32 years and their mean body mass index was 34.5 kg/m². All were treated randomly with GH, .03 mg/kg ideal body weight/day, and placebo for 5 weeks each. The women followed their usual diet and physical activity throughout the study. Dual-energy x-ray absorptiometry was used to assess body composition, and CT scanning was used to measure intra-abdominal adipose tissue. Fat biopsy specimens from the subcutaneous abdominal and gluteal regions were used to determine adipose tissue LPL activity.

Results.—The total fat mass declined by about 5% with GH treatment, from 40.5 to a mean of 38.4 kg (Fig 8–5), but the fat-free mass increased from a mean of 50.5 to a mean of 53.5 kg. Intra-abdominal adipose tissue decreased by a mean of 7%. Computed tomography scanning at the femoral level demonstrated a 7% reduction in adipose tissue and a 5% increase in muscle volume with GH treatment, signifying no apparent regional differences in GH-mediated reduction of adipose tissue mass. Adipose tissue LPL activity declined by about 50% and plasma levels of free fatty acids increased significantly during GH treatment.

Conclusion.—Short-term GH treatment significantly reduced total fat mass in obese women. The GH-induced reductions in adipose tissue mass may occur via reduced LPL activity and enhanced lipolysis. How-

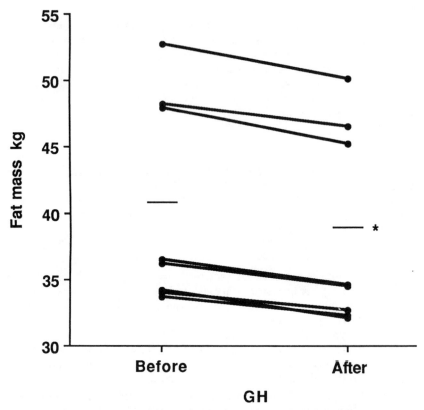

Fig 8–5.—The effect of treatment with GH on total fat mass. The total fat mass was determined by dual-energy x-ray absorptiometry. Individual data are shown for the subjects before and after 5 weeks of treatment with GH. Mean values are also given. *P < .01. (Courtesy of Richelsen B, Pedersen SB, Børglum JD, et al: *Am J Physiol* 266:E211–E216, 1994.)

ever, insulin resistance increases during GH treatment, suggesting that such treatment may not be recommended.

▶ Although the authors here were mainly interested in whether GH treatment reduced fat mass (40–38 kg), I was more impressed with the large increase in fat-free mass (51–54 kg) they observed over the relatively short 5-week time period. It is frequently difficult to achieve this degree of increase in fat-free mass with 6 months to 1 year of resistance training. It is unclear, however, how much of this latter change may have been the result of enhanced water content. The long-term benefits of GH, however, as a pharmacologic intervention to alter body composition are still unclear given its several secondary effects.—E.T. Poehlman, Ph.D.

Waist Circumference and Abdominal Sagittal Diameter: Best Simple Anthropometric Indexes of Abdominal Visceral Adipose Tissue Accumulation and Related Cardiovascular Risk in Men and Women
Pouliot M-C, Després J-P, Lemieux S, Moorjani S, Bouchard C, Tremblay A, Nadeau A, Lupien PJ (Laval Univ, Ste-Foy, Quebec)
Am J Cardiol 73:460–468, 1994   112-95-8–17

Background.—The amount of abdominal visceral adipose tissue measured by CT is a critical correlate of the potentially "atherogenic" metabolic disturbances associated with abdominal obesity. Its clinical use is limited by the cost and the use of radiation. The waist-to-hip circumferences ratio (WHR), the abdominal sagittal diameter, and the waist circumference are simple anthropometric indices of abdominal adipose tissue accumulation, and yet these indices have not been systematically compared regarding their associations with abdominal visceral adipose tissue accumulation and related metabolic variables.

Study Design.—The interrelationships between anthropometric and CT-derived measurements of abdominal visceral adipose tissue accumulation were studied in 70 women and 81 men. In addition, the anthropometric correlates of abdominal visceral adipose tissue accumulation were related to risk factors for cardiovascular disease, including triglyceride and HDL cholesterol levels, and fasting and postglucose insulin and glucose levels.

Findings.—Waist circumference and abdominal sagittal diameter correlated strongly with the level of abdominal visceral adipose tissue. Men and women had comparable levels of abdominal visceral adipose tissue for a given waist circumference or abdominal sagittal diameter. The more commonly used WHR was less closely related to the level of abdominal visceral adipose tissue. Most of the variance in waist circumference and abdominal sagittal diameter could be explained by variations in body fat mass and in abdominal visceral and subcutaneous adipose tissue area, whereas a lower proportion of the variance in WHR could be explained by these adipose variables. In women, waist circumference and abdominal sagittal diameter were more closely related with the metabolic variables than the WHR; such differences were not apparent in men. When the men and women were divided into quintiles of waist circumference, WHR, or the abdominal sagittal diameter, increasing values of waist circumference and abdominal sagittal diameter were more consistently associated with increases in fasting and postglucose insulin levels than were increasing levels of WHR, particularly in women. Waist circumference values above approximately 100 cm or abdominal sagittal diameter values of greater than 25 cm were more likely to be associated with disturbances in lipoprotein metabolism and in plasma insulin-glucose homeostasis.

Conclusion.—The waist circumference and sagittal abdominal diameter should be preferred over WHR when a single, simple anthropometric index is to be used to estimate the amount of abdominal visceral adipose tissue in both genders, as well as the related cardiovascular risk profile. Because the abdominal sagittal diameter used was measured on the abdominal scan obtained by CT, the use of waist circumference appears preferable until further studies substantiate the use of abdominal sagittal diameter for clinical purposes.

▶ Many indices have been used to estimate abdominal visceral adipose tissue accumulation. This paper compares the relation between adipose tissue distribution patterns with CT and several field methods to estimate fat distribution. The single best predictor of intra-abdominal body fat was the waist circumference in men and women. The results of this paper provide a valuable and elegantly simple index to estimate the distribution of body fat. The measurement of the waist circumference should be performed routinely in clinical settings to educate patients regarding the dangers of excessive storage of intra-abdominal body fat.—E.T. Poehlman, Ph.D.

Running and the Development of Disability With Age

Fries JF, Singh G, Morfeld D, Hubert HB, Lane NE, Brown BW Jr (Stanford Univ, Calif)
Ann Intern Med 121:502–509, 1994   112-95-8-18

Background.—Although physical activity is known to decrease mortality rates, its effects on morbidity and disability are less clear. An activity such as aerobic running might delay or prevent disability through increased fitness and training; however, it might also accelerate the development of disability as a result of osteoarthritis or cumulative trauma. An 8-year longitudinal comparison of progression of disability scores among runners vs. nonrunners was reported.

Methods.—There were 451 runners drawn from the membership of the 50+ Runners Association and 330 community controls. The average history of running among the runners was 12 years. Both groups were aged 50 to 72 years in 1984 when they responded to a questionnaire concerning exercise, medical, and dietary history; musculoskeletal injuries; and other variables. They also responded to annual questionnaires during 8 years of follow-up. The main outcome measure was disability, as indicated by responses to the previously validated Health Assessment Questionnaire, which evaluates function in the areas of dressing and grooming, arising, eating, walking, hygiene, reach, grip, and activities.

Results.—At baseline, the runners—including control subjects with a history of running—were leaner, had less frequent joint symptoms, took fewer medications, had fewer medical problems, and had fewer and less severe instances of disability. These differences, which may have reflected either improved health because of running or self-selection bias, persisted after 8 years. One third of the runners' club members had stopped running; however, the frequency of other vigorous exercise increased in both groups, particularly among runners.

During follow-up, disability levels increased steadily from .026 to .071 for runners and from .079 to .242 for controls. The difference was significant and consistent between sexes. The lower rate of disability among runners' club members persisted after adjustment for age, sex, body mass, baseline disability, smoking history, history of arthritis, and other co-morbid conditions. All age groups showed progressive increases in disability; the oldest groups showed an increase in the slope of the disability curve. Mortality was also lower in the runners' club members than in controls, 1.5% vs. 7.1%. The mortality differences remained after adjustment for age, sex, body mass, co-morbid conditions, educational level, smoking history, alcohol intake, and mean blood pressure; conditional risk ratio for controls compared with runners was 4.27.

Conclusion.—Compared with community controls, older adults who engage in aerobic running and other vigorous exercise have significantly slower development of disability. Mortality is lower in runners as well. The benefits of running most likely result from increased aerobic activity, strength, fitness, and organ reserve rather than from postponement of osteoarthritis. The findings have important implications for efforts to increase regular physical exercise throughout the life span. It is difficult to remove the influence of self-selection bias, however, and there is no way to tell whether more rigorous exercise could make controls as healthy as runners.

▶ I have always wondered whether a lifetime habit of running would result in increased disability "down the road." I was pleased to learn that long-term runners were less disabled and had lower rates of mortality. Although a selection bias could not be ruled out, the available evidence strongly favors that a lifetime habit of regular physical activity increases both the quality and quantity of life.—E.T. Poehlman, Ph.D.

Mechanism of Enhanced Insulin Sensitivity in Athletes: Increased Blood Flow, Muscle Glucose Transport Protein (GLUT-4) Concentration, and Glycogen Synthase Activity

Ebeling P, Bourey R, Koranyi L, Tuominen JA, Groop LC, Henriksson J, Mueckler M, Sovijärvi A, Koivisto VA (Helsinki Univ Central Hosp, Finland; Hungarian Heart Ctr, Hungary; Karolinska Institutet, Stockholm)
J Clin Invest 92:1623–1631, 1993   112-95-8–19

Background.—Physical training increases insulin-stimulated glucose disposal proportional to improvement in physical fitness. This increment in insulin sensitivity probably results from several contributing factors. Some of these factors, such as blood flow, capillary density, glucose transport proteins, glucose disposal and its oxidative and nonoxidative metabolism, and their interrelationship were studied in healthy subjects varying widely in physical fitness levels.

Methods.—Nine male athletes (mean age, 25 years) were compared with 10 sedentary control subjects (mean age, 28 years). Maximal aerobic power was 57.6 mL/kg per minute in the athletic group and 44.1 mL/kg per minute in the sedentary group.

Findings.—Whole body glucose disposal in athletes was 32%, and nonoxidative glucose disposal was 62% greater than in the sedentary group. During insulin clamp, muscle glycogen content rose by 39% in the athletes but was unchanged in the controls. Maximal aerobic power was associated with whole body and nonoxidative glucose disposal. Forearm blood flow in athletes was 64% greater than in controls, whereas muscle capillary density was normal. During insulin infusion, basal blood flow was associated with maximal aerobic power and glucose disposal. In athletes, forearm glucose uptake was increased by 3.3-fold in the basal state and by 73% during insulin infusion. Muscle glucose transport protein (GLUT-4) levels, 93% higher in the athletes than in controls, were correlated with maximal aerobic power and whole body glucose disposal. Muscle glycogen synthase activity was 33% higher in the athletes than in the controls. Basal glycogen synthase fractional activity was closely associated with blood flow.

Conclusion.—Athletes have increased muscle blood flow and glucose uptake. The cellular mechanisms of glucose uptake are elevated GLUT-4 protein content, glycogen synthase activity, and glucose storage as glycogen. The close association between glycogen synthase fractional activity and blood flow suggests they are related causally in the promotion of glucose disposal.

▶ This remarkably detailed and intensive study examines the mechanisms that underlie enhanced insulin sensitivity in young athletes. These investigators have nicely tied together the notion that a metabolic chain of events consisting of increased blood flow, capillarization, and glucose transporter proteins together enhance glucose disposal. The cross-sectional nature of the design, however, precludes conclusions regarding cause and effect relationships. One also wonders whether such high levels of training are necessary to achieve these metabolic adaptations given the fact that most individuals will never engage in the level of physical activity required to achieve the degree of cardiovascular fitness observed in this study.—E.T. Poehlman, Ph.D.

Suggested Reading

The following articles are recommended to the reader:

Kriska AM, LaPorte RE, Petitt DJ, et al: The association of physical activity with obesity, fat distribution and glucose intolerance in Pima Indians. *Diabetologia* 36:863–869, 1993.
   ▶ This is an interesting paper that supports the notion that regular physical

activity may be protective against the development of NIDDM by its influence on obesity and fat distribution.

Houmard JA, McCulley C, Roy LK, et al: Effects of exercise training on absolute and relative measurements of regional adiposity. *Int J Obes* 18:243–248, 1994.

▶ A thorough investigation of the effects of endurance training on measures of regional adiposity.

Franch-Arcas G, Plank LD, Monk DN, et al: A new method for the estimation of the components of energy expenditure in patients with major trauma. *Am J Physiol* 267:E1002–E1009, 1994.

▶ A new approach using indirect calorimetry and body composition methodology to examine metabolic and nutritional disorders in critically ill patients.

Poehlman ET, Scheffers J, Gottlieb SS, et al: Increased resting metabolic rate in patients with congestive heart failure. *Ann Intern Med* 121:860–862, 1994.

▶ Elevated levels of resting energy expenditure may contribute to the unexplained weight loss in heart failure patients.

Roberts SB, Fuss P, Heyman MB, et al: Control of food intake in older men. *JAMA* 272:1601–1606, 1994.

▶ These findings support the notion that with aging we lose the ability to respond to short-term perturbations to energy surfeit and deficit conditions.

Goran MI, Kaskoun M, Johnson R: Determinants of resting energy expenditure in young children. *J Pediatr* 125:362–367, 1994.

▶ As observed in adults, fat-free mass and to a lesser extent fat mass are the major determinants of resting energy expenditure in prepubertal children. Interestingly, no differences in resting energy expenditure were observed between children with lean or obese parents.

9 Lipoproteins and Atherosclerosis

Introduction

This year's selections reflect continued progress in 2 major areas: drug and dietary therapy for dyslipidemia and pathogenesis and molecular mechanisms of atherosclerosis. Progress, I might add, at a price. The price is the continuing attrition of physician scientists from the research community. The reality is that physician scientists are a luxury we can no longer afford. Deciding which research projects get funded in this field falls increasingly to basic scientists who lack sufficient clinical knowledge to judge the relevance of a given research proposal. Add to this the dismal amounts of money available at this critical juncture in medicine in addition to the number of senior members of the academic research community who have been important contributors to a given field and who simply no longer do research. There are no younger people to fill this gap.

Despite the proportions of the ongoing changes in the practice of medicine and in the academic medical community, discoveries with clinical relevance and application continue to be made that provide further rationale for various therapies and a better understanding in the case of atherosclerosis of the complexities that underlie its pathogenesis. Even with the premature passing of David Blankenhorn, who led the Cholesterol Lowering Atherosclerosis Study (CLAS), useful insights into the favorable effects of aggressive lipid modifying on arteriosclerosis continue to be published on this seminal study by his colleagues at the University of Southern California (Abstract 112-95-9-1). The same can be said for the ongoing Familial Atherosclerosis Study (FATS) in Seattle. More hard data from these 2 clinical studies support of diet and drug therapy for the afflicted (CLAS) as well as for those at risk (FATS). Lowering lipids (according to NCEP guidelines) in those at risk without disease (FATS) has the same beneficial effects with regard to lesion regression and progression as in those with symptomatic disease (Abstract 112-95-9-5). And the carotid as well as the coronary arteries (saphenous vein grafts or nonbypassed vessels) accrue the gains (CLAS). There is, at last, evidence of the adverse consequences of elevated homocysteine levels on arterial wall biology and the behavior of endothelial and smooth muscle cells, and more evidence of cigarette smoking's deleterious consequences, with new information indicating that it possibly promotes an atherogenic dyslipidemia (Abstract 112-95-9-2).

In the diet and exercise selections, n-3 fatty acids warrant continued attention. The Zutphen study points out that a modest amount of fish (surprisingly only 1 meal of fish per week) was sufficient to reduce the incidence of stroke (Abstract 112-95-9-10). It is the "mix" (the proportion of saturated and unsaturated fatty acids and cholesterol; the amount of fat in the diet relative to the total caloric content) that matters when it comes to fat intake. Dr. William Connor's group at the Oregon Health Sciences University (Abstract 112-95-9-11) shows that the beneficial effects of n-3 fatty acids on hemostasis can be dampened with increasing intake of saturated fat. Even when endurance athletes exercise acutely, their plasma lipid profile benefits (112-95-9-13) and the HDL changes involve a reduction in the activity of cholesteryl ester transfer protein.

From the burgeoning literature on pharmacotherapy for dyslipidemia and atherosclerosis, selections are included that provide pathophysiologic insights as well as evidence of possible benefit. Angiotensin-converting enzyme inhibitors, for example, have antiatherosclerotic properties, implying that angiotensin plays a role in lesion formation (Abstract 112-95-9-14). The fact that probucol and other antioxidants prevent the inhibition of endothelium-dependent relaxation by LDL (Abstract 112-95-9-15) is further evidence that oxidized lipoproteins have this deleterious consequence. Happily, lovastatin normalizes platelet function in patients with hypercholesterolemia (Abstract 112-95-9-17), presumably as a result of it altering platelet membrane eicosanoid receptors. But if modifying cellular cholesterol synthesis alters these receptors, what is it doing to others and possibly to surface-bound enzymes?

Oxidized lipoproteins and their still poorly characterized products continue to dominate research into the mechanisms of atherogenesis. Dr. Alan Fogelman, recipient of the 1994 Lyman Duff Award from the American Heart Association, and his group at UCLA have made substantial contributions to this field. It is rather astonishing that one person can wear so many hats so well (Dr. Fogelman is Chief of Medicine, Cardiology, and heads a large premier research team). He is a master at deploying basic scientists on clinically relevant problems (Abstract 112-95-9-7). The Tempere group in Finland provides us with a receptor pathway (the α_2-macroglobulin receptor/LDL receptor–related protein [α_2-MR/LRP]) that allows arterial smooth muscle cells (SMCs) to internalize a number of different atherogenic lipoproteins. We have known that macrophages have this receptor and the scavenger receptor pathway that together contribute to lipid accumulation, but SMCs do not have scavenger receptors and still become lipid-laden. The α_2-MR/LRP gives arterial SMCs the dubious distinction to do the same. All of this makes for a stimulating read, I think. Proceed.

John D. Bagdade, M.D.

Moving?

I'd like to receive my *Year Book of Endocrinology* without interruption.
Please note the following change of address, effective:

Name: _____

New Address: _____

_____

City: _____ State: _____ Zip: _____

Old Address: _____

_____

City: _____ State: _____ Zip: _____

Reservation Card

Yes, I would like my own copy of *Year Book of Endocrinology* . Please begin my subscription with the current edition according to the terms described below.* I understand that I will have 30 days to examine each annual edition. If satisfied, I will pay just $72.95 plus sales tax, postage and handling (price subject to change without notice).

Name: _____

Address: _____

City: _____ State: _____ Zip: _____

Method of Payment
○ Visa   ○ Mastercard   ○ AmEx   ○ Bill me   ○ Check (in US dollars, payable to Mosby, Inc.)

Card number: _____ Exp date: _____

Signature: _____

LS-0909

*Your *Year Book* Service Guarantee:

When you subscribe to the *Year Book*, we'll send you an advance notice of future volumes about two months before they publish. This automatic notice system is designed to take up as little of your time as possible. If you do not want the *Year Book*, the advance notice makes it quick and easy for you to let us know your decision, and you will always have at least 20 days to decide. If we don't hear from you, we'll send you the new volume as soon as it's available. And, of course, the *Year Book* is yours to examine free of charge for 30 days (postage, handling and applicable sales tax are added to each shipment.).

BUSINESS REPLY MAIL

FIRST CLASS MAIL PERMIT No. 762   CHICAGO, IL

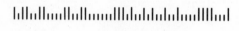

POSTAGE WILL BE PAID BY ADDRESSEE

Chris Hughes
Mosby-Year Book, Inc.
200 N. LaSalle Street
Suite 2600
Chicago, IL 60601-9981

‖|‖|‖‖|‖||‖‖‖|‖|‖|‖|‖||‖‖‖|‖|

BUSINESS REPLY MAIL

FIRST CLASS MAIL PERMIT No. 762   CHICAGO, IL

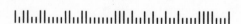

POSTAGE WILL BE PAID BY ADDRESSEE

Chris Hughes
Mosby-Year Book, Inc.
200 N. LaSalle Street
Suite 2600
Chicago, IL 60601-9981

‖|‖|‖‖|‖||‖‖‖|‖|‖|‖|‖||‖‖‖|‖|

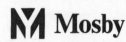

Dedicated to publishing excellence

General Interest

Beneficial Effects of Colestipol-Niacin Therapy on the Common Carotid Artery: Two- and Four-Year Reduction of Intima-Media Thickness Measured by Ultrasound

Blankenhorn DH, Selzer RH, Crawford DW, Barth JD, Liu C-r, Liu C-h, Mack WJ, Alaupovic P (Univ of Southern California, Los Angeles; California Inst Technology/Jet Propulsion Lab; Interuniversity Cardiology Inst of The Netherlands; et al)

Circulation 88:20–28, 1993   112-95-9-1

Background.—Previous clinical trials of cholesterol-lowering measures have used serial imaging of coronary and femoral but not cervical arteries. The Cholesterol Lowering Atherosclerosis Study was a randomized, placebo-controlled study of colestipol-niacin plus dietary therapy in men having coronary bypass surgery, in which arteries at all 3 of these sites were monitored by angiography. A pilot study of carotid ultrasound imaging also was included.

Methods.—Seventy-eight patients had ultrasound studies at baseline and after 2 and 4 years. Forty-six, including 24 randomized to active treatment and 22 placebo recipients, had matching cervical angiograms available. Cervical and coronary artery ultrasound images and angiograms were analyzed by computerized image-processing and compared by operators who were blind to treatment group.

Results.—The thickness of the wall of the carotid artery decreased significantly at both 2 and 4 years in actively treated patients, whereas in placebo recipients the wall thickness increased significantly. Thinning of the carotid artery wall was associated with reduced levels of apolipoprotein B and with increased levels of apolipoprotein C-III and HDL cholesterol. Ultrasound measurements of carotid wall thickness correlated with visual readings of coronary angiographic stenosis at baseline and with computerized measurements of carotid angiographic edge roughness at 2 years but not at 4 years.

Conclusion.—Atherosclerotic thickening of the common carotid arterial wall is effectively reduced by treatment with colestipol and niacin. The intima–media thickness of the carotid artery serves as a useful end point in small-scale coronary risk factor trials.

▶ There seems to be no end to the amount of useful information that can be derived from an excellent clinical trial. Here the National Institutes of Health had the good sense to provide funds to support the pilot study of carotid ultrasound (an unlikely event today because of the added cost). It is reassuring to know that aggressive lipid modification treatment had beneficial effects on arterial lesions that were generalized. Knowing that the therapy works, shouldn't we treat asymptomatic carotid disease in this way? I think so.—J.D. Bagdade, M.D.

Promotion of Vascular Smooth Muscle Cell Growth by Homocysteine: A Link to Atherosclerosis

Tsai J-C, Perrella MA, Yoshizumi M, Hsieh C-M, Haber E, Schlegel R, Lee M-E
(Harvard School of Public Health, Boston; Harvard Med School, Boston; Brigham and Women's Hosp, Boston, Mass; Massachusetts Gen Hosp, Boston)
Proc Natl Acad Sci U S A 91:6369–6373, 1994   112-95-9–2

Background.—Plasma homocysteine levels are increased in 20% to 30% of patients with premature atherosclerosis. Hyperhomocysteinemia is an independent risk factor for myocardial infarction and stroke, but how homocysteine induces atherosclerosis is not clear. Because proliferation of vascular smooth muscle cells is a prominent feature of human atherosclerotic lesions, studies were performed to determine whether homocysteine influences the growth of vascular smooth muscle and endothelial cells in culture.

Methods.—The effects of homocysteine at concentrations similar to those observed in patients on [³H] thymidine incorporation in quiescent rat aortic smooth muscle cells (RASMCs) and human umbilical vein endothelial cells were studied. Labeling with 5-bromodeoxyuridine was used to determine the distribution of cells undergoing active DNA synthesis. The induction of cyclin messenger RNA (mRNA) was studied to confirm that homocysteine induced quiescent RASMCs to reenter the cell cycle.

Results.—Homocysteine increased DNA synthesis in RASMCs in a dose-dependent manner: [³H] thymidine incorporation increased 25% with as little as .1 mM of homocysteine and increased 4.5-fold with 1 mM of homocysteine. In contrast, homocysteine decreased DNA synthesis in human umbilical vein endothelial cells in a dose-dependent manner. In RASMCs, homocysteine increased mRNA levels of cyclin D1 by threefold and cyclin A by 15-fold, indicating that homocysteine induced the mRNA of cyclins that are important for reentry of quiescent RASMCs into the cell cycle. Furthermore, homocysteine promoted proliferation of quiescent RASMCs, and this increase was amplified in the presence of 2% serum.

Discussion.—Homocysteine has opposing effects on DNA synthesis in vascular smooth muscle and endothelial cells. By promoting the proliferation of vascular smooth muscle cells and inhibiting the regeneration of injured endothelial cells, homocysteine may initiate or accelerate the progression of atherosclerosis. Homocysteine alone can induce quiescent RASMCs to reenter the cell cycle and proliferate, but it also acts synergistically with serum to promote proliferation of RASMCs.

▶ It seems that with all the interest and literature on homocysteine and its association with atherosclerosis, the effects of this metabolite of methionine on arterial wall cells would be known. Past in vitro studies dealing with homocysteine's effects have been performed at high and unphysiologic homocysteine levels. Its opposing and deleterious effects on endothelial cells and ASMCs make it double trouble.—J.D. Bagdade, M.D.

Sex Differences in Endothelial Function in Normal and Hypercholesterolaemic Subjects
Chowienczyk PJ, Watts GF, Cockcroft JR, Brett SE, Ritter JM (St Thomas' Hosp, London)
Lancet 344:305–306, 1994   112-95-9-3

Introduction.—It is still not clear how premenopausal women are protected against atherosclerosis. One link between female sex hormones

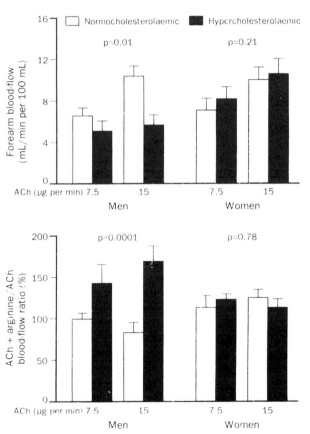

Fig 9–1.—Mean (SE) forearm blood flow during acetylcholine infusion and ratio of blood flow during acetylcholine + arginine infusion to that during acetylcholine infusion alone. *P* values refer to differences between control and hypercholesterolemic subjects calculated by analysis of variance with both doses of acetylcholine (AC*h*). (Courtesy of Chowienczyk PJ, Watts GF, Cockcroft JR, et al: *Lancet* 344:305–306, 1994.)

and atherosclerosis is the nitric oxide pathway, because sex hormones regulate constitutive nitric oxide synthase in vascular endothelium. The endothelial cell L-arginine/nitric oxide pathway is abnormal in patients with hypercholesterolemia and may be important in the pathogenesis of vascular disease. Studies were performed to determine whether sex differences exist in this pathway in which acetylcholine stimulates endothelial synthesis of nitric oxide from L-arginine.

Methods.—Twelve men and 14 women with primary hypercholesterolemia and matched controls were studied. Forearm vasodilator responses to brachial artery infusions of nitroprusside, saline, acetylcholine, saline, L-arginine alone, and L-arginine with acetylcholine were measured by venous occlusion plethysmography.

Results.—Nitroprusside increased blood flow similarly in all groups, whereas L-arginine alone did not. Although responses to acetylcholine were reduced by 55% in men with hypercholesterolemia compared with those in controls, they were the same as in controls in women with hypercholesterolemia (Fig 9-1). The infusion of L-arginine normalized responses to acetylcholine in men with hypercholesterolemia but had similar effects in women with hypercholesterolemia and control women.

Implications.—Sex affects endothelial function in human vasculature in vivo, especially in the susceptibility of the L-arginine/nitric oxide pathway to damage by hypercholesterolemia. Women are protected against the adverse effects of hypercholesterolemia on the L-arginine/nitric oxide pathway, and this may be an important mechanism by which premenopausal women are protected against vascular disease.

▶ In addition to their antioxidant properties (Sack et al: *Lancet* 343:269, 1994), estrogens have this important protective property on vascular endothelium.—J.D. Bagdade, M.D.

Effects of Cigarette Smoking and Its Cessation on Lipid Metabolism and Energy Expenditure in Heavy Smokers
Hellerstein MK, Benowitz NL, Neese RA, Schwartz J-M, Hoh R, Jacob P III, Hsieh J, Faix D (Univ of California, San Francisco; Univ of California, Berkeley)
J Clin Invest 93:265–272, 1994   112-95-9-4

Introduction.—Weight gain after cessation of cigarette smoking (CS) is a common occurrence and is one of the most common reasons for continuing or resuming CS. The mechanism for CS lowering body weight is unknown, but it appears to relate to an acute calorigenic effect in human beings. For this reason, relationships between lipolytic, calorigenic, and dyslipidemic effects of CS were examined as part of determining the metabolic effects of CS cessation.

Methods.—Heavy smokers (more than 20 cigarettes/day) were maintained on isoenergetic constant diets for 2 weeks (1 week with and 1 week without CS). Stable isotope infusions with indirect calorimetry were performed on day 7 in each phase.

Results.—Resting energy expenditure increased in all 7 subjects after acute CS, but not significantly. Smoking increased the flux of both free fatty acids and glycerol by more than 75%, but fat oxidation was unchanged. Re-esterification of free fatty acids in the liver increased more than threefold. Neither de novo hepatic lipogenesis nor hepatic glucose production was significantly altered by smoking.

Implications.—The dyslipidemic effects of smoking may result from increased entry of free fatty acids into the circulation and their increased hepatic re-esterification, which increases VLDL-triglyceride production and alters lipids in an atherogenic direction. Because the thermogenic effect of CS is small, smokers can stop without fearing a rebound accrual of body fat as long as food intake does not increase.

▶ Viva la clinical research! No molecular probes or directional blots in this one. Good use of the UCSF General Clinical Research Center, and solid science to boot. The implication of the results here is that the CS-induced hepatic re-esterification of free fatty acids from their increased flux contributes to their proatherogenic profile. It would be informative to know just what kind of triglyceride-rich particle produced under these conditions predominates. Is it apolipoprotein B only, apo B:C, or apo B:C:E (*Prog Lipid Res* 30:105, 1991)? Do they have a high affinity for cholesteryl ester transfer protein? Are they more susceptible to oxidative modification?—J.D. Bagdade, M.D.

Effects of Intensive Lipid-Lowering Therapy on the Coronary Arteries of Asymptomatic Subjects With Elevated Apolipoprotein B
Zhao X-Q, Brown G, Hillger L, Sacco D, Bisson B, Fisher L, Albers JJ (Univ of Washington, Seattle)
Circulation 88:2744–2753, 1993   112-95-9-5

Background.—Intensive lipid-lowering therapy not only reduces the frequency of cardiovascular events in patients with established coronary heart disease and in patients with hyperlipidemia, but also enhances regression and reduces the progression of preexisting atherosclerotic lesions. Data from the Familial Atherosclerosis Treatment Study (FATS) were analyzed to determine whether intensive lipid-lowering therapy benefits individuals with a high-risk profile who have never had symptoms.

Patients.—Of the 120 men who completed the 30-month FATS protocol, 91 were symptomatic with clinically proven coronary artery disease, and 29 were asymptomatic. All had apolipoprotein B greater than or

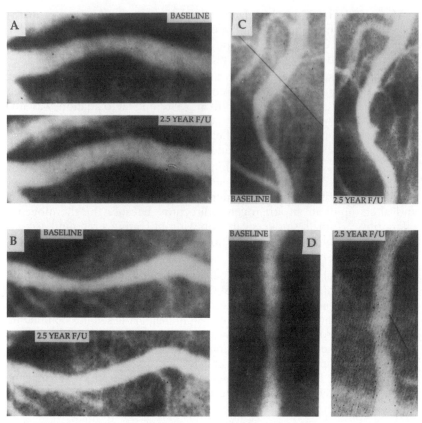

Fig 9–2.—Arteriographic examples of regression in asymptomatic patients treated intensively. **A,** proximal left anterior descending coronary artery (LAD) lesion, percent stenosis decreased from 31% to 17%. **B,** mid-LAD lesion, percent stenosis decreased from 46% to 23%. **C,** right coronary artery lesion, percent stenosis decreased from 48% to 30% with ulceration. **D,** a first diagonal lesion, percent stenosis decreased from 69% to 53%. *Abbreviation:* F/U, follow-up. (Courtesy of Zhao X-Q, Brown G, Hillger L, et al: *Circulation* 88:2744–2753, 1993.)

equal to 125 mg/dL, family history of premature cardiovascular events, and coronary atherosclerosis.

Treatment.—In a double-blind, placebo-controlled trial, the patients were randomly assigned to intensive therapy with colestipol (10 g 3 times daily) plus niacin (1 g 4 times daily); colestipol plus lovastatin (20 mg twice daily); or to conventional therapy (placebo) or colestipol if LDL cholesterol was elevated. All patients received dietary counseling. End points included quantitative arteriographic disease change and clinical events over a 2.5-year interval.

Outcome.—At baseline, symptomatic and asymptomatic patients had comparable LDL/HDL ratios, lipoprotein(a) levels, and conventional risk factors. As expected, asymptomatic patients had less severe angiographic evidence of disease than did symptomatic patients. Symptomatic patients treated intensively had less (24% vs. 48%) definite proximal lesion progression and more regression (15% vs. 36%) than did those treated conventionally. Likewise, in the intensively treated asymptomatic patients, definite progression was observed less frequently (19% vs. 38%), and evidence of regression was greater (31% vs. 0%) (Fig 9-2). The extent of the beneficial effects of intensive therapy was similar in symptomatic and asymptomatic patients. Death, myocardial infarction, or revascularization occurred in 7% of symptomatic patients treated intensively, compared with 26% of symptomatic patients in the conventional group; none of the asymptomatic patients had clinical events.

Conclusion.—Despite comparable high-risk profiles, asymptomatic patients have less coronary disease at baseline and have an excellent and better short-term clinical prognosis than symptomatic patients. However, arterial disease progresses in a similar proportion of both symptomatic and asymptomatic patients treated with conventional therapy, whereas regression of arterial disease occurs with intensive lipid-lowering therapy in a similar proportion of each group. These findings support an active treatment strategy such as the current guidelines of the National Cholesterol Education Program, which target LDL cholesterol to be less than 130 mg/dL in high-risk asymptomatic patients.

▶ Another example of the continuing yield of important and useful information from a well-designed (and well-funded) clinical trial (FATS). The bottom line here is that arterial disease is reversible in both symptomatic and asymptomatic high-risk patients. In the context of health care reform, this preventive strategy seems eminently cost-effective.—J.D. Bagdade, M.D.

Mechanisms of Atherogenesis

Intact Human Ceruloplasmin Oxidatively Modifies Low Density Lipoprotein

Ehrenwald E, Chisolm GM, Fox PL (Cleveland Clinic Research Inst, Ohio)
J Clin Invest 93:1493–1501, 1994   112-95-9–6

Background.—Ceruloplasmin is an abundant plasma protein that carries 95% of the copper found in blood. Although its elevation after inflammation and trauma has led to its classification as an acute phase protein, its physiologic role is still unclear. In the light of the observation that ceruloplasmin suppresses the oxidation of lipids, the effects of ceruloplasmin on the oxidation of plasma LDL were investigated.

Methods.—Low-density lipoprotein was isolated by sequential ultracentrifugation from freshly drawn, citrated normolipemic plasma. Immediately before use, LDL was extensively dialyzed at 4°C against saline. Low-density lipoprotein was oxidized by incubation with copper sulfate and other test materials in .05 mL phosphate-buffered saline for 20 to 24 hours at 37°C. Lipoprotein oxidation was measured as formation of thiobarbituric acid-reacting substances (TBARS).

Results.—Contrary to expectations, human ceruloplasmin was found to enhance rather than suppress copper ion–mediated oxidation of LDL. Ceruloplasmin increased the oxidative modification of LDL, estimated as at least 25-fold in 20 hours, and increased electrophoretic mobility, concentrations of conjugated dienes, and total lipid peroxides in plasma. In contrast, when ceruloplasmin was first degraded to a complex containing 115- and 19-kD fragments, it inhibited the cupric ion–induced oxidation of LDL. The antioxidant capacity of degraded ceruloplasmin in this system was similar to that of other proteins including albumin. The fact that ultrafiltration failed to remove the copper in ceruloplasmin responsible for oxidant activity suggested that it was tightly associated with the protein. Treatment of ceruloplasmin with Chelex-100, which removed 1 of 7 copper atoms per molecule, completely blocked oxidant activity. Once copper was restored to ceruloplasmin, its oxidant activity resumed.

Conclusion.—Purified, undegraded human ceruloplasmin has potent oxidant, rather than antioxidant, activity on LDL. This copper-carrying protein may play a role in the oxidation of LDL in blood or in the arterial wall, and its physiologic role may be quite different from what is commonly believed.

▶ This series of observations emphasizes the importance of laboratory technique. It seems that the notion that ceruloplasmin was an antioxidant was related to the finding that the commercially available form had this property, but (as the authors show here) not the material isolated from fresh plasma that removes a contaminating metalloproteinase that would break down ceruloplasmin into smaller fragments. Paradoxically, these fragments that were generated in the commercial preparation method had antioxidant properties and were responsible for the spurious conclusion that ceruloplasmin was an antioxidant. Its ability to oxidatively modify LDL may account for recent evidence showing that it is an independent risk factor of cardiovascular disease (*Am J Epidemiol* 136:1982, 1992).—J.D. Bagdade, M.D.

Genetic Evidence for a Common Pathway Mediating Oxidative Stress, Inflammatory Gene Induction, and Aortic Fatty Streak Formation in Mice

Liao F, Andalibi A, Qiao J-H, Allayee H, Fogelman AM, Lusis AJ (Univ of California, Los Angeles)
J Clin Invest 94:877–884, 1994   112-95-9-7

Background.—Studies of inbred mice given an atherogenic diet have shown that susceptibility to aortic atherosclerosis correlates with the accumulation of lipid peroxidation products as well as the induction of inflammatory genes and the activation of NF-kB–like transcription factors. NF-kB is activated by oxidative stress. The pattern of gene activation resembles that seen after injecting minimally modified LDL. The hypothesis that oxidized lipids stimulated processes at the gene level related to inflammation was tested.

Objective.—Studies were carried out in BXH recombinant inbred mice, derived from susceptible and resistant parental mice, to examine relationships among the activation of NF-kB–like transcription factor, the induction of hepatic inflammatory genes, and the development of fatty streaks in the aorta.

Results.—Both the induction of inflammatory genes and the activation of NF-kB–like transcription factors were found to cosegregate with the formation of atherosclerotic lesions in the aortas of recombinant inbred mice. Inflammatory gene activation correlated with the accumulation of conjugated dienes in the liver.

Implications.—The induction of inflammatory mediators secondary to oxidative stress appears to have a key role in the process of atherogenesis. In this murine model, a gene designated *Ath-1* may regulate the accumulation of lipid peroxides in tissue or the cellular response to peroxides.

▶ The concept that atherosclerosis is a local inflammatory process is not new. Now it seems likely that it is not only a local phenomenon but rather a systemic one; evidence here demonstrates in mice that conjugated diene products of only mild lipoprotein oxidation that accumulate in the liver can activate genes for monocyte chemotactic protein, inflammatory serum amyloid, and heme oxygenase. Data of this type strengthen the growing body of evidence for the "lipoprotein oxidation hypothesis" for atherosclerosis.—J.D. Bagdade, M.D.

Osteopontin mRNA Is Expressed by Smooth Muscle-Derived Cells in Human Atherosclerotic Lesions of the Aorta
Ikeda T, Shirasawa T, Esaki Y, Yoshiki S, Hirokawa K (Tokyo Metropolitan Inst of Gerontology; Tokyo Metropolitan Geriatric Hosp; Showa Univ, Tokyo)
J Clin Invest 92:2814–2820, 1993   112-95-9–8

Background.—Atherosclerosis is commonly accompanied by calcification, although the mechanism of calcification is unclear. Some noncollagenous bone matrix proteins are thought to be associated with the induction of aortic calcification because they influence the local mechanism of calcification. In fact, messenger RNA (mRNA) of osteopontin, a bone matrix protein, is found in the kidney, where calcification often occurs. Atherosclerotic lesions were analyzed for the presence of osteopontin, and the role of osteopontin in the calcification of these lesions was examined.

Method.—Aortic samples were examined for expression of osteopontin mRNA by Northern blot analysis and in situ hybridization.

Results.—The expression of osteopontin was found in 24 of 25 samples of aorta obtained from 17 autopsies, but it was not present in a single normal aortic sample. The magnitude of expression of osteopontin was seen to be proportional to the stage of atherosclerosis. Osteopontin mRNA positive cells were found scattered in the thickened intimal layer of fibro-fatty lesions of the aorta. In fibrous plaques, hybridization signals were detected around the fibrous mass. In advanced plaques, the signals were seen in the wall around atheromatous debris. At higher magnification of serial neighboring sections, the cells expressing osteopontin mRNA were found to be foam cells. Further analysis revealed that deposition of calcium and hybridization signals were seen side by side, closely associated with each other. Immunohistological analysis revealed that the foam cells expressing osteopontin mRNA were smooth muscle–derived cells.

Conclusion.—Smooth muscle–derived foam cells express osteopontin mRNA in atherosclerotic lesions of the aorta, and the magnitude of this expression is proportional to the severity of the lesion. Although the function of osteopontin in bone tissue is still not fully understood, its strong capacity to bind hydroxyapatite suggests that it plays an important role in calcification and is therefore likely to be implicated in the calcification of atherosclerotic lesions.

▶ This would appear to be a major mechanism contributing to calcification of atherosclerotic lesions. What then turns on the osteopontin gene? Aren't the products of lipoprotein oxidation obvious candidates?—J.D. Bagdade, M.D.

Expression of α_2-Macroglobulin Receptor/Low Density Lipoprotein Receptor–Related Protein and Scavenger Receptor in Human Atherosclerotic Lesions
Luoma J, Hiltunen T, Särkioja T, Moestrup SK, Gliemann G, Kodama T, Nikkari T, Ylä-Herttuala (Univ of Tampere, Finland; Univ of Oulu, Finland; Univ of Aarhus, Denmark; et al)
J Clin Invest 93:2014–2021, 1994   112-95-9-9

Background.—The first visible atherosclerotic lesions found in human beings are fatty streaks, which consist of lipid-loaded foam cells derived from macrophage and smooth muscle cells (SMCs). At least 3 receptor systems have been recognized that could be involved in the development of foam cells: α_2-macroglobulin receptor/LDL receptor–related protein (α_2MR/LRP), scavenger receptor, and LDL receptor. The role of these receptors in human arteries was investigated.

Method.—The expression of each of the above receptors was studied in human atherosclerotic lesions by in situ hybridization and immunocytochemistry.

Results.—An abundance of α_2MR/LRP messenger RNA and protein was found in both macrophage- and SMC-containing areas of both early and advanced lesions in human aortas; α_2MR/LRP was also found to be present in SMCs of normal aortas. Scavenger receptor mRNA and protein were found in lesion macrophages but not in lesion SMCs. Low-density-lipoprotein receptor was not found in the lesion area, but it was expressed in some aortas in medial SMCs around the adventitial border.

Conclusion.—The results of this study show that α_2MR/LRP is the only lipoprotein receptor expressed by lesion SMCs in vivo, whereas macrophages have both scavenger and α_2MR/LRP receptors. Both receptors may contribute to the formation of macrophage-derived foam cells. So far, α_2MR/LRP is the only receptor expressed in arterial smooth muscle cells in vivo that is capable of mediating the uptake of lipoproteins, and it is likely that it plays an important role in the formation of SMC-derived foam cells. Further studies are required to establish the role of α_2MR/LRP as a functional lipoprotein receptor in arterial cells and to clarify the regulation of its expression and scavenger receptor in lesion cells.

▶ Because human lesion SMCs do not express detectable amounts of either scavenger receptors or LDL receptors, there was much to support a role for an endocytotic receptor related to the LDL receptor that played a role in their accumulating lipid. In addition to showing that the α_2MR/LRP is indeed present in human lesions and expressed abundantly in SMCs, the findings from the group in Tampere suggest that it may play a central role in the accumulation in arterial wall cells of certain classes of lipoproteins long presumed to be atherogenic, such as apolipoprotein E–enriched chylomicron and VLDL remnants, lipoprotein lipase (LpL), and LpL-triglyceride–rich lipoprotein complexes.—J.D. Bagdade, M.D.

Effects of Diet

Fish Consumption and Risk of Stroke: The Zutphen Study

Keli SO, Feskens EJM, Kromhout D (Natl Inst of Public Health and Environmental Protection, Bilthoven, The Netherlands)
Stroke 25:328–332, 1994   112-95-9–10

Background.—The incidence of stroke in Danish individuals is lower than that of Greenland Eskimos, possibly because Danish persons consume less fish than do Eskimos. Although it is known that low-to-moderate daily fish consumption protects against coronary heart disease, its effect on stroke is unclear.

Method.—To investigate the effect of fish consumption on stroke risk, food intake data were analyzed by the cross-check dietary history method in 552 men aged 50–69 years during 1960, 1965, and 1970. Each participant was interviewed regarding usual food consumption patterns on weekdays and weekends during the months May, June, and July of each year. The association between fish consumption and stroke incidence from 1970 to 1985 was assessed by Cox proportional hazards models. Adjustments were made for confounding by age, systolic blood pressure, cigarette smoking, serum total cholesterol, energy intake, alcohol consumption, and prescribed diet.

Results.—The mean fish consumption in 1970 was 17.9 g/day. Men who consumed more than 20 g of fish per day in 1970 showed a significantly lower risk of stroke compared with those who ate less fish (hazard ratio: .49; 95% confidence interval: .24 to .99). The hazard ratio did not change, after adjustment for the above confounding variables. The 301 men who always ate fish between 1960 and 1970 had a reduced risk of stroke compared with the 251 men who never ate fish, or who changed their fish-eating habits in the same time period (hazard ratio: .63, which increased to .71 after adjustment for potential confounders).

Conclusion.—An inverse relation may exist between fish consumption and stroke incidence. More studies are required to explain this inverse relation. These findings imply that the consumption of at least 1 portion of fish per week may have a protective effect in the prevention of cerebral as well as cardiovascular disease.

▶ This is the first time that an inverse relation between fish consumption and stroke has been reported. The results here are consistent with other prospective studies showing a similar inverse dose-response relationship between small amounts of fish consumption and long-term mortality from coronary heart disease (Kromhout et al: *N Engl J Med* 312:1205, 1985). However, there can be too much of a good thing (i.e., n-3 polyunsaturated eicosapentaenoic and docosahexaenoic fatty acids); Eskimos who consume very large amounts of fish have a higher incidence of hemorrhagic strokes. One portion of fish per week may have a protective effect on both stroke and coronary heart disease.—J.D. Bagdade, M.D.

Effects of Dietary Fat Content, Saturated Fatty Acids, and Fish Oil on Eicosanoid Production and Hemostatic Parameters in Normal Men
Nordoy A, Hatcher L, Goodnight S, Fitzgerald GA, Connor WE (Oregon Health Sciences Univ, Portland; Vanderbilt Univ, Nashville, Tenn; Univ of Tromsø, Norway)
J Lab Clin Med 123:914–920, 1994   112-95-9–11

Background.—Eskimo and Japanese persons consume diets high in marine foods rich in very-long-chain polyunsaturated fatty acids of the n-3 family and have low death rates from coronary heart disease. These populations also ingest less than one half of the dietary saturated fatty acids traditionally ingested by Western societies. In contrast, even though some Western populations have a high level of fish they still have an increased intake of saturated fat, which is presumed to contribute to their high rates of coronary heart disease. To determine whether concomitant saturated fat intake counteracts the beneficial effects of n-3 fatty acids on in vivo platelet and vascular eicosanoid formation and other hemostatic parameters associated with arterial thrombosis, the following studies were performed.

Study Design.—Six normolipemic healthy men were fed diets that contained high and low levels of saturated fat (19% and 5% of total calories). During 3-week periods, with an intervening washout period of 6 weeks, the men were given diets with a low (25% of total fat energy) and high (39% of energy) fat content with and without inclusion of n-3 polyunsaturated or monounsaturated fatty acids (2% of energy). Fasting blood samples for lipid analysis, coagulation studies, and hematologic parameters were collected before and at the end of each dietary intervention.

Results.—The effects of n-3 fatty acids on the fatty acid composition of the principal plasma liquid fractions were similar, independent of the saturated-fat content of the diet. In vivo thromboxane A_2 production declined when n-3 fatty acids were added to the low-fat diet. Prostacyclin production declined on a low-fat diet, and did not change when n-3 fatty acids were added. Thromboxane A_3 and prostacyclin I_3 increased modestly on both low- and high-saturated-fat diets even when n-3 fatty acids were added. Antithrombin levels and concentrations of other coagulation factors were unchanged by n-3 supplementation to either diet. However, a moderate but significant prolongation of the bleeding time was observed in those individuals given the low saturated fat diet supplemented with n-3 fatty acids. This prolongation was paralleled, but did not correlate, with an inhibition of thromboxane synthesis, suggesting that the platelet-inhibitory effects of n-3 fatty acids were potentiated by a reduction in dietary saturated fat content.

Discussion.—The effects of eicosapentaenoic and docosahexaenoic acids on platelet and vascular function and eicosanoid production are influenced by the dietary content of saturated fatty acids. These interactions may explain the relationship between the consumption of fish and the occurrence of coronary heart disease in populations differing in their consumption of saturated fat. A low-fat diet supplemented with n-3 fatty acids most favorably affects platelet function and platelet vascular interactions.

▶ Are the results here not comparable to the situation in which patients treated with a reductase inhibitor think that their all-powerful drug can negate the adverse effects of dietary indiscretions? Of course, the dietary mix of saturated and unsaturated fatty acids is important, and those that are saturated continue to be the "bad guys;" here they attenuate the favorable effects of the n-3 fatty acids on hemostatic parameters.—J.D. Bagdade, M.D.

Dietary Cholesterol and Downregulation of Cholesterol 7α-Hydroxylase and Cholesterol Absorption in African Green Monkeys

Rudel L, Deckelman C, Wilson M, Scobey M, Anderson R (Wake Forest Univ, Winston-Salem, NC)

J Clin Invest 93:2463–2472, 1994   112-95-9–12

Introduction.—Regulation of the disposition of dietary cholesterol after absorption is not clear. The liver clears the bulk of lipoprotein cholesterol from plasma while, at the same time, secreting new lipoproteins containing cholesterol into plasma. Candidate sites in the liver for regulation of dietary cholesterol include proteins involved in lipoprotein particle clearance from plasma, such as the LDL receptor, hepatic lipase, and apolipoprotein B-100. To determine which components of cholesterol balance across the liver are responsive to dietary cholesterol, 45 male African green monkeys were studied; their lipoprotein and cholesterol metabolism is similar to that in humans. Sequential liver biopsies were taken during 3 different dietary periods containing varying amounts of cholesterol and were analyzed for cholesterol, cholesterol 7α-hydroxylase (C7H), and hepatic lipase messenger RNA (mRNA). Blood, fecal, and bile samples were collected at varying intervals, and cholesterol absorption was measured.

Results.—The percentage of cholesterol absorbed in the intestine was significantly lower when higher levels of cholesterol were fed. Liver concentrations of free and esterified cholesterol were significantly elevated by dietary cholesterol challenge and remained so even after 20 weeks of low-cholesterol diets. Cholesterol absorption percentages indicated that when more cholesterol was available for absorption, a significant link was found between cholesterol absorption percentage and total plasma cholesterol. Hepatic cholesterol and C7H mRNA abundance was significantly lower when the high-cholesterol diet was fed, with the decrease being greater than that seen for the LDL-receptor mRNA. Hepatic lipase mRNA abundance and apo B mRNA abundance were not sensitive to diet and had no correlation with C7H mRNA abundance. Bile acid activity decreased with downregulation of C7H.

Conclusion.—The liver may attempt to downregulate intestinal cholesterol absorption to maintain hepatic cholesterol balance by decreasing bile acid production when increased amounts of absorbed dietary cholesterol reach the liver. Regulation of C7H by dietary cholesterol could be a major component of hepatic bile acid production and thus of importance in premature development of coronary artery disease and cholesterol gallstones in African green monkeys.

▶ This represents this group's most recent efforts to explain the intrahepatic mechanisms that promote increased LDL concentrations induced by dietary cholesterol. The results demonstrate the importance of the primate model in studying cholesterol metabolism. Previous work in the rat led to the spurious conclusion that ingested cholesterol upregulated both C7H activity and mRNA abundance and that this was a general phenomenon. Increase the excretion of cholesterol by upregulating its conversion to bile acids, right? The primate data reported here indicate the contrary—a downregulation of C7H; reducing bile acid secretion may reflect an effort to limit cholesterol absorption. The problem for us is that we may be stuck with excessive intrahepatic cholesterol that will be incorporated into potentially atherogenic lipoproteins.—J.D. Bagdade, M.D.

Effects of Exercise

Kinetics of Lipids, Apolipoproteins, and Cholesteryl Ester Transfer Protein in Plasma After a Bicycle Marathon

Föger B, Wohlfarter T, Ritsch A, Lechleitner M, Miller CH, Dienstl A, Patsch JR (Univ of Innsbruck, Austria)
Metabolism 43:633–639, 1994   112-95-9-13

Introduction.—Although the effects of aerobic exercise on lipoprotein transport have been extensively studied, little information is available on its impact on the mass and activity of cholesteryl ester transfer protein (CETP), which is now recognized to be an important regulator of HDL cholesterol levels.

Methods.—Serum lipid studies were performed in 8 amateur endurance-trained athletes 2 days before and on days 1, 2, 3, 5, and 8 after a 230-km bicycle marathon.

Results.—Cholesterol and LDLs were significantly decreased on days 1-3. Triglycerides decreased 63% on day 1, steadily increasing to baseline by day 5. High-density lipoproteins increased during days 1 to 5, returning to baseline by day 8, as did HDL_2 and HDL_3 cholesterol. The HDL subfraction HDL_2 cholesterol demonstrated the most drastic change, with an increase of almost 100% on day 3. The HDL subfraction HDL_3 decreased below baseline. Significant increases in apolipoprotein (apo) A-I and apo A-II were noted by day 8. Mean plasma CETP mass of the athletes before the race was comparable to that of the controls. After exertion, CETP mass dropped significantly by day 2 and still had not reached baseline by day 8, with similar changes in CETP activity. The CETP mass decrease was directly related to an increase in HDL_2 and an increase in the HDL_2 to HDL_3 ratio. No correlation between CETP mass and HDL_3 cholesterol and HDL apolipoproteins was found.

Conclusion.—Major changes in plasma lipids, for the most part attributable to increases in lipoprotein lipase, occurred after strenuous exercise, requiring 5 days to return to baseline. Also contributing to the changes in lipoproteins and the increase in HDL cholesterol is the significant decrease in the mass and activity of CETP. The magnitude of the observed changes is comparable to or exceeds the therapeutic effects of the most potent antilipemic drugs.

▶ There is an important message here about lipoprotein lipase (LPL) that deserves further study. Our current perception of CETP activity is that it is proatherogenic and that it is activated by LPL (i.e., the postprandial state being the prototype situation for LPL-CETP interaction during which, by the way, those nasty postprandial modified lipoproteins are generated). The exercise paradigm shown here is that exercise-induced stimulation of LPL activity turns off CETP activity! Is this a reflection of differences in the actions of skeletal muscle and adipose tissue LPL? Or is a different (i.e., family) kind of triglyceride-rich lipoprotein metabolized during exercise?—J.D. Bagdade, M.D.

Effects of Drug Therapy

Inhibitors of Angiotensin Converting Enzyme Decrease Early Atherosclerosis in Hyperlipidemic Hamsters: Fosinopril Reduces Plasma Cholesterol and Captopril Inhibits Macrophage–Foam Cell Accumulation Independently of Blood Pressure and Plasma Lipids
Kowala MC, Grove RI, Aberg G (Bristol-Myers Squibb Pharmaceutical Research Inst, Princeton, NJ; Bristol-Myers Squibb Pharmaceutical Research Inst, Seattle)
Atherosclerosis 108:61–72, 1994   112-95-9–14

Objectives.—Angiotensin-converting enzyme (ACE) inhibitors, such as captopril, have been shown to prevent atherosclerosis in Watanabe heritable hyperlipidemic rabbits, in cholesterol-fed monkeys, and in hypertensive rats fed cholesterol. However, ACE inhibitors also reduce blood pressure, suggesting that a reduction in blood pressure protects arteries from developing lesions. Whether ACE inhibitors can modulate atherosclerosis without altering blood pressure was determined.

Study Design.—The effects of 2 ACE inhibitors, fosinopril and captopril, on ACE activity, blood pressure, plasma cholesterol, and atherosclerosis were compared in hamsters fed chow supplemented with .05% cholesterol and 10% coconut oil.

Results.—In the blood pressure studies, fosinopril reduced blood pressure acutely, whereas chronic treatment with fosinopril and captopril had no effect on blood pressure. In the pressor studies, both fosinopril and captopril inhibited the angiotensin I pressor response, indicating that these agents suppressed ACE activity in vivo. Fosinopril reduced total plasma cholesterol by 17%, VLDL plus LDL cholesterol by 27%, and total triglycerides by 45%. Captopril reduced HDL cholesterol by 20%. Neither drug altered blood pressure at 3 weeks. En face preparations of the lesion-prone aortic arch from controls were stained with oil red O for lipids and showed numerous subendothelial macrophage–foam cells embedded along the inner curvature. Fosinopril reduced the number (by

85%) and foam cell size (by 38%) of intimal macrophage–foam cells/ mm² and fatty streak area (by 90%), whereas captopril decreased these parameters by 44%, 16%, and 53% respectively.

Conclusion.—Captopril appears to decrease atherosclerosis by inhibiting ACE activity in vivo without affecting plasma LDL cholesterol or blood pressure. Inhibiting ACE appears to directly impede the accumulation and formation of arterial macrophage–foam cells. Fosinopril has the additional property of suppressing the development of the fatty streak by decreasing plasma LDL cholesterol.

▶ This adds to the growing body of evidence that angiotensin has local effects on the behavior of arterial wall cells whose activities not only contribute to foam cell formation but also have salutary effects on chronic inflammation (Schrier et al: *J Clin Invest* 69:651, 1982) and restenosis and hypertrophy of the arterial intima (Owens: *Circ Res* 56:525, 1985), independent of blood pressure.—J.D. Bagdade, M.D.

Probucol and Other Antioxidants Prevent the Inhibition of Endothelium-Dependent Relaxation by Low Density Lipoproteins
Plane F, Jacobs M, McManus D, Bruckdorfer KR (Royal Free Hosp, London)
Atherosclerosis 103:73–79, 1993   112-95-9–15

Background.—It has been proposed that increased plasma levels of LDL and its oxidative products have an important pathogenetic role in atherosclerosis. Oxidized LDL (oxLDL) has been identified in atherosclerotic lesions, and there is evidence in experimental animals that the antioxidant probucol, may prevent the disease. Vasodilation mediated by the release of endothelium-derived nitric oxide (endothelium-derived releasing factor) is impaired in atherosclerosis. The defect may be an early marker of the disease, and it correlates with increased plasma LDL.

Objective.—The effects of antioxidants including probucol and ascorbic acid on the inhibitory effect of native LDL were examined in vitro.

Findings.—Both probucol, 10 μM, and ascorbic acid, 100 μM, prevented the inhibitory effect of LDL on acetylcholine-evoked vasodilation of rabbit aortic rings. The antioxidants did not alter the inhibitory effect of oxLDL. Superoxide dismutase did not influence the effects of either native LDL or oxLDL. Low-density lipoprotein from 3 subjects who had taken probucol orally for 10 days was much less vulnerable to oxidation and no longer inhibited vascular relaxation.

Implication.—Administration of an antioxidant may well help prevent impaired coronary vasodilation, an early consequence of hypercholesterolemia and a marker of atherosclerosis.

▶ Further evidence here that products of lipid oxidation directly interfere with arterial relaxation and endothelial-dependent vasodilation. Nasty substances, aren't they? But what are they precisely? We still don't know. And besides free radical scavengers, what other protective systems are operative? Lecithin cholesterol/acyltransferase may be one. This ubiquitous plasma enzyme does a lot more than esterify. It clearly will meet Dan Steinberg's definition of being a "good guy" and will wear a white hat on those pathway slides if my colleague Subbaiah's efforts materialize (and the National Institutes of Health provides him the basic support to do so).—J.D. Bagdade, M.D.

Effect of Gemfibrozil on Adipose Tissue and Muscle Lipoprotein Lipase

Simsolo RB, Ong JM, Kern PA (Cedars-Sinai Med Ctr, Los Angeles)
Metabolism 42:1486–1491, 1993   112-95-9–16

Introduction.—Plasma triglyceride levels are lowered by decreasing VLDL triglyceride output by the liver or by increasing triglyceride-rich lipoprotein removal. Triglyceride-rich lipoproteins are catabolized by action of lipoprotein lipase (LPL), which is found primarily in adipose and muscle tissues. Gemfibrozil is believed to decrease hepatic VLDL production, but its effect on LPL are unclear. The action of gemfibrozil on adipose tissue and muscle LPL was investigated.

Methods.—Sixteen patients were divided into 3 groups, based on cause of hypertriglyceridemia (inherited, diabetes, or chronic renal disease) and were studied with adipose tissue and muscle biopsies, plasma lipids, glycosylated hemoglobin, and thyroid function before and 6 weeks after gemfibrozil treatment.

Results.—In all 3 groups, HDL levels increased and serum triglyceride and total cholesterol decreased significantly. Adipose tissue samples showed no significant change in LPL activity, LPL immunoreactive mass, LPL synthesis, or messenger RNA levels. Muscle samples showed changes in LPL activity, but they were not significant, nor were changes in immunoreactive mass. There were no changes in weight, diet, or medications during treatment.

Conclusion.—The sporadic increases in LPL muscle activity in several patients is worth further investigation regarding development of drugs that regulate lipid metabolism. Gemfibrozil therapy does not significantly change LPL expression, suggesting that its primary mechanism is inhibition of VLDL production.

▶ The triglyceride-lowering actions of the fibrate are regarded on the basis of a number of earlier clinical studies to involve both the removal and the production of VLDL. The authors' inability to show that gemfibrozil upregulates gene expression does not, however, necessarily mean that the catabolism of triglyceride-rich lipoprotein is not increased, as earlier kinetic studies show. Changes in LPL distribution in plasma, activity, and turnover, for example, could influence VLDL kinetic behavior and hence triglyceride levels without altering gene expression. The conclusion here that VLDL synthesis must be inhibited on the basis of the results of the molecular studies reflects a tendency of the "gene-jocks" to believe that if the gene doesn't show the expected change, then the gene product must not be a player, reflects their frequent inability to explain things physiologically.—J.D. Bagdade, M.D.

The Actions of Lovastatin on Platelet Function and Platelet Eicosanoid Receptors in Type II Hypercholesterolaemia
Kaczmarek D, Hohfeld T, Wambach G, Schrör K (Heinrich-Heine Universität, Düsseldorf, Germany)
Eur J Clin Pharmacol 45:451–457, 1993   112-95-9–17

Introduction.—Patients with hypercholesterolemia have an increased risk of thrombosis as a result of platelet hyperactivity. Most previous studies show that lipid lowering agents fail to reduce platelet hyperreactivity. In an uncontrolled retrospective study, the 3-hydroxy-3-methylglutaryl coenzyme A (HMG CoA) reductase inhibitor lovastatin was found to normalize platelet function in a group of hypercholesterolemic patients.

Method.—Eighteen patients with increased triglyceride and LDL-cholesterol levels were randomly assigned to double-blind treatment with lovastatin (20 mg daily) or a placebo after 1 month of a lipid-lowering diet. Platelet function was determined at 0 and 12 weeks.

Results.—In the lovastatin group, total serum and LDL-cholesterol levels declined by 20% and 25%, respectively, and washed platelets had significantly reduced aggregation and ex vivo thromboxane formation. In addition, thromboxane and prostacyclin binding sites on platelet membranes increased significantly in the lovastatin group, but not the placebo group. Those receiving placebo had no significant change in cholesterol or in any parameter of platelet function.

Conclusion.—Lovastatin normalizes platelet function in patients with hypercholesterolemia. The changes observed in receptors for thromboxane and prostacyclin suggest that the observed alterations in platelet function result from modifications in platelet membrane composition at the megakaryocyte level.

▶ Further evidence here of the pervasive effects of the HMG CoA reductase inhibitors. Of course, they're doing more than just lowering LDL levels. Although it's reassuring to know that platelet function in these patients is normalized by lovastatin, it is disturbing that this effect may result from drug-induced changes in platelet membrane composition and receptor function. What are its long-term effects on all those "normal" cells?—J.D. Bagdade, M.D.

Suggested Reading

The following articles are recommended to the reader:

Durrington PN: Can agreement be reached on cholesterol lowering? *Br Heart J* 71:125–128, 1994.

▶ An overview of a recent meeting of the Royal College of Physicians in London confirms the value of intervention in high-risk cases and identifies the outstanding areas that require consideration.

Gröne EF, Walli AK, Gröne H-J, et al: The role of lipids in nephrosclerosis and glomerulosclerosis. *Atherosclerosis* 107:1–14, 1994.

▶ An update on this timely topic that concludes that based on data from animal studies, high plasma cholesterol levels accelerate the progression of glomerular damage.

Alaupovic P, Hodis HN, Knight-Gibson C, et al: Effects of lovastatin on apo A- and apo B-containing lipoproteins: Families in a subpopulation of patients participating in the Monitored Atherosclerosis Study (MARS). *Arterioscler Thromb* 14:1906–1914, 1994.

▶ This reductase inhibitor is highly effective in reducing levels of potentially atherogenic levels of lipoprotein particles that contain apo B only, but it is less effective in reducing other apo B–containing lipoproteins that may be equally atherogenic.

Blankenhorn DH, Hodis HN: Arterial imaging and atherosclerosis reversal. *Arterioscler Thromb* 14:177–192, 1994.

▶ This Lyman Duff Memorial Lecture by the late pioneer in the field reviews evidence for the reversibility of atherosclerosis.

10 Thyroid

Introduction

As in past years, the thyroid section has been subdivided into separate areas of interest that permit basic and clinical research to complement each other and be useful to clinicians, basic scientists, fellows, and residents. The rapid progress in the use of molecular biology techniques to define the etiology of human disease is evident in almost every area of thyroidology, including the thyroid hormone resistance syndromes, the inherited abnormalities in thyroid hormone binding, inherited pituitary hypothyroidism, mutated TSH receptors, medullary carcinoma, and epithelial cell thyroid cancers.

Animal models for studying the pathogenesis of thyroid disease, including the severe combined immunodeficiency disease mouse, continue to increase. Over the past few years, extremely sophisticated methods to define the basic etiology of this common disorder have expanded; however, no unifying hypotheses as to the pathogenesis of autoimmune thyroiditis, the effects of iodine on this process, and the etiology of Graves' ophthalmopathy have been defined. In the clinical arena, many studies are briefly described in the discussion at the end of each article in an attempt to stimulate readers to further evaluate these studies, which may have an impact on their approach to the diagnosis and management of a wide variety of thyroid diseases.

Credit for the information described in this section truly belongs to the authors of the various papers, and I am indebted to them for their help in making my task easier. I do apologize to the authors of many other studies that were more than worthy of inclusion, but space does not permit us this luxury.

Lewis E. Braverman, M.D.

Metabolism, Binding, Action of Thyroid Hormones

Down-Regulation of Type II L-Thyroxine, 5′-Monodeiodinase in Cultured GC Cells: Different Pathways of Regulation by L-Triiodothyronine and 3,3′5′-Triiodo-L-Thyronine*

Halperin Y, Shapiro LE, Surks MI (Albert Einstein College of Medicine, Bronx, NY)
Endocrinology 135:1464–1469, 1994   112-95-10–1

Background.—Iodothyronines are believed to downregulate type II T_4 monodeiodinase (5'-DII) through extranuclear acceleration of enzyme inactivation. The regulation of 5'-DII in cultured GC cells, in which nuclear thyroid receptor (TR) mediates thyroid hormone responses, were studied.

Methods and Findings.—GC cells actively converted T_4 to T_3 independent of propylthiouracil and with a K_m of 1.4 nM. These are characteristic of 5'-DII. The K_m was unaffected by GC cell incubation with 10 nM T_3. However, 10 nM T_3 significantly downregulated the maximum velocity from .15 to .018 pmol/mg protein·min. Dose-response analysis demonstrated that a 50% decrease in enzyme activity was attained with .25 nM T_3 or 12 nM rT_3. In time-course analysis, a 50% decrease in enzyme activity occurred after 40 minutes of incubation with 100 nM rT_3 and after 160 minutes of incubation with 10 nM T_3.

Conclusion.—The downregulation of 5'-DII by these iodothryonines in GC cells may occur by different mechanisms, including enzyme inactivation for rT_3, in accord with the current consensus, and reduced enzyme production for T_3, probably mediated by TR.

▶ The downregulation of 5'-DII by thyroid hormones has been recognized for years, and this paper defines 2 different pathways for this decrease: enzyme inactivation by rT_3 as previously described and decreased enzyme production by T_3 as now reported. Everts et al. (*Endocrinology* 134:2490, 1994) emphasize the importance of the uptake of thyroid hormones by cultured rat anterior pituitary cells and suggest that T_4 and T_3 share a common carrier in these cultured cells.—L.E. Braverman, M.D.

3,5,3'-Triiodothyronine (T$_3$) Sulfate: A Major Metabolite in T$_3$ Metabolism in Man

LoPresti JS, Nicoloff JT (Univ of Southern California, Los Angeles)
J Clin Endocrinol Metab 78:688–692, 1994   112-95-10–2

Background.—Previous studies have shown that T_3 metabolism depends more on nondeiodinative conjugation than direct deiodinative degradation for its disposal in human beings. The qualitative aspects of T_3 to T_3S formation and whether sulfation may be influenced by variations in circulating T_3 levels were investigated.

Participants and Methods.—Five healthy males aged 32–52 years were studied. Tracer T_3 kinetic studies were undertaken before and after iopanoic acid (IA) administration to selectively impair T_3 deiodinative disposal. Low .5-g load, followed by .5 g/day for 7 days and high (3.0-g load, followed by 3.0 g/day for 7 days) dosing schedules were used to obtain varying levels of deiodinase inhibition. High IA doses were repeated with simultaneous oral T_3 administration at 100 µg daily to normalize serum T_3 levels that were decreased by IA-induced inhibition of T_4 to T_3 conversion.

Results.—A significant reduction in baseline serum T_3 and T_3/T_4 values (2.3 $\pm$ 0.1 nmol/L and 1.9 $\pm$ 0.1 $\times$ 10^{-2}, respectively) was observed for both the low IA (1.5 $\pm$ 0.1 nmol/L and 1.2 $\pm$ 0.1 $\times 10^{-2}$, respectively), and the high IA (1.5 $\pm$ 0.1 nmol/L and 0.9 $\pm$ 0.2 $\times$ 10^{-2}, respectively) dosing schedules. The addition of oral T_3 to the high IA schedule restored both T_3 and T_3/T_4 values to near-normal levels (2.9 $\pm$ 0.3 nmol/L and 1.7 $\pm$ 0.2 $\times$ 10^{-2}, respectively). Low IA also significantly decreased T_3 clearance and fractional urinary tracer recovery (30 $\pm$ 4 to 18 $\pm$ 2 L/day and 70 $\pm$ 3% to 37 $\pm$ 4%, respectively). Conversely, high IA demonstrated only a minor further decrease in clearance and urinary tracer recovery (16 $\pm$ 2 L/day and 32 $\pm$ 3%, respectively). Compared to the effects of high IA only, simultaneous oral administration of T_3 unexpectedly resulted in a significant increase of T_3 clearance (23 $\pm$ 4 L/day), without altering urinary tracer recovery (34 $\pm$ 5%).

Conclusion.—The urinary T_3 metabolite pattern showed that the major products of T_3 metabolism were T_3 sulfate and 3,3-diiodothyronine sulfate, verifying previous reports that suggest most nondeiodinative T_3 disposal occurs through T_3 sulfate formation. Nondeiodinative disposal may also be influenced by the circulating T_3 level, indicating that sulfotransferase enzyme systems could play a major role in regulating the prereceptor availability of this ligand.

▶ Chopra and colleagues used a new in vitro assay to study T_3 sulfation activity in various rat tissues and concluded that sulfation activity is rich in liver, kidney, and brain in adult rats; is very abundant in fetal rat skin early in gestation; and is unaffected by thyroid status (*Endocrinology* 133:1951, 1993). The other major conjugation pathway in the liver for thyroid hormone metabolism, glucuronidation, has been studied by Visser and co-workers (*Endocrinology* 135:1004, 1994), who emphasize the rapid rates of glucuronidation of tetrac and triac by both rat and human hepatic microsomes, at least partially explaining the short half-life and low bioactivity of triac in vivo.—L.E. Braverman, M.D.

Effect of Triidothyronine on Postischemic Myocardial Function in the Isolated Heart
Kadletz M, Mullen PG, Ding M, Wolfe LG, Wechsler AS (Med College of Virginia-Virginia Commonwealth Univ, Richmond)
Ann Thorac Surg 57:657–662, 1994   112-95-10–3

Introduction.—Thyroid dysfunction significantly affects cardiac function. Patients undergoing cardiopulmonary bypass may have a euthyroid-sick syndrome develop. It is thought that the decline in the free T_3 levels may be a cause of postoperative myocardial complications. Clinical trials have shown improvements in myocardial recovery after ischemia with T_3

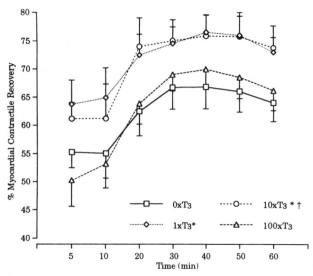

Fig 10–1.—Myocardial contractile recovery after minimal (4 mm Hg) ischemia. Triiodothyronine at both the physiologic (1 × T₃) and 10 times the physiologic (10 × T₃) concentration significantly improved myocardial function. Triiodothyronine at one hundred times the physiologic concentration (100 × T₃) had no beneficial effect. (*P < .05 compared with control values [0 × T₃]; †P < .05 compared with 100 × T₃.) (Courtesy of Kadletz M, Mullen PG, Ding M, et al: *Ann Thorac Surg* 57:657–662, 1994.)

supplementation that restores physiologic levels. It was hypothesized that myocardial recovery with T₃ may be dose-related. The effects of graduated doses of T₃ on postischemic rabbit hearts were studied.

Methods.—The isolated hearts of 57 rabbits were subjected to normothermic global ischemia until myocardial contracture reached 4 mm Hg in 1 cohort or 15 mm Hg in the other cohort. After ischemia, the hearts in each cohort were reperfused with either a physiologic concentration of T₃, 10 or 100 times the physiologic concentration of T₃, or carrier solution only. Hemodynamic variables and coronary flow were monitored regularly for 60 minutes after ischemia. After 60 minutes, the ventricular wet–dry ratio was assessed. Postischemic parameters were compared with preischemic parameters.

Results.—In the hearts with 4 mm Hg ischemic contracture, myocardial contractile recovery was significantly improved with infusions of 1 and 10 times the physiologic concentration of T₃, whereas recovery was nonsignificantly slower in the hearts treated with 100 times the physiologic concentration, compared with controls (Fig 10–1). In the hearts with 15 mm Hg ischemic contracture, myocardial contractile recovery was slightly improved with treatment with the physiologic concentration of T₃ and significantly improved with 10 times the physiologic concentration, whereas 100 times the physiologic concentration significantly decreased recovery compared with the controls. Differences in coronary flow among groups were not significant, nor were there significant differences in the wet–dry weight ratios.

Discussion.—Reperfusion with physiologic concentrations of T_3 brought significant improvements in myocardial function only in mildly ischemic hearts. Severely ischemic hearts required 10 times the physiologic concentration of T_3 to improve recovery. Myocardial function was not improved in mildly injured hearts with 100 times the physiologic concentration and was significantly impaired in severely injured hearts. These findings indicate that there is a dose-response relationship. Further study is required to elucidate the mechanism involved.

▶ This paper experimentally supports the use of thyroid hormone during cardiac surgery, an approach currently being used in some centers. However, caution must be emphasized until carefully controlled studies involving endocrinologists are carried out to determine the efficacy of using thyroid hormone during and after cardiac surgery. Gotzsche (*Eur J Endocrinol* 130:171, 1994) reported an acute increase in Ca^{2+} uptake by rat hearts after T_3 administration, which may play a role in the acute positive inotropic effect of T_3 on cardiac function in vivo. The risk of excess thyroid hormone is reported by Shammas et al. (*Am Heart J* 127:232, 1994), with myocardial dysfunction and necrosis occurring after the ingestion of 8 mg of L-thyroxine. Simple substituted phenols, such as 3,5-diiodo-4-hydroxyphenylproprionic acid, have been shown to have potent effects on myocardial function in rats similar to those observed with T_4 (Pennock et al: *J Pharm Exp Ther* 268:216, 1994). These compounds deserve further study.—L.E. Braverman, M.D.

Regulation of GLUT2 Glucose Transporter Expression in Liver by Thyroid Hormone: Evidence for Hormonal Regulation of the Hepatic Glucose Transport System
Weinstein SP, O'Boyle E, Fisher M, Haber RS (Mount Sinai School of Medicine, New York)
Endocrinology 135:649–654, 1994   112-95-10–4

Background.—It is well known that thyroid hormone increases hepatic glucose output. Thyroid hormone was thus investigated to determine whether it upregulates expression of GLUT2, the primary hepatic glucose transporter, thereby facilitating increased glucose efflux across the hepatocyte plasma membrane.

Methods and Findings.—Chronically hypothyroid, euthyroid, and hyperthyroid rats were used. GLUT2 protein concentration was twice as high in the crude liver membranes of hyperthyroid vs. hypothyroid rats. Intermediate levels were noted in euthyroid controls. Comparable results were observed for total GLUT2 protein, measured in detergent extracts of liver. Parallel changes in GLUT2 messenger RNA (mRNA) concentration per gram of tissue were observed after Northern analysis of total liver RNA. In hypothyroid rats, a rapid increase in hepatic GLUT2 mRNA concentration (2.5-fold at 1 day) was observed after daily administration of T$_3$ at 100 μg/100 g body weight. However, only a minor and gradual change in hepatic GLUT2 protein concentration occurred (+40% at 4 days). This indicated that the GLUT2 protein in liver may have a prolonged half-life.

Conclusion.—Thyroid hormone regulates hepatic GLUT2 mRNA and protein expression, as it does the enzymes of gluconeogenesis and glycocysis. The hepatic GLUT2 glucose transporter should therefore be considered a regulatory target for hormones that control hepatic glucose metabolism.

▶ The effects of thyroid hormone on regulation of glucose homeostasis have been of interest for years. This lovely study certainly suggests that the GLUT2 glucose transporter is a target for thyroid hormone action, and this mechanism may explain at least some of the effects of thyroid hormone excess on glucose regulation in man. Hyperthyroidism in human beings is associated with an increased efficiency of plasma glucose recovery from hypoglycemia caused primarily by an enhanced glucagon response (Morghetti et al: *J Clin Endocrinol Metab* 78:169, 1994).—L.E. Braverman, M.D.

Evidence That Phosphorylation Events Participate in Thyroid Hormone Action
Jones KE, Brubaker JH, Chin WW (Brigham and Women's Hosp, Boston; Harvard Med School, Boston; Howard Hughes Med Inst, Boston)
Endocrinology 134:543–548, 1994   112-95-10–5

Introduction.—Nuclear receptors regulate transcription of genes responsive to thyroid hormone. Three murine thyroid hormone receptor (TR) isoforms have been identified: TRα, TRβ$_1$, and TRβ$_2$. Studies have found that some TR isoforms can be phosphorylated, and phosphorylation of TR isoforms may modify their transcriptional activity. This hypothesis was tested by using a protein kinase inhibitor and a phosphatase inhibitor to alter the cellular phosphorylation state and studying transactivation with reporter plasmids containing a variety of thyroid hormone response elements (TREs).

Methods.—One group of monkey kidney CV-1 cells were transfected with expression plasmids containing either rat TRα, TRβ$_1$, or no TR and with luciferase plasmids containing the synthetic DR4 or the chick lysozyme F2 TREs. The transfected cells were maintained in a hypothyroid medium for 24 hours, then incubated with either T$_3$ or the phosphatase inhibitor, okadaic acid (OA), in various doses, or both. Another group of transfected cells were incubated with either T$_3$ or the proteinkinase inhibitor, H7, or both. The luciferase transcriptional activity was assayed after incubation. Rat pituitary GH$_3$ cells were incubated with T$_3$ or H7 or both, or T$_3$, OA, or both, and GH messenger RNA (mRNA) levels were assayed to investigate endogenous T$_3$ response.

Results.—Luciferase activity increased significantly after incubation with T_3, slightly after incubation with OA alone, and highly significantly after incubation with both T_3 and OA in cells transfected with all TREs, but not in cells without TREs, when compared with hypothyroid levels. Okadaic acid enhanced the T_3-mediated increase in luciferase activity in a dose-dependent manner. Incubation with H7 alone induced no change in luciferase activity from the hypothyroid levels and blocked the effects of T_3 incubation. The inhibitory effects of H7 diminished after 6 hours, although it was restored when fresh H7 was added. Growth hormone mRNA levels increased with T_3 but did not change with H7 alone. The T_3-mediated stimulation of GH mRNA was attenuated by H7. The effects of OA on GH mRNA levels were variable.

Discussion.—Protein phosphorylation of both the TRα and TRβ isoforms modifies transcriptional activation in a transfection system. Endogenous T_3 responses are also blunted by protein kinase inhibitors. Further study is required to identify the protein sequences involved in phosphorylation events.

▶ Chin and colleagues continue to make major contributions to our understanding of the cellular events leading to transcriptional activation of thyroid hormone, including phosphorylation. In another report, these workers suggest that both T_3 and TRE binding are important determinants of the formation of specific thyroid hormone receptor complexes in solution as well as on DNA (Yen et al: *Endocrinology* 134:1075, 1994).—L.E. Braverman, M.D.

▶↑ The heavy metal cadmium has been reported to decrease 5'-deiodinase activity by binding to the sulfhydryl groups of the enzyme (Paier et al: *J Endocrinol* 138:219, 1993). We have recently reported that tumor necrosis factor-α, which decreases 5'-deiodinase activity in liver and kidney, also decreases TSH-induced 5'-deiodinase activity in FRTL-5 rat thyroid cells, which may further contribute to the low serum T_3 values observed in the sick euthyroid syndrome (Ongphiphadhanakul et al: *Eur J Endocrinol* 130:502, 1994). Another possible factor in the low serum T_3 euthyroid sick syndrome may be the elevated interleukin-6 levels commonly found in illness, because administration of interleukin-6 lowers serum T_3 concentrations in human beings (Stouthard et al: *J Clin Endocrinol Metab* 79:1342, 1994).

Hennemann and co-workers have restudied a family with euthyroid hyperthyroxinemia that they previously reported (1982) to be the result of either decreased entry of T_4 into T_3-producing tissues or decreased 5'-deiodination of T_4. They now suggest that the syndrome in this family is the result of decreased transport of T_4 into the liver, resulting in lower T_3 production (*J Clin Endocrinol Metab* 77:1431, 1993). Three studies have described various aspects of the developmental maturation of thyroid hormone economy. Galton and colleagues (*Endocrinology* 133:2488, 1993) reported that the c-*erb* Aα gene encodes a thyroid hormone receptor and that only the α-gene is expressed in tadpole red blood cells, subject to regulation during development and by thyroid hormone as well. The rat small intestine becomes increasingly

T_3 responsive during postnatal development, occurring in parallel with a decline in c-*erb* Aα-2 levels, suggesting that this T_3 receptor variant may play a role in this hormonal responsiveness (*Endocrinology* 135:564, 1994).

Finally, Chanoine et al. have evidence that the postnatal serum T_3 surge in the rat is primarily the result of enhanced thyroidal T_3 secretion (*Endocrinology* 133:2604, 1993). In an interesting study, Reed and associates have reported that swine exposed to the cold for 25 days have increased energy intake, thyroid size, T_3 plasma appearance rate, and hepatic 5'-deiodinase activity with little change in serum TSH (*Am J Physiol Endocrinol Metab*) 29:E786, 1994). This section could not be completed without some reference to the thyroid hormone binding proteins. Thus, the Australian–New Zealand group (Curtis et al: *J Clin Endocrinol Metab* 78:459, 1994) has suggested that the TTR met[119] mutation leads to secretion of a normal concentration of transthyretin with an enhanced affinity for T_4, and the Boston group (Rosen et al: *Endocrinology* 134:27, 1994) have data suggesting that a subtle change in the structure of the T_4-binding channel of transthyretin alters its binding affinity for the various iodothyronines.—L.E. Braverman, M.D.

Thyrotoxicosis

Thyrotropin Receptor Antisera for the Detection of Immunoreactive Protein Species in Retroocular Fibroblasts Obtained From Patients With Graves' Ophthalmopathy

Burch HB, Sellitti D, Barnes SG, Nagy EV, Bahn RS, Burman KD (Walter Reed Army Med Ctr, Washington, DC; Uniformed Services Univ of the Health Sciences, Bethesda, Md; Mayo Clinic and Found, Rochester, Minn)
J Clin Endocrinol Metab 78:1384–1391, 1994   112-95-10–6

Introduction.—Studies have definitively demonstrated that autoimmunity against the TSH receptor (hTSH-R) is the primary etiologic factor in the development of hyperthyroidism in patients with Graves' disease. There is some evidence that autoimmunity against the hTSH-R is also involved in the development of ophthalmopathy in these patients, because messenger RNA for the TSH-R has been detected in retro-ocular fibroblasts. However, the presence of antigenically active hTSH-R protein has not been proved. Therefore, hTSH-R-specific antibody was used to identify hTSH-R or immunologically related protein in retro-ocular fibroblasts from a patient with Graves' disease.

Methods.—Two hTSH-R peptides were synthesized: the immunogenic peptide, P1, consisting of amino acids 352–367, and the less immunogenic peptide, P2, consisting of amino acids 377–397. Each peptide was injected intradermally into 2 rabbits, and blood samples were collected. Cultured retro-ocular fibroblasts from patients with Graves' disease with and without ophthalmopathy and control fibroblasts cultured from cells obtained from abdominal wall and pretibial regions were incubated with the synthetic antibodies and examined with immunofluorescence studies and immunoblotting.

Results.—The serum from the rabbits immunized with P1, but not with P2, had specific immunoreactivity with the targeted immunogenic hTSH-R segment. Anti-P1 staining was abundant and specific in the retro-ocular fibroblasts obtained from patients with Graves' ophthalmopathy, whereas there was no significant staining indicating anti-P2 activity. The staining in abdominal wall and pretibial fibroblasts was reduced and nonspecific. Immunoblot analysis of retro-ocular fibroblast protein with anti-P1 sera revealed prominent bands at 95, 71, 41, and 18 kDa.

Discussion.—These findings suggest that TSH-R may be the antigen that functions in the pathogenesis of both the extra-thyroidal and eye manifestations of Graves' disease. The highly immunogenic protein portion of the hTSH-R was identified in retro-ocular fibrocytes of patients with Graves' ophthalmopathy. Its immunofluorescence pattern in these cells corresponded to that seen in thyrocytes, and it was clearly different than the pattern seen in control fibroblasts. Immunity against the 95-kDa protein band is common to patients with Graves' disease with both manifestations.

▶ Although this publication suggests a possible etiology for Graves' ophthalmopathy, the mystery still remains. Many theories have been proposed during the past decades, and the 3 more recent examples are briefly mentioned. Bahn et al. report a genomic point mutation in the extracellular domain of the TSH receptor in 2 patients with severe eye disease, pretibial dermopathy, and acropachy and also suggest that the TSH receptor may be an important fibroblast autoantigen in Graves' ophthalmopathy (*J Clin Endocrinol Metab* 78:256, 1994). McLachan, Rapoport, and co-workers suggest that interleukin-4, but not interferon-α, messenger RNA expression in orbital tissue supports a role for humoral autoimmunity in Graves' eye disease (*J Clin Endocrinol Metab* 78:1070, 1994). They also suggest from analysis of the genes for antibodies secreted by orbital-tissue-infiltrating plasma cells that particular germline genes may be associated with autoimmunity in this condition and autoimmunity in general (*J Clin Endocrinol Metab* 78:348, 1994). Finally, the Mayo Clinic group has reported the favorable outcome of transantral orbital decompression followed, in some patients, by eye muscle and lid operations, performed primarily for cosmetic indications (Fatourechi et al: *Ophthalmology* 101:938, 1994).—L.E. Braverman, M.D.

Does Early Administration of Thyroxine Reduce the Development of Graves' Ophthalmopathy After Radioiodine Treatment?
Tallstedt L, Lundell G, Blomgren H, Bring J (Huddinge Hosp, Stockholm; Karolinska Hosp, Stockholm; Univ of Uppsala, Sweden)
Eur J Endocrinol 130:494–497, 1994   112-95-10–7

Background—Graves' ophthalmopathy develops more frequently in the hypothyroid state after ^{131}I therapy for hyperthyroidism than in patients treated with an antithyroid drug or thyroidectomy. Although T$_4$

may be protective against exophthalmos, increased TSH levels may have adverse effects. The effects of early T_4 administration after ^{131}I treatment for hyperthyroidism caused by Graves' disease were evaluated retrospectively.

Methods.—Records from patients with Graves' disease treated with ^{131}I were reviewed. Two hundred forty-eight patients (group A) received T_4 when serum TSH concentration or T_4 indicated hypothyroidism; T_4, .05 mg, was initiated 2 weeks after therapy with a dosage increase to .1 mg after 2 weeks in 244 patients (group B).

Results.—Ophthalmopathy developed or worsened after treatment in 18% of patients in group A and 11% in group B. The average increases in Hertel readings were comparable for the groups: 3.5 mm in group A and 3.2 mm in group B. Twenty-six patients in group A and 11 in group B required specific therapy for progressive eye changes despite increased T_4 treatment. In group A, 23 required antithyroid drugs; 8, glucocorticoids; 6, glucocorticoids plus retrobulbar radiation; 3, orbital decompression; and 1, retrobulbar radiation only. In group B, 10 patients received antithyroid drugs; 6, glucocorticoids; 2, glucocorticoids plus retrobulbar radiation; 1, orbital decompression.

Conclusion.—Early administration of T_4 after ^{131}I treatment reduces the occurrence of Graves' ophthalmopathy. Therapy with T_4 should be started 2 weeks after the ^{131}I therapy in all patients with hyperthyroidism caused by Graves' disease, especially in those receiving larger doses of [131]I.

▶ These workers previously reported that Graves' ophthalmopathy worsened after radioactive iodine (RAI) therapy (*N Engl J Med* 326:1733, 1992). They now suggest that post-RAI hypothyroidism may have played a role in this progression because early administration of L-T_4 after RAI therapy decreased the occurrence and progression of eye disease. However, they still suggest that RAI therapy may enhance this risk. Kung et al. also reported that an elevated serum TSH is an important adverse factor for the development or exacerbation of Graves' eye disease, that methimazole plus L-T_4 administration after RAI therapy did not prevent Graves' ophthalmopathy, and that levels of thyroid receptor antibodies after RAI therapy had no role in Graves' eye disease (*J Clin Endocrinol Metab* 79:542, 1994). Smoking has again been implicated as an associated finding in patients with Graves' ophthalmopathy (Tallstedt et al: *Acta Endocrinol* 129:147, 1993).—L.E. Braverman, M.D.

Treatment of Graves' Disease by Carbimazole: High Dose With Thyroxine Compared to Titration Dose
Edmonds CJ, Tellez M (Northwick Park Hosp, Harrow, England)
Eur J Endocrinol 131:120–124, 1994   112-95-10–8

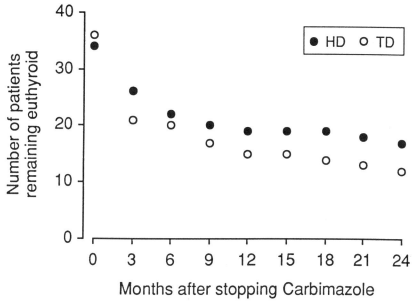

Fig 10–2.—The number of patients remaining euthyroid related to the time elapsing after finishing the 12-month course of carbimazole. Thirty-four patients were treated with the high-dose (HD) regimen and 36 patients treated with the titration-dose (TD) regimen. (Courtesy of Edmonds CJ, Tellez M: *Eur J Endocrinol* 131:120–124, 1994.)

Introduction.—Antithyroid drugs are usually administered with a titration regimen, beginning with a large dose and reducing gradually to the smallest dose capable of maintaining a euthyroid condition. However, a high dose can be maintained throughout the length of the treatment with T_4 added to maintain normal serum thyroid hormone concentration. It was hypothesized that a consistent high-dose regimen of antithyroid medication with T_4 would increase the length of remission. The long-term efficacy of the 2-dose regimens in controlling Graves' disease was compared.

Methods.—Seventy patients with Graves' disease were randomly assigned to receive either a titration-dose (TD) or high-dose (HD) regimen of carbimazole. They were treated for 1 year and followed up for 2 years after treatment was completed. The patients were monitored with measurements of plasma free T3 serum thyroglobulin, serum thyroid microsomal and thyroglobulin antibodies, pertechnetate uptake on thyroid scintigraphy and with classification of goiter size and ophthalmopathy.

Results.—Relapses occurred in 35% of the HD group and in 44% of the TD group within 6 months of treatment completion, in 55% of the HD group and 58% of the TD group by 1 year, and in 50% of the HD group and 66% of the TD group by 2 years after the end of treatment (Fig 10–2). The differences between treatment responses were not statistically significant. During treatment, reductions in pertechnetate uptake, serum thyroglobulin, and thyroid antibodies and the rate of thyroid microsomal antibody positivity were not significantly different in the 2 groups. The prevalence of ophthalmopathy and of cigarette smoking was similar in both groups and did not correlate significantly with the relapse rate. Pertechnetate uptake and the number of patients having undetectable TSH and small goiters in patients relapsing later than 6 months after treatment ended were similar to the same parameters in patients who did not relapse at all, whereas patients who relapsed within 6 months had significantly higher pertechnetate uptake, a greater proportion with suppressed plasma TSH, and larger goiters.

Discussion.—An advantage to routine high-dose treatment regimens with carbimazole in patients with Graves' disease was not demonstrated. However, it may be advantageous to use the HD regimen in patients who cannot be sufficiently monitored, in patients with fluctuating hyperthyroidism, and in patients with severe ophthalmopathy. The clinical significance of the differences in thyroid function parameters between patients who relapse early and late will require further study.

▶ The issue of whether combination therapy with L-T$_4$ and antithyroid drugs increases the remission rate of Graves' disease compared with antithyroid drugs alone is still not answered. In their study done in England, Edmonds and Tellez found no difference in remission rates and a wide variety of other variables using their version of these 2 protocols. Kuo et al., in a report from Taiwan, did not address the remission rate of Graves' disease after therapy, but they did observe a greater fall in TSH receptor-ab and triglyceride levels in patients treated with combined methimazole and L-T$_4$ than with methimazole alone (*Eur J Endocrinol* 131:125, 1994). Using a thyroid hormone synthesis block (large dose of carbimazole)–L-T$_4$ replacement regimen for 6 or 12 months in the treatment of Graves' disease, Weetman et al. observed a similar remission rate (65% vs. 59%, respectively) and suggested that the 6-month regimen was probably sufficient (*Q J Med* 87:337, 1994).—L.E. Braverman, M.D.

Treatment of Methimazole-Induced Agranulocytosis Using Recombinant Human Granulocyte Colony-Stimulating Factor (rhG-CSF)

Tamai H, Mukuta T, Matsubayashi S, Fukata S, Komaki G, Kuma K, Kumagai LF, Nagataki S (Kyushu Univ, Fukuoka, Japan; Kuma Hosp, Kobe, Japan; Nagasaki Univ, Japan; et al)
J Clin Endocrinol Metab 77:1356–1360, 1993   112-95-10-9

Introduction.—Agranulocytosis is a rare but serious complication of antithyroidal drug therapy in patients with Graves' disease. Treatment with purified recombinant human granulocyte colony-stimulating factors (rhG-CSF) or granulocyte macrophage colony-stimulating factors (rhGM-CSF) has increased neutrophils in patients undergoing chemotherapy or in those with AIDS. The effect on recovery time of the ad-

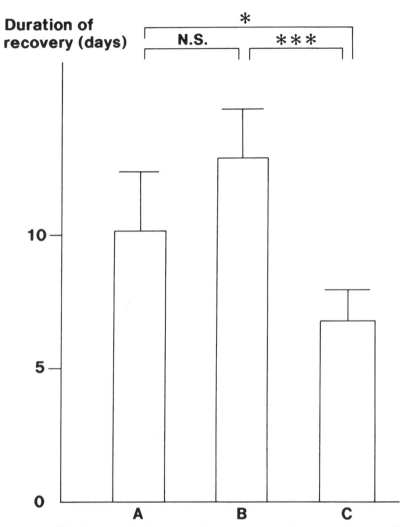

Fig 10–3.—The duration in days for peripheral granulocytes to reach greater than $1.0 \times 10^9/L$ among the 3 agranulocytosis groups that received different therapeutic regimens. *Group A* ($n = 11$), antibiotics only, *group B* ($n = 11$), antibiotics and steroids; *group C* ($n = 12$), antibiotics and recombinant human granulocyte colony-stimulating factors (75 μg/day). *Significant at 5% level; ***Significant at .1% level. (Courtesy of Tamai H. Mukuta T, Matsubayashi S, et al: *J Clin Endocrinol Metab* 77:1356–1360, 1993.)

ministration of purified rhG-CSF to patients with agranulocytosis induced by methimazole treatment was compared with that of antibiotic treatment alone or with steroids.

Methods.—Thirty-four patients with methimazole-induced (MMI) agranulocytosis were divided into 3 treatment groups. Group A received antibiotics only and group B received antibiotics and dexamethasone;

both were studied retrospectively. Group C was studied prospectively and received antibiotics and intramuscular injections of rhG-CSF. Sternal punctures were performed in the patients in group C; this group was subdivided into 2 groups determined by their ratios of granulocytes to erythrocytes. The recovery times in each group were compared.

Results.—Recovery occurred in a mean of 10.1 days, 12.3 days, and 6.8 days in groups A, B, and C, respectively (Fig 10–3). Within group C, the patients with a granulocyte to erythrocyte ratio of less than .5 had a recovery time of 9.8 days, whereas those with a ratio of at least .5 had a recovery time of 2.2 days. The granulocyte to erythrocyte ratio was strongly correlated with leukocyte counts. Patients treated with rhG-CSF experienced no adverse side effects and did not evidence serum toxicity.

Discussion.—Treatment with rhG-CSF can significantly reduce the recovery time in patients with MMI agranulocytosis. However, steroid treatment did not reduce recovery time. There does not appear to be dose-limited toxicity with rhG-CSF treatment as there is with rhGM-CSF. Therefore, agranulocytosis in patients undergoing antithyroidal drug therapy should be treated with antibiotics, when indicated, and rhG-CSF administration.

▶ Although uncommon, antithyroid drug agranulocytosis is a serious complication. Granulocyte colony-stimulating factor appears to enhance granulocyte recovery time, certainly an asset in our frenzy to decrease the length of hospital stay. Two other reports also support the use of G-CSF in antithyroid drug–induced agranulocytosis (Magner, Snyder: *Thyroid* 4:295, 1994; Balkin et al: *Thyroid* 4:305, 1993).—L.E. Braverman, M.D.

Changes in Bone Mass During Prolonged Subclinical Hyperthyroidism Due to L-Thyroxine Treatment: A Meta-Analysis
Faber J, Galloe AM (Frederiksberg Hosp, Denmark; Herlev Univ Hosp, Denmark)
Eur J Endocrinol 130:350–356, 1994
112-95-10–10

Introduction.—Subclinical hyperthyroidism is a state of euthyroidism with reduced serum TSH but normal T_4 and T_3 values. Reduced serum TSH resulting from L-T_4 treatment may adversely affect bone mass and increase the risk of premature development of osteoporosis. Several recent studies, however, fail to show such a detrimental effect. A meta-analysis was performed to determine whether L-T_4 in doses large enough to suppress serum TSH concentrations reduces bone mass in treated patients relative to healthy controls.

Methods.—Thirteen studies were identified in which bone mass was measured in the distal forearm, femoral neck, or lumbar spine in a cross-sectional manner. For each study, the differences in the reductions in bone mass at these sites were calculated for either premenopausal or postmenopausal women because of the protective role of preserved estrogen production.

Results.—A combination of the studies yielded 441 measurements performed in premenopausal women treated for an average of 8.51 years with an average dose of L-T$_4$ of 164 µg/day; 317 measurements were performed in postmenopausal women treated for an average of 9.93 years with an average dose of 171 µg/day. The excess loss of bone mass at the 3 sites in treated premenopausal women relative to healthy premenopausal women was nonsignificant. Measurements obtained in premenopausal women were used to construct a theoretical bone. A premenopausal woman at an average age of 39.6 years, with a duration of treatment of 8.51 years and suppressed TSH, would have an excess loss of bone mass of 2.67% or .31% annually as compared to healthy premenopausal women. The excess loss of bone mass for postmenopausal women, however, proved to be significant. The theoretical bone in a postmenopausal woman with an average age of 61.2 years and suppressed serum TSH during 9.93 years of treatment would have an excess loss of bone mass of 9.02%, or .91% annually as compared to healthy postmenopausal women.

Conclusion.—Reduced serum TSH as a sign of subclinical hyperthyroidism was not detrimental to bone mass in premenopausal women. The total loss with 10 years of treatment would not be clinically significant. In contrast, postmenopausal women have a significant and probably clinically relevant excess bone loss during suppressive L-T$_4$ treatment.

▶ This meta-analysis suggests that TSH-suppressive doses of L-T$_4$ do increase bone loss in postmenopausal but not in premenopausal women, but I believe that premenopausal women may also be at risk over a long period of time. Two studies again report the adverse effects of thyrotoxicosis on bone metabolism and reversal by restoration of the euthyroid state (Garnero et al: *J Clin Endocrinol Metab* 78:955, 1994; Diamond et al: *Ann Intern Med* 120:8, 1994). In mixed cultures of osteoblasts and osteoclasts, addition of T$_3$ acted on osteoblasts to indirectly stimulate osteoclastic bone resorption (Britto et al: *Endocrinology* 134:169, 1994). Thyrotoxic doses of T$_3$ administered to adult rats induced bone loss greatest at the distal femur subregion, and diphosphonate administration (as we have reported earlier) prevents the thyroid hormone–induced bone loss (Rosen et al: *Calcif Tissue Int* 55:173, 1994).—L.E. Braverman, M.D.

A Comparison of Propylthiouracil Versus Methimazole in the Treatment of Hyperthyroidism in Pregnancy
Wing DA, Millar LK, Koonings PP, Montoro MN, Mestman JH (Los Angeles County/Univ of Southern California Med Ctr, Los Angeles)
Am J Obstet Gynecol 170:90–95, 1994   112-95-10–11

Introduction.—Hyperthyroidism in pregnancy is generally treated with either propylthiouracil or methimazole. Because methimazole has been associated clinically with neonatal aplasia cutis, propylthiouracil has been used more frequently. The therapeutic efficacy and pregnancy outcomes in patients treated with these 2 agents were reviewed retrospectively.

Methods.—The records of 185 pregnant patients with a history or diagnosis of hyperthyroidism seen in an obstetrics clinic between 1974 and 1990 were reviewed. The maternal and fetal outcomes, including the time to normalization of the free T_4 index, the incidence of congenital anomalies, and the incidence of congenital hypothyroidism, were measured in patients treated with propylthiouracil and compared with those measured in patients treated with methimazole.

Results.—Of the 185 hyperthyroid patients, 99 were treated with propylthiouracil and 36 were treated with methimazole. At the time of delivery, 32% of the propylthiouracil-treated group and 33% of the methimazole-treated group were still hyperthyroid. Among those who were euthyroid at delivery, the median time to normalization of the free T_4 index was 7 weeks in the group treated with propylthiouracil and 8 weeks in the group treated with methimazole. The incidence of major congenital anomalies was 3% among patients treated with propylthiouracil and 2.7% among patients treated with methimazole. This was consistent with the incidence in the general population. No infants were born with aplasia cutis.

Discussion.—There were no significant differences between the 2 treatment groups in the maternal and fetal outcomes measured. The safety and efficacy of propylthiouracil and methimazole are comparable.

▶ This report strongly suggests that methimazole in appropriate doses is as effective and as safe as propylthiouracil in hyperthyroidism in pregnancy, contradicting the generally accepted preference for propylthiouracil. The importance of good drug control of hyperthyroidism during pregnancy is emphasized by Kriplani et al. (*Eur J Obstet Gynecol Reprod Biol* 54:159, 1994), who reported an increased incidence of maternal and fetal complications.—L.E. Braverman, M.D.

Low Serum Thyrotropin Concentrations as a Risk Factor for Atrial Fibrillation in Older Persons
Sawin CT, Geller A, Wolf PA, Belanger AJ, Baker E, Bacharach P, Wilson PWF, Benjamin EJ, D'Agostino RB (Boston Veterans Affairs Med Ctr; Evans Mem Department of Clinical Research, Boston; Boston Univ; et al)
N Engl J Med 331:1249–1252, 1994   112-95-10–12

Background.—Atrial fibrillation is a well-recognized manifestation of hyperthyroidism. Although low serum TSH concentrations are an established indicator of hyperthyroidism, they may also be found in individu-

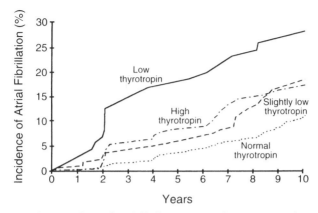

Fig 10–4.—Cumulative incidence of atrial fibrillation among subjects 60 years of age or older, according to serum thyrotropin values at baseline. (Courtesy of Sawin CT, Geller A, Wolf PA, et al: N Engl J Med 331:1249–1252, 1994.)

als without clinical evidence of this disorder. Clinically euthyroid elderly individuals were investigated to determine whether low serum TSH concentrations are a risk factor for subsequent atrial fibrillation.

Participants and Methods.—A total of 2,007 individuals, including 814 men and 1,193 women aged 60 years or older, were studied. None of the participants had atrial fibrillation. Serum TSH levels were used to classify all participants. Sixty-one were placed in a low value group, defined as ≤ 0.1 mU per liter; 187 were placed in a slightly low value group, defined as > 0.1 to 0.4 mU per liter; 1,576 were placed in a normal value group, defined as > 0.4 to 5.0 mU per liter; and 183 were placed in a high value group, defined as > 5.0 mU per liter. The frequency of atrial fibrillation was determined over a 10-year period.

Results.—Thirteen participants with low initial values, 23 with slightly low values, 133 with normal values, and 23 with high values experienced atrial fibrillation during the follow-up period. At 10 years, the cumulative incidence of atrial fibrillation was 28% among those with low values, compared with 11% among individuals with normal values (Fig 10–4). The age-adjusted incidence of atrial fibrillation was 28 per 1,000 person-years among participants with low values and 10 per 1,000 person-years among those with normal values. After adjusting for other established risk factors, participants with low values had a 3.1 relative risk of atrial fibrillation compared to those with normal values. The 10-year incidence of atrial fibrillation did not differ significantly between individuals with slightly low and high values and those with normal values.

Conclusion.—Low serum TSH concentrations are associated with an increased risk for atrial fibrillation among elderly individuals aged 60 years and older.

▶ This observation certainly suggests that subclinical hyperthyroidism is more common in the elderly than previously suspected and that atrial fibrillation may be one clinical manifestation of a suppressed serum TSH. In the same issue of the *New England Journal of Medicine* (331:1302, 1994), my colleague, Robert Utiger, wrote an editorial on this paper and concluded as follows: "If the patient already has atrial fibrillation, other atrial arrhythmias, other cardiac disorders, or accelerated bone loss, to which small degrees of thyroid hormone excess might contribute, antithyroid therapy should be seriously considered. For the remainder of patients, no intervention should be undertaken unless subclinical hyperthyroidism persists for several months. Even if the patient's serum thyrotropin concentration remains low, balancing the risks of the disease against the problems of antithyroid therapy leads me to the conclusion that careful follow-up rather than intervention is the most prudent policy."—L.E. Braverman, M.D.

Serum Interleukin-6 in Amiodarone-Induced Thyrotoxicosis
Bartalena L, Grasso L, Brogioni S, Aghini-Lombardi F, Braverman LE, Martino E (Univ of Pisa, Tirrenia-Pisa, Italy; Univ of Massachusetts, Worcester)
J Clin Endocrinol Metab 78:423–427, 1994   112-95-10-13

Introduction.—About 10% of cardiac patients treated with the iodine-rich drug, amiodarone, develop either hyperthyroidism or hypothyroidism. Patients with amiodarone-induced thyrotoxicosis (AIT) may or may not have an underlying thyroid abnormality. Increased serum interleukin-6 (IL-6) levels have been found in patients with acute or subacute thyroiditis. The significance of IL-6 levels in the pathogenesis of AIT was explored.

Methods.—Serum free T_4, T_3, and IL-6 levels, urinary iodine excretion, and thyroidal radioiodine uptake (RAIU) were measured in a cross-section of patients. The patients included 15 patients with AIT and a normal thyroid gland (AIT−), 12 patients with AIT and goiter (AIT+), 14 euthyroid patients who had received chronic amiodarone treatment, 10 patients with amiodarone-induced hypothyroidism, 56 patients with spontaneous hyperthyroidism caused by Graves' disease or toxic goiter, 20 patients with nontoxic goiter, and 50 healthy controls. Two of the AIT− patients received either methimazole followed by prednisone or prednisone only.

Results.—Serum IL-6 concentrations were significantly higher in AIT− patients than in all the other groups, but they were only slightly higher in AIT+ patients than in patients with Graves' disease- or toxic goiter–induced spontaneous hyperthyroidism (Fig 10–5). Serum free T_4 and T_3 were comparable in patients with AIT or spontaneous hyperthy-

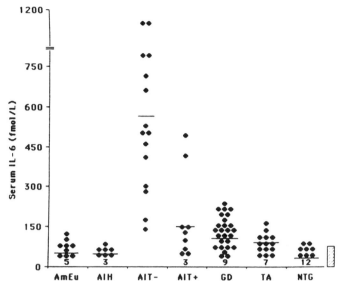

Fig 10–5.—*Abbreviations: AmEu,* euthyroid patients who received chronic amiodarone treatment; *AIH,* amiodarone-induced hypothyroidism; *AIT−,* amiodarone-induced thyrotoxicosis without thyroid abnormalities; *AIT+,* amiodarone-induced thyrotoxicosis with nodular goiter and/or thyroid autoimmune disease; *GD,* Graves' disease; *TA,* toxic goiter; and *NTG,* nontoxic goiter. Serum interleukin-6 (IL-6) levels in AmEu, AIH, AIT−, AIT+, GD, TA, and NTG patients. *Figures below the individual values* indicate the number of patients in each group with undetectable (< 25 fmol/L) serum IL-6 levels. *Horizontal lines* indicate the mean value in each group. The *hatched bar* indicates the range of IL-6 values in healthy controls. (Courtesy of Bartalena L, Grasso L, Brogioni S, et al: *J Clin Endocrinol Metab* 78:423-427, 1994.)

roidism. The AIT− patients had very low thyroidal RAIU, whereas it was inappropriately normal or high in the AIT+ patients. Prednisone treatment quickly corrected serum IL-6 and free T_3 values even though urinary iodine excretion remained high, whereas methimazole treatment did not reverse thyrotoxicosis.

Discussion.—Measuring serum IL-6 levels identifies 2 subgroups of patients with AIT. Patients with thyroid abnormalities have normal or high thyroidal RAIU and only slightly higher serum IL-6 levels than patients with spontaneous hyperthyroidism, suggesting amiodarone-induced thyroiditis. Patients with no thyroid abnormalities have markedly low thyroidal RAIU and serum IL-6 values much higher than patients with spontaneous hyperthyroidism. Methimazole and potassium perchlorate, because they prevent thyroid trapping of iodine and release inorganic iodine trapped in the gland, may be effective in managing some patients with AIT who have normal or only slightly elevated serum IL-6 levels. However, the efficacy of glucocorticoid treatment suggests that, in some patients with significantly elevated serum IL-6 levels, the AIT may be caused by an inflammatory process.

▶ This group continues to study amiodarone-induced thyroid dysfunction, and they now suggest that elevations in serum IL-6 levels in amiodarone-induced thyrotoxicosis suggest thyroiditis as the underlying pathology. In vitro studies have demonstrated the cytotoxicity of amiodarone on rat FRTL-5 cells and primary cultures of human thyroid follicles (Chiovata et al: *Endocrinology* 134:2277, 1994), confirming the in vivo study described above. Surgical therapy for amiodarone-induced thyrotoxicosis is a viable option, provided an extremely capable surgical team is available (Mulligan et al: *Surgery* 114:1114, 1993). The mechanism of action of amiodarone has been explored in a series of studies, and it has become evident that the major metabolite of amiodarone, desethylamiodarone, rather than amiodarone, binds to the thyroid hormone β_1-receptor protein, perhaps inducing a state of tissue hypothyroidism, especially in the myocardium (Bakker et al: *Endocrinology* 134:1665, 1994; Gotzche: *Acta Endocrinol* 129:337, 1993; Barlow et al: *Eur J Endocrinol* 130:417, 1994); Gotzsche, Orskov: *Eur J Endocrinol* 130:281, 1994). Finally, DeJong et al. have proposed that amiodarone induces the low T_3 syndrome by decreasing transport of T_4 into the perfused liver as well as impairing 5'-deiodination of T_4 (*Am J Physiol Endocrinol Metab*) 266:E44, 1994).—L.E. Braverman, M.D.

▶↑ Many workers have suggested that measurement of TSH receptor antibodies (TRAb) during antithyroid drug therapy for Graves' disease predicts remission and relapse after drug withdrawal. Feldt-Rasmussen et al. (*J Clin Endocrinol Metab* 78:98, 1994) carried out a meta-analysis of many studies and, although the absence of TRAb is significantly protective against relapse, "the available methods of TRAb do not allow a sufficiently high prediction of relapse or remission after antithyroid drug therapy for the individual patient." I agree, because I essentially never measure TRAb levels to determine when to discontinue drug therapy. The intensity of lymphocytic infiltration of the thyroid in patients with Graves' disease is better predicted by microsomal antibody titers than TRAb (Paschke et al: *J Clin Endocrinol Metab* 77:939, 1993).

Although many of us believed that thyroid surgery would induce an increase in release of hormone in untreated patients with Graves' hyperthyroidism, Hermann et al. (*Surgery* 115:240, 1994) disproved this untested hypothesis. The concentration of free T_3 and free T_4 concentrations in the venous effluent during surgery for untreated hyperthyroid Graves' disease did not exceed peripheral blood levels, and these authors suggest that immediate thyroidectomy could be considered for emergency therapy of imminent thyroid storm. Surgeons are much braver than we mortal souls! In a prospective controlled study, hyperthyroidism resulted in abnormal liver function studies that resolved upon restoration of euthyroidism even though transient asymptomatic propylthiouracil-induced hepatotoxicity occurs in one third of patients (Huang et al: *Am J Gastroenterol* 89:1071, 1994).

The toxic effects of thyrotoxicosis on muscle were studied in the *mdx* muscular dystrophy mouse. Thyroxine-induced thyrotoxicosis produced greater dystrophy in both cardiac and soleus muscles (Anderson, Kardami: *Muscle Nerve* 17:64, 1994). Momotani and associates studied postpartum hyperthyroidism in women with a history of Graves' disease and found that silent thyroiditis commonly develops concomitantly with the recurrence of active Graves' disease and delays or masks the development of Graves' hyperthyroidism (*J Clin Endocrinol Metab* 79:285, 1994). Finally, human chorionic gonadotropin (hCG) has been suggested as playing an important role in the aggravation of Graves' hyperthyroidism during the first trimester of pregnancy (Tamaki et al: *Thyroid* 3:189, 1993), further confirming the in vitro data that hCG is a human thyroid stimulator (Kraiem et al: *J Clin Endocrinol Metab* 79:595, 1994).—L.E. Braverman, M.D.

Hypothyroid

The Influence of the Maternal Thyroid Hormone Environment During Pregnancy on the Ontogenesis of Brain and Placental Ornithine Decarboxylase Activity in the Rat

Pickard MR, Sinha AK, Ogilvie L, Ekins RP (Univ College London, England)
J Endocrinol 139:205–212, 1993   112-95-10–14

Introduction.—Although it has previously been thought that the placenta is impermeable to maternal thyroid hormones, these substances may play a possible role in fetal brain development. The influence of maternal hypothyroxinemia on early brain and placental development was investigated.

Methods.—A partially thyroidectomized (parathyroid-spared; TX) and normal Sprague–Dawley rat dam model was used. Ornithine decarboxylase (ODC)-specific activity and other more general indicators of cell growth were assessed in prenatal whole brain at 15, 19, and 22 days of gestation, in postnatal brain regions at 5, 10, and 14 days, and in placenta.

Results.—Reduced fetal body weight, brain weight, brain DNA content, and brain total protein content occurred as a result of maternal hypothyroxinemia at 15 days of gestation. The latter effect was maintained until 19 days of gestation. Additional changes in brain cell growth were noted near term, including an increase in the DNA concentration accompanied by a decrease in the total protein:DNA ratio. Postnatal brain region growth appeared normal, although an isolated increase in the protein content of the cerebellum was observed at postnatal day 5. The specific activity of brain ODC showed an intricate pattern of change in the offspring of TX dams, superimposed upon the normal ontogenetic decline. Fetal brain activity was initially deficient at 15 days of gestation but increased at 22 days in relation to controls. During the postnatal period, ODC-specific activity was transiently reduced in the brain stem, the subcortex, and the cerebral cortex. Placental development was less consistently affected. In the TX dam, wet weight and gross indices of cell growth, such as DNA content and concentration and total protein:DNA ratio, were normal. However, reductions in cytosolic concentrations were noted at 15 days, and reductions in total protein were noted at 19 days.

Conclusion.—Maternal hypothyroxinemia leads to abnormal fetal brain cell development. Damage extends into the neonatal period long after the onset of fetal thyroid hormone synthesis. The reduced supply of maternal T_4 to the fetal brain may play an important role in this dysgenesis. However, other factors such as the impairment of placental function also need to be considered.

▶ These workers demonstrate that maternal hypothyroxinemia affects fetal brain development in the rat, suggesting the possibility that this phenomenon might occur in human beings. This is an important reason for maintaining normal serum T_4 values during early pregnancy. The detection of thyroid hormones in human embryonic cavities during the first trimester of pregnancy, before fetal thyroid function is present, also suggests that thyroid hormones do cross the developing placenta from mother to fetus during early life (Contempre et al: *J Clin Endocrinol Metab* 77:1719, 1993). The Escobar group published a technical paper comparing different methods for detecting thyroid hormones in rat fetuses (*Endocrinology* 134:2410, 1994). No explanation was found for the far different values reported by others, attesting to the difficulty in accurately measuring thyroid hormones in whole body tissues.—L.E. Braverman, M.D.

Effects of Dioxins and Polychlorinated Biphenyls on Thyroid Hormone Status of Pregnant Women and Their Infants
Koopman-Esseboom C, Morse DC, Weisglas-Kuperus N, Lutkeschipholt IJ, Van Der Paauw CG, Tuinstra LGMT, Brouwer A, Sauer PJJ (Erasmus Univ, Rotterdam, The Netherlands; Univ Hosp, Rotterdam, The Netherlands; Sophia Children's Hosp, Rotterdam, The Netherlands; et al)
Pediatr Res 36:468–473, 1994   112-95-10–15

Background.—The potentially hazardous compounds known as dioxins, including polychlorinated dibenzo-p-dioxin (PCDD), dibenzofuran (PCDF), and polychlorinated biphenyl (PCB), have been shown to alter thyroid hormone homeostasis in previous animal studies. The effects of PCDD, PCDF, and PCB on the thyroid hormone status of pregnant women and their infants were evaluated as part of the larger prospective longitudinal Dutch PBC/Dioxin Study, which is considering the possible adverse effects of these compounds on human beings.

Participants and Methods.—A total of 105 healthy mother-infant pairs were enrolled between June 1990 and February 1992. Four nonplanar PCB congeners were measured in maternal plasma during the last month of pregnancy to determine maternal exposure. The same PCB congeners were measured in a blood sample of the umbilical cord to estimate prenatal exposure. During the second week after delivery, mothers collected a 24-hour representative sample of breast milk, which was used to measure 17 PCDD and PCDF congeners, 3 planar PCB congeners, and 23 nonplanar PCB congeners.

Results.—A significant correlation was noted between higher PCDD, PCDF, and PCB levels in human milk (expressed as toxic equivalents), and lower plasma levels of maternal total T_3 and total T_4, and in higher plasma levels of TSH in infants during the second week and third month after delivery. Moreover, lower plasma free T_4 and total T_4 levels were noted during the second week after delivery in infants exposed to higher toxic equivalents levels.

Conclusion.—Increased levels of dioxins and PCB can effect the human thyroid hormone status. Studies addressing the impact of PCDD, PCDF, and PCB on the development of the fetus and infant will be further investigated.

▶ This provocative study should be confirmed by others, especially in areas of dioxin excess in the United States. Polychlorinated biphenyls and other hepatic microsomal enzyme inducers were studied in the rat and found to increase uridine diphosphate–glucuronosyltransferase activity toward T_4, decreasing serum T_4 levels (Barter and Klaassen: *Toxicol Appl Pharmacol* 128:9, 1994). Pregnant women perhaps should be screened for asymptomatic autoimmune thyroid disease during the first trimester, because such thyroid antibody–positive women are at risk for hypothyroidism developing later in pregnancy, despite a marked reduction in antibody titers (Glinoer et al: *J Clin Endocrinol Metab* 79:197, 1994). I am not sure that such testing would meet with the approval of our managed care businesspeople because it might not be cost-effective!—L.E. Braverman, M.D.

A 20-Basepair Duplication in the Human Thyroid Peroxidase Gene Results in a Total Iodide Organification Defect and Congenital Hypothyroidism
Bikker H, (Den) Hartog MT, Baas F, Gons MH, Vulsma T, De Vijlder JJM (Children's Hosp, Amsterdam; Academic Med Ctr, Amsterdam)
J Clin Endocrinol Metab 79:248–252, 1994   112-95-10–16

Background.—Thyroid peroxidase (TPO), a primary enzyme in the synthesis of thyroid hormones, catalyzes both the iodination and the coupling of iodotyrosine residues in thyroglobulin. Linkage studies have shown that TPO gene defects result in TPO deficiency in a number of families. A novel mutation resulting in TPO deficiency was described.

Case Report.—The patient was born in 1968 after a pregnancy of 45 weeks. The neonatal period was complicated by extended neonatal icterus. Hypothyroidism was diagnosed at 4 months of age. All signs of thyroid hormone deficiency were demonstrated. Thyroid peroxidase activity and the iodination degree of thyroglobulin were under detection parameters. In addition, Northern blot analysis failed to detect TPO messenger RNA. After subjecting the TPO gene to denaturing gradient gel electrophoretic analysis, a homozygous mutation on exon 2 was identified. Sequence analysis revealed the presence of a 20-basepair duplication, 47 basepairs downstream of the ATG start codon. The mother and father were heterozygous for the same duplication, verifying the recessive mode of inheritance of the mutation.

Conclusion.—The total iodide organification defect found in this patient is a result of a homozygous mutation in the TPO gene. This mutation generates a frame shift, leading to a termination signal in exon 3, which is compatible with the complete absence of TPO. The parents of this patient were carriers of 1 TPO allele with the insertion, but they did not demonstrate any clinical evidence of hypothyroidism. This suggests that a single operative TPO allele is adequate for thyroid function.

▶ This is yet another example of bringing basic science to the bedside.—L.E. Braverman, M.D.

Evidence for the Secretion of Thyrotropin With Enhanced Bioactivity in Syndromes of Thyroid Hormone Resistance

Persani L, Asteria C, Tonacchera M, Vitti P, Chatterjee VKK, Beck-Peccoz P (Inst of Endocrine Sciences, Milan, Italy; Univ of Milan, Italy; Centro Auxologico Italiano IRCCS, Milan, Italy; Inst of Endocrinology, Pisa, Italy; Univ of Pisa, Italy)
J Clin Endocrinol Metab 78:1034–1039, 1994   112-95-10–17

Introduction.—Patients with resistance to thyroid hormone (RTH) exhibit a wide spectrum of clinical expression. However, they typically have elevated serum free thyroid hormones and goiter, even when TSH secretion is normal. Circulating TSH may exhibit elevated biological activity in these patients. The bioactivity of TSH derived from the sera of patients with RTH with different clinical presentations was measured.

Methods.—Fifteen patients with normal thyroid function, 6 euthyroid patients with simple goiter, and 11 patients with RTH of 8 kindreds underwent a TRH challenge to determine serum TSH and free thyroid hormone response. The TSH bioactivity was analyzed in the blood samples obtained 20 to 180 minutes after the injection of TRH in 7 patients with RTH and in 5 normal controls. The TSH was isolated, and Chinese hamster ovary cells and FRTL-5 cells were incubated with the purified TSH receptor, and the ratio of biological to immunoreactive TSH (TSH B/I) was calculated. Circulating TSH from 4 patients with RTH and 4 controls was analyzed with concanavalin A lectin affinity chromatography.

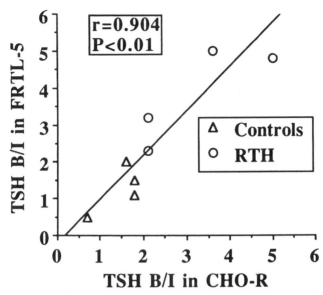

Fig 10–6.—Highly significant correlation between the ratios of biologically active vs. immunoreactive (B/I) immunoconcentrated TSH measured in Chinese hamster ovary cells transfected with the recombinant human TSH receptor (CHO-R) and FRTL-5 bioassays, using TSH IRP 80/558 as standard in both methods. (Courtesy of Persani L, Asteria C, Tonacchera M, et al: *J Clin Endocrinol Metab* 78:1034–1039, 1994.)

Results.—All but 1 of the patients with RTH had normal circulating TSH levels. Genetic analysis confirmed mutations in the TRβ gene in patients with 5 of the 8 RTH kindreds. The TSH response to TRH injection was similar in all of the patient groups, but RTH patients had significantly higher free thyroid hormone responses than did normal and goitrous patients. The mean TSH B/I was 1.3 in the controls and 4.2 in RTH, with significantly higher bioactivity in all of the RTH patients. Bioactivity in the goitrous patients was similar to that in the controls. The FRTL-5 bioassays measured B/I ratios that correlated well with these findings (Fig 10-6). The TSH bioactivity was not significantly altered by TRH treatment, but supraphysiologic doses of T_3 normalized TSH B/I. Baseline chromatography of TSH from RTH and control patients revealed similar unbound fraction, but significantly lower weakly bound fraction and significantly higher firmly bound fraction in RTH patients. After T_3 treatment, the unbound fraction decreased and the weakly bound fraction increased.

Discussion.—Circulating immunoreactive TSH levels may be normal in patients with thyroid hormone resistance, and these patients secrete TSH with enhanced bioactivity. The increased bioactive TSH levels may cause the hypersecretion of free thyroid hormones and goiter seen in these patients. The role of TSH bioactivity in the pathogenesis of the various clinical expressions of this genetic syndrome requires further study.

▶ This study certainly provides an explanation for the thyroid gland hyperfunction in patients with thyroid hormone resistance and normal serum TSH values. The important role of altered TSH carbohydrate content and sialylation is emphasized by Helton and Magner in their study demonstrating an increase in β-galactoside α-36-sialyltransferase messenger RNA content in hypothyroid mouse thyrotrophs and corticotrophs (*Endocrinology* 134:2347, 1994).—L.E. Braverman, M.D.

Mutations of CpG Dinucleotides Located in the Triiodothyronine (T₃)-Binding Domain of the Thyroid Hormone Receptor (TR) β Gene That Appears to Be Devoid of Natural Mutations May Not Be Detected Because They Are Unlikely to Produce the Clinical Phenotype of Resistance to Thyroid Hormone

Hayashi Y, Sunthornthepvarakul T, Refetoff S (Mental Retardation Research Ctr, Chicago; Univ of Chicago)

J Clin Invest 94:607–615, 1994   112-95-10–18

Background.—Resistance to thyroid hormone (RTH) is characterized by a variable tissue hyposensitivity to thyroid hormone. Thyroid hormone receptor (TR) β gene mutations detected in patients with this disorder have demonstrated 2 clusters or "hot areas" of mutations (RTHmut) in the T_3-binding domain. Moreover, 45% of RTHmuts and 90% of recurring mutations are situated in CpG dinucleotides (hot areas). It was determined why the region between the 2 hot areas fails to demonstrate RTHmuts.

Methods.—Ten artificial mutant TRβs (ARTmut) were produced in the "cold" region, based on the hot spot rule (cytosines with thymidines $[C \rightarrow T]$ or guanines with adenines $[G \rightarrow A]$ substitutions in CpGs). Comparisons between the properties of ARTmuts and 6 RTHmuts were made.

Results.—Among the RTHmuts, R320H exhibiting a mild form of RTH demonstrated the least impairment of T_3-binding affinity (K_a). In comparison, K_a was normal in 6 ARTmuts (group A) and reduced to a lesser extent than R320H in 3 (group B). T_3 binding did not occur in 1 that was truncated (R410X). Each RTHmut showed impaired ability to transactivate T_3-responsive elements. In addition, all RTHmuts demonstrated a strong dominant negative effect on cotransfected wild-type TRβ. Minimal impairment or normal transactivation was noted for group A ARTmuts, and weak or no dominant negative effect was noted for B ARTmuts. Transactivation and dominant negative effect were not demonstrated in R410X.

Conclusion.—Mutations expected to occur with the most frequency in the cold region of the ligand-binding domain of TRβ are not likely to be detected. This is because of the small or no alteration of T$_3$ binding and transactivation function and little or no dominant negative effect. The insensitivity to amino acid changes indicates that the cold region of the putative ligand-binding domain may not directly interact with T$_3$.

▶ The RTH syndrome continues to be studied in ever greater detail. Weiss and co-workers provide data that "do not support the genetic linkage of attention deficit hyperactivity disorder (ADD) and RTH, but do suggest that RTH is associated with lower IQ scores that may confer a high likelihood of exhibiting ADD symptoms" (*J Clin Endocrinol Metab* 78:1525, 1994). Further point mutations of TRβ gene in RTH continue to appear (Magaya et al: *J Clin Endocrinol Metab* 77:982, 1993; Weiss et al: *J Clin Endocrinol Metab* 78:1253, 1994). Finally, the presence of thyroid dysfunction itself in patients with RTH should not be overlooked. For example, Robinson et al. report a patient with RTH and autoimmune hypothyroidism (*South Med J* 86:1395, 1993).—L.E. Braverman, M.D.

Familial Unresponsiveness to Thyrotropin by Autosomal Recessive Inheritance
Takamatsu J, Nishikawa M, Horimoto M, Ohsawa N (Osaka Med College, Takatsuki, Japan; Kansai Med Univ, Moriguchi, Osaka, Japan)
J Clin Endocrinol Metab 77:1569–1573, 1993   112-95-10–19

Background.—Resistance of the thyroid gland to TSH is not a well-recognized phenomenon. To date, the incidence of TSH unresponsiveness has only been reported and sufficiently investigated in 3 patients. Siblings in whom this defect was diagnosed were reported, representing the first documentation of familial occurrence.

Case Report.—Female, 26, was given a diagnosis of congenital hypothyroidism at infancy. The thyroid was atrophic. Thyroid function tests without T$_4$ replacement revealed serum free T$_4$ levels of less than 3 pmol/L, serum TSH of 125 mU/L, and serum thyroglobulin of less than 5 mg/L. A ^{123}I scintigram demonstrated reduced uptake (5% at 24 hours). However, normal shape at the proper position in the neck was observed. No autoantibodies against thyroglobulin, thyroid peroxidase, and TSH receptor in serum were identified. The amount of cyclic adenosine monophosphate (cAMP) released into FRTL-5 cell culture in the presence of TSH did not differ from that released by the same amount of TSH from normal individuals. This indicated that the TSH bioactivity in this patient was normal. Congenital hypothyroidism was also diagnosed in the patient's brother. Data on his thyroid function were comparable to those of his sister. A consanguineous marriage had taken place between the parents of these siblings (mother and father were first cousins). Although the mother had a normal serum free T_4 level, slightly elevated serum TSH and thyroglobulin levels were detected, suggesting subclinical hypothyroidism.

Conclusion.—A mutation of the TSH receptor gene, abnormality in transcription-regulating factor, abnormality in GTP-binding protein, and/or inhibition of the action of cAMP may account for the pathogenesis of TSH unresponsiveness in these patients. The family history indicates that the manner of inheritance is autosomal recessive.

▶ The genetic defect responsible for this syndrome is certain to be described soon.—L.E. Braverman, M.D.

Decreased Levothyroxine Requirement in Women With Hypothyroidism During Androgen Therapy for Breast Cancer
Arafah BM (Univ Hosps of Cleveland, Ohio)
Ann Intern Med 121:247–251, 1994   112-95-10–20

Introduction.—Patients with no thyroid disease undergoing androgen treatment have decreasing serum T_4-binding globulin levels and circulating total thyroid hormone levels but maintain a clinically euthyroid state. However, there have been no reports of the effects of androgen treatment on patients requiring thyroid hormone replacement. Postmenopausal women with and without hypothyroidism who were being treated with androgens for metastatic, hormone-dependent breast cancer were studied.

Methods.—Four women with stable levothyroxine-controlled primary hypothyroidism and 7 women with no thyroid disease were treated with androgens for as long as they controlled tumor growth. Blood samples were drawn regularly during and for 6 to 12 weeks after androgen therapy. Serum levels of T_4, T_4-binding globulin, TSH, and T_3 resin uptake were monitored.

Results.—In control patients, total T_4 and T_4-binding globulin decreased and T_3 resin uptake levels increased proportionally by the 4th week of androgen therapy and then remained steady. Serum TSH decreased slightly until 8 weeks, then remained stable. Free T_4 levels did not change. By 6 to 12 weeks after the discontinuation of androgen treatment, all values returned to baseline. In patients receiving thyroid hormone replacement regimens, TSH levels declined and free T_4 increased significantly by week 8, producing clinical thyrotoxicity (Fig 10–7). The T_4 dose was reduced in 3 patients, and a euthyroid condition was restored. Serum values returned to baseline 8–10 weeks after androgen treatment ended.

Discussion.—Androgen treatment in postmenopausal women caused significant changes in serum total thyroid hormone concentrations. Women without thyroid disease exhibited changes and remained euthyroid. However, women receiving thyroid hormone replacement therapy

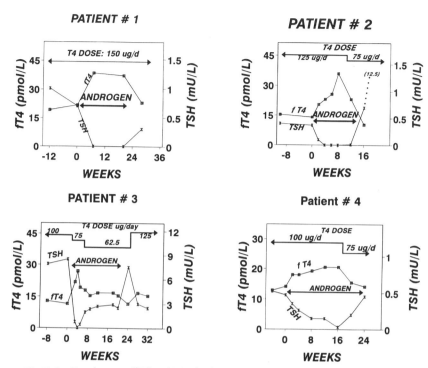

Fig 10–7.—Free thyroxine *(fT4)* and TSH levels in 4 women who received long-term treatment for primary hypothyroidism measured before, during, and after androgen therapy for breast cancer. The *upper portion* of each graph shows the levothyroxine dose used; the *arrows* indicate the beginning and duration of androgen therapy. Levothyroxine dose was not altered in patient 1 but was reduced during androgen administration to patients 2, 3, and 4 to maintain euthyroidism. (Courtesy of Arafah BM: *Ann Intern Med* 121:247–251, 1994.)

became thyrotoxic until their levothyroxine dose was reduced by 25% to 50%. The changes were reversible in both groups after discontinuation of androgen therapy.

▶ Fortunately, the administration of androgens to women with hypothyroidism is not too common. Although not new, the decreased absorption of L-T$_4$ by sucralfate and aluminum hydroxide is called to the reader's attention (Sherman et al: *Am J Med* 96:531, 1994; Liel et al: *Am J Med* 97:363, 1994). Hays and Nielson report a small decrease in the absorption of L-T$_4$ in the elderly (*Thyroid* 4:55, 1994).—L.E. Braverman, M.D.

▶↑ Acquired hypothyroidism caused by Hashimoto's thyroiditis with high thyroglobulin and TPO antibodies is described in 4 infants under age 2 years, certainly an unexpected finding (Foley et al: *N Engl J Med* 330:466, 1994). Primary open-angle glaucoma and hypothyroidism appear to be associated (Smith et al: *Ophthalmology* 100:1580, 1993). Should serum TSH concentrations be measured in all patients with open-angle glaucoma? Elevations of serum skeletal muscle creatine kinase are commonly present in hypothyroid patients (Burnett et al: *N Z Med J* 107:355, 1994), and serum cardiac muscle creatine kinase levels may also be elevated when measured by highly sensitive assays (Miyamoto et al: *Eur J Clin Chem Clin Biochem* 32:589, 1994) and may remain elevated during the first 6–8 weeks of thyroid hormone therapy.—L.E. Braverman, M.D.

Cancer, Nodules, Growth Factors

Comparison Between Preoperative Cytology and Intraoperative Frozen-Section Biopsy in the Diagnosis of Thyroid Nodules

Rodríguez JM, Parrilla P, Sola J, Bas A, Aguilar J, Moreno A, Soria T (Virgen de la Arrixaca Univ Hosp, El Palmar, Murcia, Spain)
Br J Surg 81:1151–1154, 1994   112-95-10–21

Introduction.—Fine-needle aspiration cytology (FNAC) is routinely performed in patients with thyroid nodules. Intraoperative biopsy is also routinely performed, although it adds to the surgical time and expense and has uncertain diagnostic accuracy. The results of FNAC and intraoperative biopsy were compared in patients who had both procedures to assess the value of intraoperative biopsy.

Methods.—During a 5-year period, 175 consecutive patients underwent both FNAC before surgery for thyroid nodules and intraoperative frozen-section biopsy. Both FNAC and biopsy diagnostic results were recorded as benign, suspicious, or malignant. These results were compared with the definitive histological diagnosis of the excised nodules in each patient. The sensitivity, specificity, and diagnostic accuracy of each procedure was calculated.

Results.—Of 143 patients with benign lesions, FNAC correctly diagnosed 76 of 77 patients, and intraoperative biopsy correctly diagnosed 75 of 77 patients. The FNAC diagnosed suspicious lesions in 76 patients, of which 67 were benign and 9 were malignant. Intraoperative biopsy in these 76 patients diagnosed benign lesions in 69 patients and malignant lesions in 7. All 17 malignant FNAC diagnoses were confirmed histologically, but only 13 of 17 biopsy diagnoses of malignancy were correct. The overall sensitivity of FNAC vs. intraoperative biopsy was 94.4% vs. 77.7%; specificity was 53.9% vs. 98.6%; diagnostic accuracy was 58% vs. 95.2%. The diagnostic accuracy of FNAC vs. intraoperative biopsy was 98% vs. 97% in the benign group, 12% vs. 96% in the suspicious group, and 100% vs. 76% in the malignant group.

Discussion.—The value of intraoperative biopsy varies depending on the results of FNAC. Intraoperative biopsy is less accurate than FNAC in diagnosing malignancy and adds little to the cytologically benign diagnosis. Biopsy is indicated when the cytologic findings are suspicious of malignancy.

▶ It is evident from this and other papers (Tielens et al: *Cancer* 73:424, 1994; van Zuidewijn et al: *World J Surg* 18:506, 1994; McHenry et al: *Am J Surg* 166:353, 1993) that the routine use of frozen section examination to determine the correct diagnosis of the thyroid nodule should probably be reconsidered, especially in view of the usefulness of the fine-needle aspiration biopsy. Although we do not do ultrasound-guided needle aspiration biopsies of "nonpalpable or difficult to palpate" thyroid nodules, Sanchez et al. (*J Am Coll Surg* 178:33, 1994) reported that diagnostic biopsies were obtained in 26 of 32 patients, but only 1 was malignant. Proton MR spectroscopy of fine-needle biopsies and surgical specimens was able to differentiate between benign and malignant follicular neoplasms (Delbridge et al: *World J Surg* 18:512, 1994). If this technique proves as efficacious on fine-needle biopsies in other centers, unnecessary surgery can be avoided.

It is well recognized that x-ray exposure to the head and neck during infancy increases the occurrence of thyroid cancer and hyperparathyroidism in adulthood. Fedorak et al. (*Am Surg* 6:428, 1994) now report an increased incidence of thyroid cancer in patients with primary hyperparathyroidism but no history of previous irradiation. There might be an increased association between lymphocytic thyroiditis and thyroid cancer (McKee et al: *Br J Surg* 80:1303, 1993; Haapala et al: *APMIS* 102:390, 1994), suggesting that the presence of hypofunctioning nodules in patients with Hashimoto's thyroiditis should not be overlooked. Primary thyroid lymphoma responds well to radiotherapy but is often difficult to distinguish from chronic thyroiditis by needle aspiration biopsy (Brownlie et al: *N Z Med J* 107:301, 1994).—L.E. Braverman, M.D.

Diagnostic Use of Recombinant Human Thyrotropin in Patients With Thyroid Carcinoma (Phase I/II Study)

Meier CA, Braverman LE, Ebner SA, Veronikis I, Daniels GH, Ross DS, Deraska DJ, Davies TF, Valentine M, DeGroot LJ, Curran P, McEllin K, Reynolds J, Robbins J, Weintraub BD (Natl Inst of Diabetes and Digestive and Kidney Diseases, Bethesda, Md; Univ of Massachusetts, Worcester; Massachusetts Gen Hosp, Boston; et al)
J Clin Endocrinol Metab 78:188–196, 1994   112-95-10–22

Background.—Radioiodine uptake and serum thyroglobulin (Tg) levels are the currently used studies to detect residual or metastatic thyroid tissue in patients with differentiated thyroid carcinoma. Both of these studies require that the subject be sufficiently hypothyroid for endogenous TSH stimulation; nearly all patients have clinical hypothyroid symptoms during this period. With the use of recombinant human TSH (rhTSH), ^{131}I uptake and Tg release can be stimulated from residual thyroid tissue in euthyroid patients.

Methods.—The safety, dosage, and efficacy of rhTSH in 19 patients with differentiated thyroid carcinoma were examined in this preliminary study. The patients had recently undergone thyroidectomy and were receiving suppressive doses of T_3. The patients received 10- to 40-unit doses of rhTSH for 1–3 days. The day after the last dose, they were given 1–2 mCi of ^{131}I, followed 48 hours later by a neck and whole-body scan. T_3 was discontinued for a median of 19 days, resulting in marked elevation of endogenous serum TSH levels, and then given a second dose of ^{131}I, followed 48 hours later by a repeat whole-body scan.

Results.—There were no major adverse effects of rhTSH, although 16% of patients receiving the higher doses reported nausea. Psychometric measures of quality of life were much better during rhTSH treatment than after T_3 withdrawal. Serum TSH peaked 2–8 hours after rhTSH injection, to 127 mU/L with the 10-unit dose, 309 mU/L with the 20-unit dose, and 510 mU/L with the 30-unit dose. Twenty-four hours after injection, TSH levels decreased to 83, 173, and 463 mU/L, respectively.

In 63% of patients, both thyroid scans were of similar quality and showed a similar number of abnormal ^{131}I uptake sites. Sixteen percent of patients showed additional uptake sites in the chest or thyroid bed on the rhTSH scan that were not visible on the hypothyroid scan. Another 16% had additional lesions shown only after T_3 withdrawal. One patient had an uptake focus that was better demonstrated after rhTSH than after withdrawal. The scan made after rhTSH showed a lower amount of radioiodine uptake in the thyroid bed in 68% of patients. After correction for the increased whole-body retention of ^{131}I during hypothyroidism, however, uptake was comparable to that after T_3 withdrawal. Nearly three fourths of patients had at least doubled serum Tg levels in response to rhTSH; the same patients had a similar Tg response to T_3 withdrawal. In all but 1 of these, the increase was quantitatively lower after rhTSH.

Conclusion.—Preliminary data suggest that rhTSH is a safe and effective method of stimulating ^{131}I uptake and Tg secretion without causing symptoms of hypothyroidism. The optimal dose regimen of rhTSH would appear to be 10–20 units/day given over 1 or more days before radioiodine administration. Proof of the efficacy of rhTSH awaits a phase III trial.

▶ Recombinant human TSH will hopefully be available within 18 months and should prove to be useful, avoiding the hypothyroid symptoms following thyroid hormone withdrawal. It has been suggested that scanning doses of 3 to 10 mCi ^{131}I might decrease subsequent thyroid uptake after therapeutic doses of [131]I (Park et al: *Thyroid* 4:49, 1994). This "stunning" phenomenon should be further evaluated. Comtois et al. suggest that 30 mCi of ^{131}I successfully ablates residual thyroid bed uptake after surgery for thyroid cancer, but only 27% had successful ablation at this outpatient ^{131}I dose (*J Nucl Med* 34:1927, 1993). We do not use the low-dose ^{131}I regimen. Finally, the best documented study of the usefulness of large doses of ^{131}I to decrease the size of large, locally compressive, nontoxic goiters has been reported by Huysmans et al. (*Ann Intern Med* 121:757, 1994). Potentiation of ^{131}I uptake by using recombinant TSH might be helpful in increasing the efficacy of the

[131]I in treating these bulky goiters. Surgery still remains the best therapy if the patient is reasonably healthy.—L.E. Braverman, M.D.

Long-Term Impact of Initial Surgical and Medical Therapy on Papillary and Follicular Thyroid Cancer

Mazzaferri EL, Jhiang SM (Ohio State Univ, Columbus)
Am J Med 97:418–427, 1994   112-95-10–23

Objective.—The long-term effects of treatment were examined in a series of 1,355 patients seen in the past 4 decades with well-differentiated papillary and follicular cancers of the thyroid gland. The median follow-up was 15.7 years; 42% of patients were followed for 20 years, and 14% for 30 years.

Outcome.—Papillary cancers were present in 79% of patients and follicular cancers in 21%. A total of 215 patients (16%) died. More of the patients with follicular cancer died, but the difference was not significant when the data were adjusted for patients having distant disease when diagnosed. Tumors recurred in 289 (21%) of patients; 45 (16%) of these patients died of cancer. Distant metastases developed in 88 (7%) of pa-

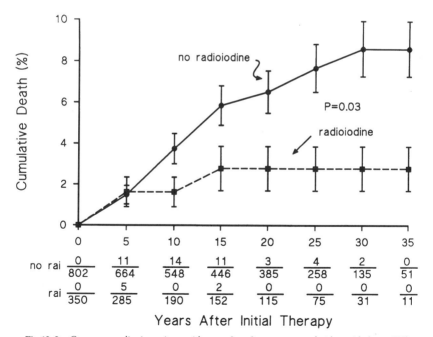

Fig 10–8.—Cancer mortality in patients with stage 2 or 3 tumors treated either with (*n* = 350) or without (*n* = 802) [131]I. Of those treated with ^{131}I, more were males (38% vs. 30%, *P* = .02) and more had lymph node metastases (53% vs. 45%, *P* < .05) and stage 3 tumors (23% vs. 16%, *P* < .01). The 2 groups were comparable with respect to other risk factors. The *P* values are all less than the values shown. (Courtesy of Mazzaferri EL, Jhiang SM: *Am J Med* 97:418–427, 1994.)

tients. Mortality rates for follicular and papillary cancers at 30 years were 10% and 6%, respectively.

Treatment Factors.—Treatment was delayed for a median of 18 months in patients who died of cancer, compared with 4 months for those who survived. Mortality from cancer was 4% when patients were treated within a year of diagnosis and 10% in others. The respective 30-year mortality rates were 6% and 13%. More aggressive surgical treatment was associated with lower recurrence and mortality rates. In patients given medical treatment initially, those receiving external radiation had the highest recurrence rates and cancer mortality rates, and those given radioiodine had the lowest (Fig 10–8). Time to treatment, thyroid surgery beyond lobectomy, and ^{131}I therapy remained significant factors on multivariate analysis.

Conclusion.—Along with tumor-related features, initial treatment has a long-term influence on the outcome of well-differentiated thyroid cancers, with the best results seen in patients treated with near total thyroidectomy followed by ^{131}I therapy and long-term L-T$_4$ therapy.

▶ Although Dr. Mazzaferri and colleagues have come under attack by others, this paper is the most convincing that near total thyroidectomy followed by ^{131}I and thyroid hormone therapy results in the best prognosis for both recurrence and mortality from differentiated thyroid cancer. This is our approach to this disease. Another less comprehensive paper (DeGroot et al: *World J Surg* 18:123, 1994) agrees with the Mazzaferri data, and Pacini et al. (*World J Surg* 18:600, 1994) report a favorable outcome of the treatment of metastatic thyroid cancer with ^{131}I. Shah et al. reached a different conclusion and reported that lobectomy in "low-risk" patients with thyroid cancer did as well as those undergoing total thyroidectomy (*Am J Surg* 166:331, 1993).—L.E. Braverman, M.D.

Serum Thyroglobulin in the Follow-Up of Patients With Treated Differentiated Thyroid Cancer
Ozata M, Suzuki S, Miyamoto T, Liu RT, Fierro-Renoy F, Degroot LJ (Univ of Chicago, Ill)
J Clin Endocrinol Metab 79:98–105, 1994   112-95-10–24

Background.—Measuring serum thyroglobulin (Tg) is a sensitive way to detect recurrence or metastases in patients treated for differentiated thyroid cancer. However, discrepancies have been reported between the serum Tg level and disease activity. The critical value of serum Tg measurement in determining the presence or absence of cancer was investigated.

Methods.—Serum Tg data obtained while patients were on and off T$_4$ treatment were evaluated. The 180 patients were followed for up to 18 years. Radioiodine scanning, radiography, and clinical examination were performed to establish the presence of cancer.

Findings.—Among patients with no evidence of active disease after therapy, the presence of Tg did not indicate cancer in patients with a partial thyroidectomy with or without ablation. In those patients, Tg levels often exceeded 5 or 10 ng/mL. The presence of residual normal thyroid tissue reduced the diagnostic value of serum Tg assay. Among patients undergoing near total (NTT) or total thyroidectomy (TT) and ^{131}I ablation, 5.5% of patients had Tg levels exceeding 5 ng/mL, and 1.8% had Tg levels exceeding 10 ng/mL. Without therapy, 22.8% of the patients had Tg exceeding 5 ng/mL, and 10.5% had levels exceeding 10 ng/mL. In this group, a Tg level below 10 ng/mL during suppressive treatment indicated absence of apparent tumor in 98.2%. Assay sensitivity was increased by hormone withdrawal, whereas false positive results increased especially at lower cutoff levels. There was no cutoff value that properly classified all patients.

Among patients with recurrent or continued disease, Tg levels ranged from 2 to 21,000 ng/mL during T_4 treatment. Without treatment, Tg levels ranged from 6 to 10,700 ng/mL. A Tg level exceeding 10 ng/mL without treatment indicated the presence of active disease in 76.9% of the patients. In patients undergoing NTT and TT and ^{131}I ablation, Tg levels were uniformly lower during T_4 treatment. However, TSH levels below the normal range were unrelated to lower TG values. Thyroglobulin values and amount of ^{131}I used for ablation were uncorrelated in these patients.

Conclusion.—Thyroglobulin and ^{131}I scans are complementary in the follow-up of patients with differentiated thyroid cancer. In most patients, Tg assay cannot be used to exclude the presence of cancer. However, recurrent cancer is very rare in patients who have had NTT or TT and ^{131}I ablation, a negative postablation scan, and Tg values below 2 ng/mL on replacement or 3 ng/mL off replacement therapy.

▶ This paper is difficult to interpret, but the message is loud and clear: the serum Tg is extremely useful in following patients with treated thyroid cancer. Two papers use the identification of ^{131}I-labeled T_4 in serum after a scanning dose of ^{131}I to determine the presence of functioning thyroid tissue in patients with previously treated thyroid cancer even in the absence of uptake on scan (Bianchi et al: *J Nucl Med* 34:2032, 1993; Hays and McDougall: *Thyroid* 4:195, 1994). Although a bit cumbersome, this method, along with serum Tg levels (unless Tg antibodies preclude their measurement), appears to be helpful in determining whether ^{131}I should be given in the absence of uptake on scan. Some of the cardiac effects of the larger TSH suppressive doses of L-T_4 used in patients with thyroid cancer can be alleviated by using a long-acting β-blocker (Bianchi et al: *J Clin Endocrinol Metab* 78:1028, 1994).—L.E. Braverman, M.D.

Clinical Meaning of DNA Content in the Long Term Behaviour of Follicular Thyroid Tumours: A 12-Year Follow Up

Lukács GL, Balázs G, Zs-Nagy I, Mikó T (Univ Med School, Debrecen, Hungary)
Eur J Surg 160:417–423,1994   112-95-10–25

Background.—The best method of diagnosing and establishing the prognosis of neoplastic and non-neoplastic follicular thyroid tumors has not been determined. Possible correlations between DNA aneuploidy in benign and malignant follicular tumors of the thyroid and disease progression were investigated.

Methods.—The retrospective analysis included 71 of 75 patients who had had cytofluorimetric nuclear DNA studies done on their follicular thyroid tumors between 1977 and 1980 and for whom clinical follow-up data were available. Patients had been followed for 12 years. The main outcome measure was the association between clinical course and the finding of aneuploidy in original histologic specimens.

Findings.—Aneuploidy was identified in 6 of 40 follicular adenomas, 3 of 17 adenomatous goiters, and 13 of 14 follicular carcinomas. During follow-up, there were no benign tumor recurrences. Five patients with carcinoma had died of distant metastases during follow-up. All had aneuploid stemlines. Eight patients with carcinomas and aneuploidy are still alive with no recurrences or metastases.

Conclusion.—Deoxyribonucleic acid aneuploidy of follicular thyroid tumors apparently does not predict subsequent invasion and metastases. Furthermore, DNA analysis of tumor cells does not distinguish between minimally invasive and extremely invasive carcinomas.

▶ This paper certainly puts a damper on the enthusiasm for using DNA aneuploidy to determine thyroid cancer virulence. Ozama et al. (*Hum Pathol* 25:271, 1994) agree with these conclusions. The p53 gene is a tumor suppressor gene, and p53 mutations have been reported in human cancers, including the thyroid. Zou et al. report p53 point mutations in some thyroid cancers that were not associated with tumor stage or histology (*J Clin Endocrinol Metab* 77:1054, 1993). High-molecular-weight cytokeratins have now been reported to be markers for papillary and the follicular variant of papillary thyroid cancer, distinguishing these lesions from benign and malignant follicular neoplasms and nodular hyperplasia (Raphael et al: *Mod Pathol* 7:295, 1994). Black pigmentation of the thyroid is found after minocycline administration. Now, dark red staining of the thyroid has been reported during antidepressant therapy, perhaps as a result of lysosomal accumulation of the drugs (Pastolero and Asa: *Arch Pathol Lab Med* 118:79, 1994).—L.E. Braverman, M.D.

Novel Mutations of Thyrotropin Receptor Gene in Thyroid Hyperfunctioning Adenomas: Rapid Identification by Fine Needle Aspiration Biopsy

Porcellini A, Ciullo I, Laviola L, Amabile G, Fenzi G, Avvedimento VE (Centro di Endocrinologia ed Oncologia Sperimentale del CNR, Napoli, Italy; Facoltà di Medicina a Catanzaro, Italy; Cattedra di Endocrinologia, Napoli, Italy)

J Clin Endocrinol Metab 79:657–661, 1994   112-95-10-26

Background.—Hyperfunctioning adenomas of the thyroid gland grow autonomously and overproduce thyroid hormones. In theory, constitutive activation of any component in the cyclic adenosine monophosphate (cAMP) cascade should lead to an adenoma of this type. Hyperfunctioning adenomas recently were encountered that carried somatic mutations in the III cytoplasmic loop of the TSH receptor (TSH-R) gene. The mutations appear to lead to clonal growth and activation of the cAMP pathway and, ultimately, hyperthyroidism.

Objective.—The messenger RNA encoding TSH-R of 11 adenomas sampled by fine-needle aspiration biopsy was analyzed and sequenced. The lesions were typical single hyperfunctioning nodules.

Findings.—Seven mutants were found, all of them located in the sixth membrane-spanning domain of the TSH-R within a cluster of 3 amino acids. All were somatic mutations that were specifically present in tumor tissue. Sequencing of DNA demonstrated that 80% to 90% of these mutations may be rapidly screened for and identified by restriction enzyme analysis of amplified cDNA obtained from aspiration biopsy samples. When the mutation Thr→Ile was introduced in the wild-type receptor and expressed in murine fibroblasts, the basal value of cAMP-dependent transcription increased significantly.

Implications.—Somatic mutations are found in a limited region of the TSH-R gene in a number of hyperfunctioning thyroidal adenomas. If further studies confirm a high prevalence of such mutations, it may be possible to detect lesions that ultimately will lead to hyperfunctioning adenomas at an early stage.

▶ This finding of mutated TSH receptors in thyroid hyperfunctioning nodules offers a logical explanation for their autonomy and hyperfunction and expands upon the earlier observations by Parma et al. (*Nature* 365:649, 1993). These workers have also reported germline mutations in the TSH-R gene in nonautoimmune autosomal dominant hyperthyroidism (Duprez et al: *Nature Gene* 7:396, 1994). In contrast to these findings, no mutations in the TSH receptor in thyroid tissue from 10 patients with Graves' disease were detected (Ahmad et al: *Thyroid* 4:151, 1994). The pathology of hot nodules from 17 patients revealed that 2 were malignant, and some had papillary architecture without malignancy (Mizukami et al: *Am J Clin Pathol* 101:29, 1994). This is an unusually high proportion of cancers. Finally, Nygaard et al. (*Thyroid* 4:167, 1994) confirm what some of us have believed, namely, that

[131]I therapy of solitary hot nodules does not usually completely ablate the nodule. Some of these solitary nodules continue to suppress the remaining tissue and some remain as cold or inhomogeneous nodules on scan. For these reasons, we prefer surgery in most of these patients.—L.E. Braverman, M.D.

Divergent Patterns of Immediate Early Gene Expression in Response to Thyroid-Stimulating Hormone and Insulin-Like Growth Factor I in Wistar Rat Thyrocytes

Tominaga T, Dela Cruz J, Burrow GN, Meinkoth JL (Univ of California, San Diego, La Jolla; Yale Univ, New Haven, Conn)
Endocrinology 135:1212–1219, 1994   112-95-10–27

Background.—Thyrotropin (TSH) and IGF-I both stimulate markers of thyroid cells, and both together stimulate DNA synthesis and cell proliferation in follicular cells of the thyroid. Stimulation of quiescent cells by mitogens leads to the induction of immediate early gene expression. Thyrotropin uses cyclic adenosine monophosphate (cAMP) as a second messenger, whereas the IGF-I receptor possesses protein tyrosine kinase activity.

Objective.—An attempt was made to learn whether different patterns of immediate early gene expression are induced by these mitogens. The expression of c-*fos*, *egr*1, c-*jun*, and *jun*B in response to TSH and IGF-I was quantified in Wistar rat thyroid cells.

Findings.—The expression of all 4 genes studied was stimulated by IGF-I. In contrast, TSH stimulated the expression of c-*fos* and *jun*B but not that of *egr*1. Thyrotropin suppressed the serum- and IGF-I-stimulated expression of c-*jun*, c-*fos*, and *egr*1, and it also repressed serum- and phorbol ester–stimulated AP-1 activity.

Interpretation.—Although TSH and IGF-I each stimulate DNA synthesis in thyroid cells, they have opposed effects on the expression of some immediate early genes. One possible explanation is the existence of distinct signaling pathways.

▶ There is increasing evidence to indicate that growth factors play a role in goiter formation. Insulin-like growth factor binding proteins are synthesized by ovine thyroid follicles, and their local release may modulate the actions of IGFs, perhaps playing a role in the TSH regulation of iodide transport and organification (Phillips et al: *Endocrinology* 134:1238, 1994). A series of papers describe the expression of fibroblast growth factor in thyroid tissue (Bechtner et al: *Acta Endocrinol* 129:458, 1993; Shingu et al: *World J Surg* 18:500, 1994; Hill et al: *Thyroid* 4:77, 1994), its stimulatory effect on growth and inhibition of iodide uptake and organification (Hill et al: *Thyroid* 4:77, 1994), and its inhibitory effect on type I-5′deiodinase activity in FRTL-5 rat thyroid cells (Tang et al: *Endocrinology* 135:493, 1994). Finally, epidermal growth factor stimulates the growth and invasion of differentiated thyroid cancer cells in vitro and in nude mice (Hoelting et al: *J Clin Endocrinol Metab* 79:401, 1994).—L.E. Braverman, M.D.

▶ ↑ The problems arising from the Chernobyl nuclear disaster continue. Radiation exposure to the thyroid has recently been estimated in the Kiev population for the first 2 months after Chernobyl and has led to the prediction that almost 200 cases of thyroid cancer will occur: 66 among those born before 1971 and 130 in the younger inhabitants (Likhtarev et al: *Health Phys* 66:137, 1994). Tezelman et al. have suggested that radioiodine therapy of Graves' disease may increase the risk of developing cancer years later (*World J Surg* 18:522, 1994), a suggestion that has not been born out in previous, much larger studies. Also, the mean dose of ^{131}I used in their study was 25.3 mCi, which probably would have ablated the thyroid. External beam radiotherapy was used in 113 patients with advanced local thyroid disease, and the results suggest that radiotherapy may be helpful in some patients (*Eur J Cancer* 30A:733, 1994). Anaplastic thyroid cancer has a terrible prognosis, but preoperative combined Adriamycin and radiotherapy, debulking surgery, and postsurgical Adriamycin and radiotherapy resulted in 4 of 33 patients surviving disease-free for more than 2 years (Tennvall et al: *Cancer* 74:1348, 1994). We have carried out a similar protocol in 1 patient who is alive and disease-free 4 years after therapy. Early discharge from the hospital after thyroid surgery is now necessary in our health care system, whether we like it or not. Next-day discharge with routine oral calcium supplementation is reported by Moore (*J Am Coll Surg* 178:11, 1994), and we also routinely discharge patients the next day and, occasionally, the night of surgery (Patwardhan et al: *Surgery* 114:1108, 1993). Total thyroidectomy should only be performed by surgeons who became proficient at this procedure during their residency training (Reeve et al: *Arch Surg* 129:834, 1994).

Kozol et al. (*Surgery* 114:1108, 1993) have reported that not all lateral aberrant thyroid tissue is malignant. Another bit of dogma may have been refuted. Insular thyroid cancer has been rarely reported and its prognosis is poor. Recently, Ashfaq et al. reported 41 patients with insular cancer as a minor or predominant component of papillary or follicular cancer. They found no correlation between the quantity of insular cancer and tumor stage, follow-up status, or ploidy, suggesting that the presence of insular cancer within papillary and follicular carcinoma does not adversely affect prognosis (*Cancer* 73:416, 1994). Two patients experienced rapid growth of papillary thyroid cancer early in pregnancy, probably caused by the thyroid stimulatory effects of human chorionic gonadotropin (Kobayashi et al: *J Surg Oncol* 55:61, 1994). Transient facial nerve palsy has been reported in 2 patients after the administration of large doses of ^{131}I, probably the result of transient radiation injury to the facial nerve from ^{131}I concentrated in the parotid gland (Levenson et al: *Ann Intern Med* 120:576, 1994). A study from a region in Italy with mild iodine deficiency strongly suggests that L-T_4 administration definitely decreases the recurrence of nodules in the remaining lobe after a lobectomy for benign nodular disease (Miccoli et al: *Surgery* 114:1097, 1993).

I am delighted to see this report because postlobectomy L-T$_4$ therapy has been our practice for years. On the other hand, Kima et al. (*World J Surg* 18:495, 1994) recommended no medical or surgical therapy for aspiration biopsy–proven benign nodules as long as the nodules do not increase in size. However, approximately 22% of the nodules in their series did increase in size! The Bern group continues to study the pathogenesis of benign multinodular goiter and reports that polyclonal and monoclonal nodules coexist in the same goiter (Kopp et al: *J Clin Endocrinol Metab* 79:134, 1994). The functional status of such nodules were also evaluated, and a dissociation was found in 3 enzyme activities measured (TPO, NADPH-cytochrome-c reductase, MAO) and iodide transport and organification, suggesting that factors other than TSH could be responsible for abnormal thyroid growth (Masini-Repiso et al: *J Clin Endocrinol Metab* 79:39, 1994).

Could these stimuli be some of the growth factors described earlier? In earlier YEAR BOOKS, it was reported that endemic goiter was an autoimmune disease with thyroid growth-stimulating antibodies as the etiology. This has been controversial, and recently Vitti and associates have failed to detect either growth-stimulating or thyroid-stimulating antibodies in the sera of either Peruvian or Italian patients with iodine-deficiency goiter (*J Clin Endocrinol Metab* 78:1020, 1994). Each year we should be reminded of another unusual constellation of abnormalities. Try Cowden's disease: rare inherited disease with mucocutaneous lesions, gastrointestinal polyposis, and benign or malignant thyroid and breast tumors (Smid and Zargi: *J Laryngol Otol* 107:1063, 1993).—L.E. Braverman, M.D.

Autoimmunity and Iodine

Recombinant Thyroid Peroxidase Autoantibodies Can Be Used for Epitopic "Fingerprinting" of Thyroid Peroxidase Autoantibodies in the Sera of Individual Patients
Nishikawa T, Costante G, Prummel MF, McLachlan SM, Rapoport B (VA Med Ctr, San Francisco; Univ of California, San Francisco)
J Clin Endocrinol Metab 78:944–949, 1994   112-95-10–28

Background.—Most patients with active autoimmune thyroid disease, including Graves' disease, have polyclonal autoantibodies to thyroid peroxidase (TPO). Such antibodies are associated with a wide range of clinical disease, and there is evidence that complement-fixing IgG1 TPO autoantibodies are associated with thyroid dysfunction and hypothyroidism. Four human monoclonal antibodies map the immunodominant region on TPO that is recognized by autoantibodies in patient sera.

Objective.—A pool of these monoclonal antibodies, expressed in bacteria as antigen-binding fragments [F(ab)], was used to compete for TPO autoantibody binding to radiolabeled TPO. Sera were obtained from 32 patients with Graves' disease.

Results.—The F(ab) inhibited TPO binding by patient sera by a mean of 82%. A wide range of binding inhibition was observed when the sera were considered individually, and a given serum could be characterized by an epitopic "fingerprint." There was close correlation between the proportions of TPO autoantibodies to the TR1.8 and TR1.9 epitopes, and also between the SP1.4 and WR1.7 epitopes, corresponding to the A and B epitopic domains in the immunodominant region of TPO. No particular epitope was associated with ophthalmopathy, and the epitopes did not correlate with patient age or sex.

Conclusion.—The demonstration of individual patterns of TPO epitopes should make it possible to determine whether there are specific disease-related epitopes.

▶ It will be of interest to see whether this group will be able to determine whether disease-associated TPO epitopes truly exist. Rapoport and colleagues have also published 2 back-to-back papers further defining the heavy and light chains of the TPO autoantibodies (Jaume et al: *J Clin Endocrinol Metab* 135:16, 1994; Costante et al: *J Clin Endocrinol Metab* 135:25, 1994).—L.E. Braverman, M.D.

Extrathyroidal Release of Thyroid Hormones From Thyroglobulin by J774 Mouse Macrophages
Brix K, Herzog V (Institut für Zellbiologie, Rheinische Friedrich-Wilhelms Universität, Bonn, Germany)
J Clin Invest 93:1388–1396, 1994   112-95-10–29

Background.—Thyroglobulin reaches the circulation as an intact molecule by TSH-regulated transepithelial vesicular transport. Thyroglobulin clearance from the circulation varies with the state of glycosylation. There have been no reports on the cells involved in native Tg clearance. The rates, kinetics, and mechanisms of thyroid hormone release by mouse macrophages—J774 cells—were analyzed.

Methods and Findings.—J774 cells were incubated with bovine Tg, resulting in the release of thyroid hormones T_3 and T_4. This release was fast, with an initial rate of about 20 pmol T_4/mg/min and about .6 pmol T_3/mg/min. Thus, macrophages preferentially released T_4. Most of the released thyroid hormones appeared after 5 minutes of macrophage incubation with Tg. Protein degradation was detected only after several hours. During Tg internalization, endocytic vesicles and endosomes were reached at 5 minutes and lysosomes at 1 hour. Release of T_4 began extracellularly by secreted proteases and continued along the endocytic pathway of Tg. Release of T_3 primarily occurred intracellularly when Tg reached the lysosomes. Thus, the release of both hormones occurred at distinct cellular sites (Fig 10–9).

Conclusion.—Unexpectedly, partial Tg hydrolysis with T_4 release occurs mainly extracellularly and in the early stages of endocytosis. By contrast, T_3 release and the proteolysis of Tg are slow processes in lyso-

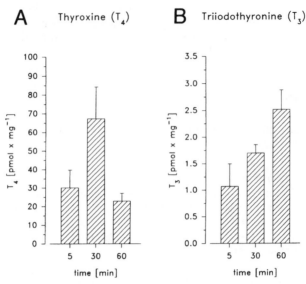

A Thyroxine (T₄)   **B** Triiodothyronine (T₃)

Fig 10–9.—Accumulation of T₃ and export of T₄ by J774 cells. Thyroid hormone levels (mean ± SE) of cell lysates after incubation of vital J774 cells with T₃ and T₄ for 5–60 minutes at 37°C. Note that T₃ levels of cell lysates increased with time (**B**), indicating intracellular accumulation of T₃. In contrast, T₄ levels in the cell lysates increased within 30 minutes and decreased again at 60 minutes (**A**), indicating that T₄ is exported into the medium. (Courtesy of Brix K, Herzog V: *J Clin Invest* 93:1388–1396, 1994.)

somes. Thus, macrophages are an extrathyroidal source for thyroid hormones from circulating Tg.

▶ This is a fascinating paper defining another peripheral source of T₄ and T₃. Kuliawat and Arvan have devised a system (filter-polarized thyrocytes) to study the pathways of Tg iodination leading to T₄ synthesis and concluded that intracellular iodination of Tg initiates the process of T₄ formation, before apical extracellular iodination (*J Biol Chem* 269:4922, 1994).—L.E. Braverman, M.D.

Engraftment of Human Lymphocytes and Thyroid Tissue into *scid* and *rag2*-Deficient Mice: Absent Progression of Lymphocytic Infiltration

Martin A, Valentine M, Unger P, Yeung SW, Schultz LD, Davies TF (Mount Sinai School of Medicine, New York; Jackson Lab, Bar Harbor, Me)
J Clin Endocrinol Metab 79:716–723, 1994   112-95-10–30

Objective.—In an attempt to develop an animal model of human autoimmune thyroid disease, the survival of transplanted human thyroid tissues and the functional status of human lymphocytes were studied in mice with severe combined immunodeficiency (*scid*), and also in a strain of "knockout" mice made deficient for recombination-activating gene-2 (*rag2*) by gene targeting. The latter mice are characterized by defective recombination of T- and B-cell receptor genes, and they lack mature T and B cells.

Observations.—Human thyroid tissues were successfully engrafted in both *scid* and *rag2*-deficient mice. When peripheral blood mononuclear cells were transplanted intraperitoneally, the *rag2*-deficient animals produced relatively little human immunoglobulin. When thyroid tissue from patients with Graves' disease or Hashimoto's thyroiditis was transplanted into *scid* mice, thyroid hormone levels increased transiently and autoantibodies to human thyroglobulin, thyroid peroxidase, and TSH receptor were detected. Lymphocytic infiltration was not more marked than in the original donor tissue, and thyroid follicles remained intact. In many transplants the extent of infiltration decreased over time. Neither T cells nor thyrocytes expressed HLA-DR antigen. Allogeneic thyroid tissues transplanted at the same time showed no unusual changes.

Conclusion.—It appears that a factor or factors that are present in patients with autoimmune thyroid disease that activate their thyroid-specific T cells may be lacking in this murine model.

▶ Davies and associates have also demonstrated in the *scid* mouse that in vivo thyroid follicle formation is TSH- and extrathyroidal growth factor–independent and is likely dependent on intrathyroidal growth factor secretion and cell-to-cell interaction (*Endocrinology* 134:1225, 1994). Volpé and colleagues also used the same model to study human Graves' thyroid xenografts to elucidate the pathogenesis of autoimmune thyroid disease in human beings (*J Clin Endocrinol Metab* 78:367, 1994).—L.E. Braverman, M.D.

The Degree of Inhibition of Thyroid Follicular Cell Proliferation by Iodide Is a Highly Individual Characteristic of Each Cell and Differs Profoundly In Vitro and In Vivo
Aeschimann S, Gerber H, von Grünigen C, Oestreicher M, Studer H (Inselspital, Bern, Switzerland)
Eur J Endocrinol 130:595–600, 1994   112-95-10-31

Background.—In vitro studies have demonstrated both growth-inhibiting and stimulating effects of iodide on follicular thyroid cells. In vivo, excessive iodide may inhibit cell growth and rarely has a stimulating effect, but most often it does not affect the proliferation of thyroid cells.

Objective.—The effects of iodide on the growth of FRTL-5 cells from different passages, and on various subclones of this cell line, were examined. In addition, the inhibiting effect of iodide on FRTL-5 cell proliferation in monolayer cultures was compared with its effect on 3-dimensionally growing cells transplanted onto nude mice.

In Vitro Studies.—Iodide in a concentration of 10^{-4} mol/L inhibited the growth of FRTL-5 cells in different passages by 11% to 67%. The extent of iodide-induced growth inhibition of 5 subclones of FRTL-5 cells, when compared with wild type cells, ranged from 25% to 46%. The degree by which each clone was inhibited proved to be reproducible in subsequent passages.

In Vivo Studies.—A much stronger growth-inhibiting effect of iodide was found when FRTL-5 cells growing as transplants in nude mice were exposed to a serum iodide concentration as low as 5.7×10^{-7} mol/L. Cells in the animal's own thyroid were unaffected. Cell lines prepared from autonomously growing hyperthyroid multinodular goiters in cats were nearly totally resistant to the growth-inhibiting effect of iodide.

Implications.—The extent to which pharmacological doses of iodide inhibit the growth of thyroid follicle cells is a characteristic of an individual strain of cells. The growth-inhibiting effects of iodide observed in vitro and in vivo are fundamentally different processes.

▶ Smerdley et al. used the FRTL-5 thyroid cell line and showed that the inhibitory effects of iodide on thyroid cell proliferation are caused by organified iodide arresting cell growth in the G2M phase and inorganic iodide in the cell cycle phase GOGI (*Endocrinology* 133:2881, 1993). Using human thyroid slices, Corvilain et al. reported that the inhibitory effect of iodide on iodide organification (acute Wolff-Chaikoff effect) is probably mediated through an inhibition of the inositol triphosphate response to TSH and of the H_2O_2 response to Ca^{2+} (*Endocrinology* 79:152, 1994). It is well recognized the excess iodine ingestion in patients with Hashimoto's thyroiditis often induces hypothyroidism. Konno et al. now describe iodine-induced hypothyroidism in patients residing in coastal regions of Japan in the absence of autoimmune thyroid disease (*J Clin Endocrinol Metab* 78:393, 1994).—L.E. Braverman, M.D.

▶↑ It has been suggested over the years that infection with *Yersinia enterocolitica* leads to autoimmune thyroid disease, especially Graves' disease. A recent report from Canada found no evidence for seroreactivity to *Y. enterocolitica*, *Escherichia coli*, or *Staphylococcus aureus* in patients with autoimmune thyroid disease (Resetkova et al: *Thyroid* 4:269, 1994). In another study, Lin et al. (*J Clin Endocrinol Metab* 79:62, 1994) reported that thyroid hormone potentiates the antiviral action of interferon-α in cultured human fibroblasts but has no effect on its own. The TSH receptor was visualized on the cell surface of human thyroid cells, FRTL-5 rat thyroid cells, and Chinese hamster ovary cells by clear granular surface staining using 2 potent TSH receptor antibody–rich sera (De Forteza et al: *J Clin Endocrinol Metab* 78:1271, 1994).

In a long-term prospective study, women with IDDM were at a threefold higher risk for experiencing postpartum thyroiditis than women without IDDM (Alvarex-Marfany et al: *J Clin Endocrinol Metab* 79:10, 1994). The incidence of chronic lymphocytic thyroiditis is far lower in black and Japanese women and men than it is in their white counterparts as determined in an autopsy study (Okayasu et al: *Am J Clin Pathol* 101:698, 1994).

A palm-tree coconut fruit (Babassu) mixed with madioca is a staple food in an endemic goiter area in Brazil with adequate iodine intake. These substances have antithyroid effects in vitro and in the rat in vivo, which could explain the prevalence of endemic goiter in this iodine-sufficient region (Gaitan et al: *Eur J Endocrinol* 131:138, 1994). A dry spot assay for thyroglobulin (Tg) has been described by Milfler et al. (*Eur J Clin Chem Clin Biochem* 32:137, 1994), and elevations in Tg are a more sensitive indicator of iodine deficiency than TSH. In this regard, iodine supplementation (200 μg daily) of pregnant women in a region in Denmark with modest iodine deficiency (50 μg daily) decreased serum TSH and Tg concentrations and thyroid size in the mothers and cord blood Tg only at delivery (Pedersen et al: *J Clin Endocrinol Metab* 77:1078, 1993). Rendl et al. (*Eur J Endocrinol* 130:498, 1994) observed a large increase in serum and urine iodine values after the use of radiographic contrast agents for endoscopic retrograde cholangiopancreaticography, placing susceptible patients at some risk for the development of iodine-induced thyroid dysfunction. In contrast to earlier studies demonstrating increased serum iodine concentrations after douching with betadine solution, povidone–iodine pessaries and obstetric cream did not significantly increase systemic iodine values, suggesting that these 2 forms of povidone iodine do not pose a risk of iodine-induced thyroid dysfunction (Darwish and Shaarawy: *Postgrad Med J* 69:39S, 1993; Sakakura et al: *Postgrad Med J* 69:49S, 1993). Further study of these 2 preparations appears warranted.—L.E. Braverman, M.D.

Miscellaneous

The Risk Factor for Development of Thyroid Disease During Interferon-α Therapy for Chronic Hepatitis C

Watanabe U, Hashimoto E, Hisamitsu T, Obata H, Hayashi N (The Inst of Gastroenterology, Tokyo Women's Med College, Japan)
Am J Gastroenterol 89:399–402, 1994   112-95-10–32

Background.—Interferon is becoming standard treatment for chronic hepatitis C. However, many side effects have been associated with interferons. The risk factors for thyroid disease development during interferon-α treatment were analyzed.

Methods.—One hundred nine patients aged 20–72 years with chronic hepatitis C were included in the study. The duration of interferon-α treatment ranged from 14 to 40 weeks. Thyroid function tests and 7 autoantibodies were evaluated at the beginning and end of treatment and every other month.

Findings.—Thyroid disease developed in 9 of the 106 patients with normal pretreatment thyroid function tests (table). However, interferon treatment did not exacerbate thyroid disease in 3 patients with abnormal thyroid function tests. In a multiple regression model, positivity for microsome antibody was a significant risk factor for thyroid disease development. Compared with patients without microsome antibody at treat-

Clinical Features and Results of Autoantibodies in 9 Patients Who Had Thyroid Dysfunction During Interferon-α Therapy

Case #, Sex, Age (yr), Preparation	Before Tx Onset	TRAb (%)	TSAb (μU/ml)	MCHA Titer	TGHA Titer	ANA Titer	AMA Titer	ASMA Titer	DNA Titer	RA Titer
1. M, 34 IFN-α2a	Before	0.0	<0.3	(−)	(−)	(−)	(−)	20	(−)	(−)
	Wk 16	0.0	<0.3	(−)	(−)	(−)	(−)	20	(−)	(−)
2. F, 62 IFN-α	Before	0.0		100	200	(−)	(−)	(−)	(−)	(−)
	Wk 18			200	400	(−)	(−)	(−)	(−)	(−)
3. F, 57 IFN-α2a	Before	0.0	<0.3	(−)	(−)	(−)	(−)	(−)	(−)	(−)
	Wk 20	5.0*	0.3	(−)	(−)	(−)	(−)	(−)	80	(−)
4. M, 46 IFN-α	Before	0.0	0.0	400	(−)	(−)	(−)	(−)	(−)	(−)
	Wk 27	20.4		1,600	(−)	(−)	(−)	(−)	(−)	(−)
5. F, 37 IFN-α2a	Before	0.0	<0.3	100	100	(−)	(−)	(−)	(−)	(−)
	Wk 30	0.0*	<0.3*	1,600	400	(−)	(−)	(−)	(−)	(−)
6. F, 52 IFN-α2a	Before	*		(−)	(−)	(−)	(−)	(−)	(−)	(−)
	Wk 30			800	(−)	(−)	(−)	(−)	(−)	(−)
7. F, 54 IFN-α2a	Before	0.0		1,600	200	(−)	(−)	(−)	(−)	(−)
	Wk 8	0.0		25,600		(−)	(−)	(−)	(−)	(−)
8. F, 56 IFN-α2a	Before			1,600	(−)	(−)	(−)	(−)	(−)	(−)
	Wk 16	0.0		6,400		(−)	(−)	(−)	(−)	(−)
9. M, 33 IFN-α2a	Before	0.2		1,600	100	(−)	(−)	(−)	(−)	(−)
	Wk 23	9.0		12,800	800	(−)	(−)	(−)	(−)	(−)
Normal		<15	<0.3	(−)	(−)	(−)	(−)	(−)	(−)	(−)

Abbreviations: TRAb, TSH receptor antibody; TSAb, thyroid-stimulating antibody.
Note: Cases 1–6, hyperthyroidism; cases 7–9, hypothyroidism.
* Became positive after several weeks.
(Courtesy of Watanabe U, Hashimoto E, Hisamitsu T, et al: Am J Gastroenterol 89:399-402, 1994.)

ment initiation, the incidence of thyroid diseases in patients with pretreatment microsome antibody was very high, those values being 3.3% and 60%, respectively. Hyperthyroidism developed in 6 patients, and hypothyroidism developed in 3. Patients with hyperthyroidism had atypical clinical findings.

Conclusion.—Positivity for microsome antibody at the start of interferon-α treatment is a risk factor for thyroid dysfunction. All patients should be screened for microsome antibodies and have thyroid function tests before this therapy is begun. Patients should also be monitored every 2–3 months during their treatment.

▶ The more common use of interferon-α for treatment of chronic hepatitis C is certain to result in an increased frequency of thyroid dysfunction. This is good for the thyroidologist but not for the patient!—L.E. Braverman, M.D.

Thyroid Dysfunction in Rheumatoid Arthritis: A Controlled Prospective Survey
Shiroky JB, Cohen M, Ballachey M-L, Neville C (Montreal Gen Hosp)
Ann Rheum Dis 52:454–456, 1993   112-95-10-33

Objective.—Because many have suggested an association between rheumatoid arthritis (RA) and Hashimoto's thyroiditis or other forms of thyroid dysfunction, 91 women and 28 men with RA from a hospital clinic and a private rheumatology practice were studied prospectively. They were compared with 108 demographically similar control subjects from the same sources, who included patients having osteoarthritis or fibromyalgia. Consecutive patients seen in a 6-month period were evaluated.

Findings.—Thyroid disease was identified in 30% of the women with RA and in 7% of men. Eleven percent of control subjects had evident thyroid disease, including 10% of patients with osteoarthritis and 12% of those with fibromyalgia. The prevalence of thyroid disease was 3.5-fold greater in women with RA than in control women. The difference resulted entirely from hypothyroidism or Hashimoto's thyroiditis. The women with both RA and thyroid disease were not demographically or clinically dissimilar to those having RA alone except for a shorter duration of arthritis in the former group.

Conclusion.—Thyroid dysfunction in the form of hypothyroidism or Hashimoto's thyroiditis is much more frequent than expected in patients with RA.

▶ Arnaout et al. extend these findings to patients with a variety of other connective tissue disorders and also conclude that thyroid dysfunction, especially autoimmune thyroid disease, is common in these patients (*Scand J Rheumatol* 23:128, 1994). Laboratory and clinical features of Sjögren's syndrome are frequently observed in younger women (mean age, 36 years) with a history of postpartum thyroiditis 5 years earlier, yet another example of overlapping autoimmune diseases (Gudbjornsson et al: *J Rheumatol* 21:215, 1994). Celiac disease and autoimmune thyroid disease, especially hypothyroidism, also coexist more frequently than expected (Counsell et al: *Gut* 35:844, 1994). Alopecia areata may be associated with autoimmune thyroid disease, especially Hashimoto's thyroiditis, and all patients with alopecia areata should probably be evaluated for hypothyroidism and chronic thyroiditis (Ueki et al: *Eur J Dermatol* 3:454, 1993). Surprisingly, hypothyroidism occurred with an increased prevalence in patients with gout, which is not an autoimmune disorder (Erickson et al: *Am J Med* 97:231, 1994). Finally, Rosenmann and Yarom report an increased incidence of abnormal thyroid pathology at autopsy in patients who died of dissecting aneurysm, and they report a patient with hypothyroidism and a dissecting aneurysm of the aorta, suggesting that abnormal glycosaminoglycan metabolism is the common event (*Isr J Med Sci* 30:510, 1994).—L.E. Braverman, M.D.

Comparison of Second and Third Generation Methods for Measurement of Serum Thyrotropin in Patients With Overt Hyperthyroidism, Patients Receiving Thyroxine Therapy, and Those With Nonthyroidal Illness
Franklyn JA, Black EG, Betteridge J, Sheppard MC (Univ of Birmingham, Edgbaston, England; Queen Elizabeth Hosp, Edgbaston, Birmingham, England)
J Clin Endocrinol Metab 78:1368–1371, 1994   112-95-10–34

Background.—The development of assays for serum TSH with improved sensitivity has been a major achievement in the assessment of thyroid status. Now even greater strides have been made with the description of third generation assays for TSH, with an approximately 10-fold increase in sensitivity. The clinical usefulness of such heightened sensitivity was investigated by comparing serum TSH results determined in second and third generation assays in patients with overt hyperthyroidism before and during treatment, in those receiving T_4 therapy, and in patients with nonthyroidal illnesses.

Method.—Serum samples were obtained from 19 patients seen with untreated overt hyperthyroidism, and from 12 patients studied serially at monthly intervals for up to 7 months after commencing carbimazole treatment. Samples were also obtained from 153 patients undergoing long-term T_4 therapy, and from 300 inpatients with nonthyroidal illnesses. Serum TSH was measured in all samples using a second-generation immunometric assay together with a free T_4 and free T_3. Samples showing subnormal TSH (less than .5 mU/L) were reassayed using a third-generation chemiluminescent immunometric method.

Results.—Both assays revealed undetectable serum TSH levels in 18 of 19 overtly hyperthyroid patients. Similarly, both assays showed undetectable TSH values in 30 of 33 patients with low serum TSH levels who were being treated for hyperthyroidism, in association with normal thyroid hormone levels in 11. Undetectable TSH was evident in patients receiving T_4, as well as in those with nonthyroidal illnesses. However, use of the more sensitive assay resulted in a reduction in the number of patients with undetectable TSH compared with the second-generation results (T_4-treated, 55 vs. 77 cases; nonthyroidal illness, 13 vs. 19 cases). A significant correlation was seen between serum TSH and free T_4 in the whole group treated with T_4, and in those receiving T_4 with low TSH. No significant correlation was seen in subjects with low serum TSH levels associated with nonthyroidal illnesses.

Conclusion.—The heightened sensitivity in TSH assay brought a reduction in the number of patients treated with T_4 or with nonthyroidal illnesses in whom circulation TSH was undetectable, and subsequently, an increase in the number of patients in whom overt hyperthyroidism can be excluded. It is clear, however, that undetectable TSH results are not diagnostic of overt hyperthyroidism but are also found in patients with treated thyroid disease and nonthyroidal diseases. In these patients, additional information in the form of clinical evaluation, measurement of circulating thyroid hormone, and knowledge of any nonthyroidal illness or drug therapy is required for accurate interpretation of results.

▶ This report and that of Taimela et al. (*Clin Chem* 40:101, 1994) are important and emphasize that even a nondetectable serum TSH measured in new generation assays do not definitively differentiate between thyrotoxicosis and nonthyroidal illness. Nelson et al. emphasize that serum free T_4 concentrations in nonthyroidal illness measured by immunoassays not infrequently underestimate the true values (Nelson et al: *J Clin Endocrinol Metab* 79:76, 1994).—L.E. Braverman, M.D.

▶ ↑ The inhibitory effect of sleep on TSH secretion appears to oppose the nocturnal peak of the circadian TSH drive, a lovely study carried out in a sleep disorder laboratory (Allan and Czeiseler: *J Clin Endocrinol Metab* 79:508, 1994). Finally, Bruhn et al. (*Endocrinology* 134:826, 1994) report that T_3 increases pro-TRH gene expression in cultured anterior pituitary cells and glucocorticoids greatly potentiate this T_3 effect.—L.E. Braverman, M.D.

Suggested Reading

The following articles are recommended to the reader:

Brent GA: The molecular basis of thyroid hormone action. N *Engl J Med* 331:847–853, 1994.

Burrow GN, Fisher DA, Larsen PR: Maternal and fetal thyroid function. N *Engl J Med* 331:1072–1078, 1994.

Klein I, Becker DV, Levey GS: Treatment of hyperthyroid disease. *Ann Intern Med* 121:281–288, 1994.

Fatourechi V, Pajouhi M, Fransway AF: Dermopathy of Graves' disease (pretibial myxedema). *Medicine* 73:1–7, 1994.

Toft AD: Thyroxine therapy. N *Engl J Med* 331:174–180, 1994.

Volpe R: Evidence that the immunosuppressive effects of antithyroid drugs are mediated through actions on the thyroid cell, modulating thyrocyte-immunocyte signaling: A review. *Thyroid* 4:217–223, 1994.

11 Diabetes

Introduction

My selection of basic and clinical research articles for the 1995 YEAR BOOK OF ENDOCRINOLOGY can only be described as eclectic. This reflects the lack of overwhelming advances in any one area compared with another. Although the power of molecular biology to unravel the genetic causes of inherited disease such as diabetes is self-evident, there have not been any major significant advances in the past year compared with the telling of the glucokinase story in the previous 2 years.

Transgenic studies continue to contribute to our understanding of the role of specific gene products, but whether the conditions induced by transgenic experiments are relevant to human disease remains an open question. Moreover, although gene therapy will probably provide a cure for single-gene disorder diseases and other diseases that are remediable by increasing expression of a specific protein, neither diabetes nor any other disease has yet enjoyed any of the benefits that gene therapy may eventually offer. However, the field is still young.

With regard to diabetes therapy, several insulin analogues are likely to be available soon, and the biguanide, metformin, has finally been approved by the Food and Drug Administration and will soon be available for the treatment of NIDDM. Transplantation of isolated islets, in the absence of encapsulation, continues to be a generally unsuccessful venture; however, studies of encapsulated islets in humans are proceeding and may ultimately be the endocrine replacement treatment of choice for IDDM. After the excitement of the Diabetes Control and Complications Trial (DCCT), relatively little has changed in our understanding of long-term complications and their treatment. Trials of aminoguanidine, the agent that blocks cross-linking of glycation end-products, have been initiated. A number of new and more detailed manuscripts emanating from the DCCT have begun to appear, expanding the insights provided in the original report.

Whether the lack of a dominant theme in diabetes research this year reflects slow progress on all fronts or a modicum of new and exciting studies on all fronts is not clear. I prefer the latter interpretation, and I hope that this choice of articles provokes thought, discussion, and perhaps more studies.

David M. Nathan, M.D.

Relationships Between Angiotensin I Converting Enzyme Gene Polymorphism, Plasma Levels, and Diabetic Retinal and Renal Complications
Marre M, Bernadet P, Gallois Y, Savagner F, Guyene T-T, Hallab M, Cambien F, Passa P, Alhenc-Gelas F (Univ Hosp, Angers, France; INSERM SC7, Paris; Hosp Saint-Louis, Paris, et al)
Diabetes 43:384–388, 1994   112-95-11-1

Background.—Nephropathy secondary to IDDM is a major cause of morbidity and mortality, much of which is cardiovascular. The occurrence of nephropathy is probably determined by renal hemodynamic abnormalities and a genetic predisposition. Through angiotensin II formation and kinin metabolism, angiotensin I–converting enzyme (ACE) regulates systemic and renal circulation, with high levels of ACE causing intraglandular hypertension. Levels of plasma and cellular ACE are determined genetically. An insertion/deletion polymorphism of the ACE gene is highly associated with ACE. Those who are homozygotic for insertion have the lowest plasma values. The relationship between the ACE gene polymorphism or plasma levels and microcirculatory disorders of diabetes were assessed in 2 independent IDDM study populations.

Methods.—In the first study, 57 research subjects with or without diabetic retinopathy were compared. In the second study, 62 patients with IDDM and diabetic nephropathy were compared with 62 diabetic control patients with the same characteristics but with normal kidney function.

Findings.—The distribution of the ACE genotype did not differ between diabetic patients with or without retinopathy and healthy controls. By contrast, there was an imbalance of ACE genotype distribution, with a low proportion of II genotype patients, in those with IDDM and diabetic nephropathy compared with their control group. All diabetic groups had mildly increased plasma ACE levels, independent of retinopathy. However, these levels were greater in patients with nephropathy than in those without.

Conclusion.—Compared with patients without nephropathy, patients with IDDM and nephropathy had an imbalance of ACE insertion polymorphism. The II genotype, a genetic basis for low ACE activity in the general population, may protect against the onset of diabetic nephropathy in IDDM.

▶ The repeated observation that diabetic nephropathy, which results in end-stage renal disease, occurs in 40% or less of the diabetic population has suggested that only a minor, vulnerable fraction of the IDDM population will have nephropathy develop. The factors that predispose that segment of the population to nephropathy remain undefined; however, the usual suspects—including environmental and genetic variables—have been rounded up.

The 2 factors that have been clearly identified in either epidemiologic or interventional studies as playing a significant role in the genesis and/or progression of nephropathy are glycemia and blood pressure.

The Diabetes Control and Complications Trial and the Steno and Stockholm studies have all demonstrated that intensive diabetes therapy will decrease the development of microalbuminuria and/or decrease the progression from microalbuminuria to clinical grade albuminuria. Numerous other studies have also demonstrated the beneficial effect of controlling hypertension with regard to the rate of progression of diabetic nephropathy. The ACE inhibitors appear to have a unique salutary effect other than their antihypertensive effects.

This study suggests that specific genotypes of converting enzyme may predispose patients with IDDM to nephropathy. In the past, the observation that blood pressure levels, angiotensin I or II levels, or ACE levels were different in patients who had complications compared with patients who did not have complications could be attributed to changes in the circulation of patients with complications that resulted in secondary changes.

This study, by taking advantage of the cloning and identification of various genotypes of the converting enzyme, identifies a specific polymorphism that was disproportionately represented in patients with nephropathy compared with IDDM patients without nephropathy. The data are tantalizing, although inconclusive, and they support the ACE genotype as being one of the additive factors in the development of diabetic nephropathy.—D.M. Nathan, M.D.

Restoration of Hypoglycaemia Awareness in Patients With Long-Duration Insulin-Dependent Diabetes

Cranston I, Lomas J, Maran A, Macdonald I, Amiel SA (Guy's Hosp, London; Cattedra di Malattle del Ricambio, Padova, Italy; Univ of Nottingham, England)
Lancet 344:283–287, 1994   112-95-11-2

Background.—Unexpected hypoglycemia is a dangerous complication of IDDM. It limits the use of intensified insulin treatment to decrease chronic diabetic complications. The possibility of restoring patient awareness of hypoglycemia in a group with long-duration insulin-dependent diabetes was investigated.

Methods.—Symptomatic, cognitive, and hormonal responses to controlled hypoglycemia were assessed in 6 diabetic patients with good glycemic control and 6 with poor control. Assessments were made before and after hypoglycemia avoidance.

Findings.—Initially, all patients had a loss of hypoglycemia awareness. Responses to the first challenge were minimal and began only when plasma glucose was significantly lower than 2.8 mmol/L, at which time cognitive function deteriorated. After 4.1 months of scrupulous hypoglycemia avoidance, hormonal and symptom responses to the challenge were elevated, beginning at plasma glucose levels that were significantly greater than those that caused cognitive dysfunction. No significant deterioration in glycosaylated hemoglobin was noted.

Conclusion.—By avoiding hypoglycemia, the normal hierarchy of subjective awareness before cognitive dysfunction during hypoglycemia can be restored; this occurs independent of the duration of disease or initial metabolic control.

▶ In addition to the labor-intensive and time-consuming aspects and the expense of intensive therapy, the increased frequency of hypoglycemia remains the major barrier to its widespread implementation in IDDM. Previous work has established the loss of counterregulation with the longer duration of diabetes as glucagon and epinephrine responses to hypoglycemia wane. This creates a situation in which the threshold for adrenergic warning symptoms draws closer to the glucose level at which CNS function is affected. Alternatively, warning symptoms can disappear entirely.

In addition to a longer duration of IDDM, intensive therapy itself appears to alter the counterregulatory defense against hypoglycemia, explaining in part the increased frequency of severe hypoglycemia that was demonstrated with intensive therapy in the Diabetes Control and Complications Trial. Although several studies have suggested that changes in glucose transport in the CNS may be responsible for the alteration in counterregulation with intensive therapy, the idea that hypoglycemia begets hypoglycemia has been supported by recent studies (Veneman et al: *Diabetes* 42:1233, 1993).

In this study, a 3-week period of hypoglycemia-free therapy, in which there was only a small (.5%) nonsignificant drift upward in hemoglobin A_{1c} levels, resulted in improvement, albeit not normalization of counterregulation in 12 IDDM patients, half of whom were treated intensively. The improvement included increases in epinephrine, norepinephrine, and GH secretion to a hypoglycemic clamp. The hormonal change was accompanied by restoration of some of the adrenergic warning symptoms that occurred at a relatively higher blood glucose level.

This news is heartening, because patients may not be forever consigned to being at risk for severe hypoglycemia, but it is also frustrating, because it once again places the burden on patients to control their blood glucose levels to as close to the normal range as possible but not to cross the line into hypoglycemia (notably, it took 3–4 months to achieve a 3-week hypoglycemia-free period in the study patients). This once again demonstrates that although glucagon is the primary defense mechanism against hypoglycemia, epinephrine responses can serve in a protective capacity, even in the absence of glucagon.

Whether the biochemical changes and improvement in adrenergic symptom scores that occurred with the hypoglycemia-free period will be sufficient to prevent or significantly decrease the frequency of severe hypoglycemia has yet to be demonstrated.—D.M. Nathan, M.D.

Effects of Long-Term Enalapril Treatment on Persistent Microalbuminuria in Well-Controlled Hypertensive and Normotensive NIDDM Patients

Sano T, Kawamura T, Matsumae H, Sasaki H, Nakayama M, Hara T, Matsuo S, Hotta N, Sakamoto N (Chubu-Rosai Hosp, Japan, Nagoya Univ, Japan)
Diabetes Care 17:420–424, 1994   112-95-11-3

Background.—Diabetic patients who have nephropathy develop often become hypertensive at the same time. Hypertension accompanies progressive nephropathy in rats that are made diabetic with streptozocin. Improving glomerular hyperfiltration appears to counter the progression of nephropathy in rats. Treatment with an angiotensin-converting enzyme (ACE) inhibitor limits the development of proteinuria and glomerular lesions in this setting.

Objective.—The value of long-term treatment with enalapril, an ACE inhibitor, was examined in 52 patients with NIDDM who had persistent microalbuminuria of as great as 300 mg/24 hr and a serum creatinine of less than 1.2 mg/dL.

Study Plan.—Twenty-six initially normotensive patients and 26 whose blood pressure had been well controlled by nifedipine, 30 mg/day, for 4-6 years were randomly assigned to receive or not receive 5 mg of enalapril daily.

Results.—Urinary albumin excretion was higher after 4 years than at baseline in controls, but it was markedly reduced in those who were given enalapril. Arterial blood pressure and renal function remained stable in both groups, and there were no significant changes in creatinine clearance, serum lipids, or urinary excretion of β_2-microglobulin. There were no side effects from either nifedipine or enalapril.

Conclusion.—An ACE inhibitor can limit urinary albumin excretion over the long term in patients with NIDDM, both those who are normotensive and those in whom hypertension is controlled by medication.

▶ The beneficial effect of ACE inhibitors in diabetic nephropathy has become increasingly clear with longer duration studies in different types of diabetes and at different stages of nephropathy. In IDDM, ACE inhibitors slow the progression of microalbuminuria to clinical grade albuminuria (albumin > 300 mg/24 hr) in both normotensive and hypertensive patients. The rate of progression of the later stages of nephropathy is also decreased. The concern in NIDDM has been whether the efficacy of ACE inhibition that has been demonstrated for IDDM would be limited in NIDDM, because of the fixed resistance of the renal circulation secondary to afferent and efferent atherosclerosis.

In this study, which is admirable because of its long duration, the benefits of low-dose ACE inhibition were documented in hypertensive and normotensive patients with NIDDM. Albumin excretion was decreased, and there was no increase in urine albumin excretion in the controls in this study over time, which is not the usual course. Whether this Japanese NIDDM population is similar enough to the United States population with NIDDM to extrapolate its results is not certain; however, it does demonstrate a fairly uniform effect of ACE inhibition in the NIDDM population.

Although the clinical significance of microalbuminuria in NIDDM has been questioned because it is not as reliable a risk predictor of nephropathy as it is of IDDM, the beneficial effect of ACE inhibition demonstrated in this study supports screening patients with NIDDM for microalbuminuria and treating them with ACE inhibition.—D.M. Nathan, M.D.

Effect of Metformin on Postprandial Lipemia in Patients With Fairly to Poorly Controlled NIDDM
Jeppesen J, Zhou M-Y, Chen Y-D, Reaven GM (Stanford Univ, Calif; Geriatric Research Education and Clinical Ctr, Palo Alto, Calif)
Diabetes Care 17:1093–1099, 1994   1 12-95-11–4

Objective.—The effects of metformin on the metabolism of triglyceride (TG)-rich lipoprotein of intestinal origin were studied in 16 patients with NIDDM whose fasting plasma glucose had decreased more than 2.2 mmol/L when they were given glipizide but who continued to have fasting levels greater than 8.3 mmol/L.

Methods.—The patients (mean age, 57 years) had diabetes for a mean of 7 years. Plasma glucose, insulin, and TG levels were measured at frequent intervals during treatment with a mean daily dose of 2.3 g of metformin. Six of the patients had hypoglycemic symptoms during treatment, and a dose reduction was necessary in 2 instances. Vitamin A was administered to quantify the postprandial concentrations of intestinal TG-rich lipoprotein in plasma and in chylomicron and chylomicron remnant fractions.

Results.—Metformin treatment was associated with significant reductions in the fasting plasma glucose, GHb, and day-long plasma glucose concentrations as well as in the steady-state plasma glucose. Postprandial levels of glucose, insulin, free fatty acids, and TG all were lower after metformin treatment. Postprandial plasma and chylomicron levels of intestinal TG-rich lipoprotein were reduced by 33%.

Conclusion.—In sulfonylurea-treated patients who continue to have uncontrolled NIDDM, adding metformin should help lower the risk of vascular complications.

▶ Because it is possible and even likely that metformin, a biguanide that has no significant risk of lactic acidosis, may be approved for use in the United States, I thought it appropriate to include an article that describes its action. Metformin has been used throughout Europe and Canada for more than a decade with interesting results.

Although its mechanism of action remains somewhat unclear, metformin is well recognized as decreasing glycemia with relatively little hypoglycemia or weight gain. These 2 features distinguish metformin from both sulfonylurea and insulin therapy. The absence of weight gain with improved glycemia, as demonstrated again in this study, is especially intriguing.

This study demonstrates a significant decrease in glucose when metformin was added to sulfonylurea therapy in near maximal doses. Insulin levels decreased, reflecting in part decreased insulin resistance as measured by a modification of the insulin suppression test. Finally, treatment with metformin decreased postprandial concentrations of TG-rich lipoproteins. All the changes mediated by metformin appear to be beneficial with regard to cardiovascular risk. The availability of metformin will be a welcome addition to the treatment of NIDDM in the United States.—D.M. Nathan, M.D.

Declining Incidence of Nephropathy in Insulin-Dependent Diabetes Mellitus
Bojestig M, Arnqvist HJ, Hermansson G, Karlberg BE, Ludvigsson J (Univ Hosp, Linköping, Sweden; Eksjö Hosp, Sweden)
N Engl J Med 330:15–18, 1994   112-95-11–5

Introduction.—Diabetic kidney disease is the predominant reason for the high relative mortality of patients with IDDM. From 1950 to the early 1980s, the cumulative incidence of nephropathy among patients with a 25-year history of diabetes remained relatively stable at 25% to 30%. However, a number of important changes in diabetes management have occurred in recent years, including self-monitoring, better education, and better adjustment of treatment to the patient's lifestyle.

Methods.—Recent trends in the incidence of diabetic nephropathy were examined. The study included 213 Swedish patients who were given a diagnosis of IDDM between 1961 and 1980. One hundred ninety-seven of these patients were followed up from the onset of their diabetes until 1991 or until death. Diabetic nephropathy was considered to be present in patients who had persistent albuminuria, as indicated by a positive Albustix text. After 1980, all patients had periodic measurements of glycosylated hemoglobin.

Findings.—For patients with a 25-year history of diabetes, the cumulative incidence of persistent albuminuria fell from 30% in those who were diagnosed between 1961 and 1965 to 9% in those who were diagnosed from 1966 to 1970. For patients with a 20-year history, the cumulative incidence was 28% for those who were diagnosed between 1961 and 1965 vs. 6% for those who were diagnosed between 1971 and 1975. None of the study patients who were diagnosed in 1976 or later had persistent albuminuria by 1991. The average glycosylated hemoglobin measurement fell from 7.4% in 1980–1985 to 7% in 1986–1991. Mean values for patients with and without persistent albuminuria were 8% vs. 7%, respectively.

Conclusion.—For patients with long-standing IDDM, the cumulative incidence of diabetic nephropathy appears to have fallen dramatically in the last decade. The difference seems to be the result of improvements in glycemic control and are not related to antihypertensive treatment.

▶ Careful attention to follow-up, relatively stable populations, and provision of care in centralized health care facilities provide a fertile environment for long-term epidemiologic studies in Sweden. Previous long-term follow-up studies at the Steno Hospital in Copenhagen (Deckert et al: *Diabetologia* 14:363, 1978) have provided much of our understanding of the long-term course of IDDM in the "insulin era."

Although we may carp about several shortcomings in this study, including changing methodologies with regard to glycosylated hemoglobin and the surrogate end point of dipstick-positive proteinuria, it provides important information regarding a temporal decrease in the development of diabetic nephropathy over the past several decades.

The life-table analyses demonstrate a decreasing cumulative incidence of clinically significant nephropathy for populations diagnosed from 1966 through 1976 compared with the population that was diagnosed before 1966. The follow-up of the most recent cohort of patients, who were diagnosed between 1976 and 1980, was too brief to provide data that were convincing as to a decrease in nephropathy.

Notably, this study provides further support for some of the earlier observations regarding the natural history of diabetic nephropathy (Kussman et al: *JAMA* 236:1861, 1976), that is, the development of gross proteinuria as the first indicator of clinical nephropathy occurs between the 10th and 20th year after the onset of diabetes, and the development of nephropathy after 20–25 years' duration appears to be unusual. In addition, the severe consequences of developing nephropathy in IDDM were also documented, with a tenfold increase in mortality in patients who had nephropathy compared with those who did not.

What is unconvincing about this article is the proposition that lowered glycemia was responsible for the change in nephropathy. The only data presented with regard to glycemia include a modest decrease in hemoglobin A_{1c} in the most recent decade. The authors do not suggest and cannot demonstrate a significant difference in glycemic levels in patients whose onset of diabetes was between 1966 and 1976, when intensive therapy was unusual, even in Sweden.

Because the most potent effect of intensive therapy appears to be during the early and mid-portions of the course of disease (preventing or delaying the development of microalbuminuria and/or the progression of microalbuminuria to clinical grade proteinuria), it is unlikely that the demonstration of a decrease in hemoglobin A_{1c} in the recent past has much relevance for the older cohorts.

The Diabetes Control and Complications Trial data (DCCT Research Group: *N Engl J Med* 329:977, 1993) suggest that we should begin to see a significant decrease in nephropathy now, because more intensive treatment regimens have been widely introduced in the past decade. Factors other than glycemic control may still play a significant role in determining which patients with IDDM have nephropathy and which do not.—D.M. Nathan, M.D.

References

1. Deckert, et al: *Diabetolgia* 14:363, 1978.
2. Kuseman M, et al: *JAMA* 236:1861, 1976.
3. DCCT Research Group: N *Engl J Med* 329:977, 1993.

The Effects of Dietary Protein Restriction and Blood-Pressure Control on the Progression of Chronic Renal Disease
Klahr S, Levey AS, Beck GJ, Caggiula AW, Hunsicker L, Kusek JW, Striker G, for the Modification of Diet in Renal Disease Study Group (Natl Inst of Diabetes and Digestive and Kidney Diseases, Bethesda, Md; Washington Univ, St Louis, Mo; New England Med Ctr, Boston; et al)
N Engl J Med 330:877–884, 1994   112-95-11–6

Objective.—Animal studies have found that protein restriction and control of hypertension can delay the progression of renal disease. Studies in humans have been hampered by methodologic problems. The results of the Modification of Diet in Renal Disease (MDRD) Study, in which 840 patients with various renal diseases were randomized as to dietary protein intake and blood pressure control, were reported.

Methods.—The MDRD Study consisted of 2 randomized, multicenter trials. The first included 585 patients, all with glomerular filtration rates of 25–55 mL/min/1.73 m^2. They received either a usual protein or a low-protein daily diet, consisting of 1.3 vs. .58 g/kg. They were also assigned to a usual or low blood pressure group with mean arterial pressure values of 107 and 92 mm Hg, respectively. In the second study, glomerular filtration rates were lower: 13–24 mL/min/1.73 m^2. One group received a daily low-protein diet of .58 g/kg, whereas the other received a very-low-protein daily diet of .28 g/kg. Blood pressure groups were the same as in the first study. The patients were evaluated monthly over a mean follow-up of 2.2 years, based on intention to treat.

Results.—The first study showed no difference between diet or blood pressure groups in the mean projected 3-year decline in the glomerular filtration rate. The low-protein group and the low–blood pressure group showed a more rapid decline in the glomerular filtration rate during the first 4 months of the study, after which the decline slowed. The second study revealed a marginally slower decline in the very-low-protein group than in the low-protein group. However, no difference was observed in time to end-stage renal disease or death. Patients in the low–blood pressure group of both studies who had more advanced proteinuria at baseline showed a significantly slower rate of decline in the glomerular filtration rate. All the protein restriction and blood pressure interventions were well tolerated.

Conclusion.—A low-protein diet may slow the decline in renal function somewhat in patients with moderate renal insufficiency. In patients with more severe renal insufficiency, a very-low-protein diet does not even offer this small benefit. In patients with urinary protein excretion greater than 1 g/day, maintaining blood pressure at a low level may be of some benefit.

▶ Although the MDRD Study specifically excluded insulin-treated diabetic patients and therefore had only a small number of diabetic patients, the overall results of this study, albeit generally negative, may have implications for the treatment of diabetic patients with end-stage renal disease.

The arguments to include or exclude diabetic patients from the MDRD Study must have been fierce during its planning, because diabetes represents the major cause of end-stage renal disease in the United States. In any case, protein restriction had very little effect on the progression of moderately severe and severe nephropathy. Remember that the controls' "usual" protein diet was considerably lower in protein than the usual United States diet, and it may have had a beneficial effect on the progression of nephropathy. This would explain the relatively low rate of progression in the control group.

Although this study does not abrogate the short-term beneficial effects of *lower* protein diets, as demonstrated in studies of IDDM (Cohen et al: *BMJ* 294:1443, 1987; Ciavarella et al: *Diabetes Care* 10:407, 1987; Zeller et al: *N Engl J Med* 324:78, 1991), it certainly dampens enthusiasm for very-low-protein or formula diets. (In a way, I am glad that these experimental diets did not work. They are difficult to implement and distasteful to patients. Diabetic patients also require more carbohydrates to provide adequate calories. When I have monitored protein intake with 24-hour urine measurements, remarkably few patients demonstrably restricted their protein intake as much as they thought or said they had.)—D.M. Nathan, M.D.

Weight Loss in Severely Obese Subjects Prevents the Progression of Impaired Glucose Tolerance to Type II Diabetes: A Longitudinal Interventional Study

Long SD, Swanson MS, O'Brien K, Pories WJ, MacDonald KG Jr, Caro JF, Leggett-Frazier N (East Carolina Univ, Greenville, NC; Thomas Jefferson Univ, Philadelphia)

Diabetes Care 17:372–375, 1994   112-95-11–7

Background.—The prevalence of type II diabetes and impaired glucose tolerance (IGT) is known to be increased by obesity. Although short-term improvement in glucose tolerance by caloric restriction or weight loss has been seen in individuals with IGT, the long-term implications of these interventions on the development of clinical diabetes are unknown. Whether weight loss prevents the progression of IGT to type II diabetes was investigated.

Methods.—A total of 136 individuals with IGT and clinically severe obesity were followed for an average of 5 years. The experimental group comprised 109 patients who underwent gastric bypass surgery for weight loss. A control group consisted of 27 individuals who did not undergo surgery but had a similar follow-up. The principal outcome measure was the incidence, density, or number of reported cases of diabetes divided by the time of exposure to risk.

Results.—Diabetes developed in 6 of the 27 patients in the control group during an average of 4.8 years of post-diagnosis follow-up, yielding a rate of conversion to diabetes of 4.72 cases per 100 person-years. Based on the 95% confidence interval of the comparison group, it would be expected that diabetes would develop in 22 to 36 patients in the experimental group. However, the disease developed in only 1 of the 109 experimental group patients, which resulted in a conversion rate for the experimental group of only .15 cases per 100 person-years, which is significantly lower than that of the control group.

Conclusion.—These results provide evidence that weight loss prevents the development of type II diabetes in an extremely high-risk population for the disease. Patients with impaired glucose tolerance who did not lose weight had type II diabetes at a rate of 4.72 cases per 100 person-years, whereas loss of around 50% of body weight resulted in a significant reduction in the conversion rate to type II diabetes to .15 cases per 100 person-years.

▶ Despite the nonrandomized design of this clinical study (it is notoriously difficult to perform randomized, controlled trials when surgical procedures are involved), I included it because it demonstrates an important principle. Obesity is one of the best-recognized risk factors for all levels of glucose intolerance and for the progression of IGT to NIDDM.

Despite this well-recognized association and the major public health problem posed by IGT and NIDDM, there are startlingly few studies that demonstrate the long-term (greater than 1 year) efficacy of treatment of obesity in preventing the development of NIDDM. The importance of this study is twofold: It demonstrates the efficacy of gastric bypass procedures in ameliorating morbid obesity and the potent effect of weight loss on reducing the progression of IGT to NIDDM.

Although the study was poorly controlled, using a nonrandomly assigned control group, the almost nonexistent progression from IGT to NIDDM after gastric bypass was dramatically lower than in most studies of the natural history of IGT, where progression to NIDDM has ranged from 2% to 10% per year.

A multicenter national study on the prevention of NIDDM will soon begin. Gastric bypass surgery is certainly not a realistic solution to weight loss for most patients who are moderately overweight and at risk for IGT and

NIDDM; nevertheless, this article demonstrates the impressive efficacy of weight loss and encourages study of other, more widely applicable methods.—D.M. Nathan, M.D.

Ophthalmic Examination Among Adults With Diagnosed Diabetes Mellitus

Brechner RJ, Cowie CC, Howie LJ, Herman WH, Will JC, Harris MI (Ctrs for Disease Control and Prevention, Atlanta, Ga; Social and Scientific Systems Inc, Bethesda, Md; Natl Inst of Diabetes and Digestive and Kidney Diseases, Bethesda, Md; et al)
JAMA 270:1714–1718, 1993   112-95-11–8

Introduction.—Early laser photocoagulation therapy can significantly reduce the risk of visual loss in patients with diabetes. Symptoms of diabetic retinopathy may not appear until the disease is advanced and less amenable to laser treatment. It is unknown whether diabetic patients are having their eyes examined in accordance with current recommendations: an annual dilated examination after 5 years of IDDM and an annual dilated examination at diagnosis of NIDDM.

Methods.—Data from the 1989 National Health Interview Survey (NIHS) was used to determine whether adult diabetic patients are having recommended eye examinations and what factors are associated with meeting the recommendations. The NIHS is a cross-sectional, nationwide survey of the civilian, noninstitutionalized population. Of a representative sample of 84,572 research subjects who were identified by multistage probability sampling, 2,405 diagnosed diabetic patients responded to a questionnaire on their disease.

Findings.—Only 49% of patients with diabetes had undergone a dilated eye examination in the previous year, including 57% of those with IDDM, 55% of those with NIDDM, and 44% of those with NIDDM who were not receiving insulin therapy. The figures were only somewhat better in research subjects who were at high risk of visual loss—61% in those with retinopathy and 57% in those with diabetes of long duration. According to logistic regression analysis of research subjects with NIDDM, the likelihood of having had a dilated examination in the past year increased with greater age, higher socioeconomic status, and attendance at a diabetes education class. There was no association with race, duration of disease, frequency of physician visits, or insurance.

Conclusion.—Approximately half of adult patients with diabetes do not appear to be receiving recommended regular eye examinations for the detection and prompt treatment of retinopathy. Patient and professional educational efforts are needed to correct this situation, with a particular focus on younger patients and those in lower socioeconomic brackets.

▶ Diabetic retinopathy progresses through a series of stages that can culminate in macular edema or proliferative retinopathy, either of which can lead to substantial loss of vision.

Appropriately timed laser photocoagulation will decrease the development of vision loss. Because the majority of patients are asymptomatic during the development of retinopathy, screening for eye disease is critical if we are to identify patients who require more frequent follow-up and/or laser therapy.

Moreover, identification of the early stages of eye disease in diabetic patients might motivate them to intensify their diabetes management, which would also have a beneficial effect on their long-term outcome.

It is not very surprising that a significant portion of the diabetic population escapes examination, despite the recommendations by the American Diabetes Association and American College of Ophthalmology, which suggest an annual dilated examination for all patients with NIDDM and for patients with IDDM after 5 years' duration of diabetes.

Although it seems obvious that more careful attention to the need for an ophthalmologic examination is required, I am not ready to automatically sign on to the somewhat arbitrary choice of screening frequency. Although it is true that there are patients who experience otherwise preventable vision loss because of inadequate detection and screening, the financial cost of implementing the annual examination strategy would be extraordinary. Whether there are sufficient resources (ophthalmologists and perhaps optometrists and well-trained internists) capable of providing an adequate examination is also questionable.

Whereas the desire to provide improved eye screening and follow-up is laudable, it may well be that only a fraction of the diabetic population requires an annual examination by an ophthalmologist and that internists and optometrists can provide adequate screening. In addition, a more efficient means of screening, such as fundus photography, may be appropriate (Singer et al: *Ann Intern Med* 116:660, 1992).

There has been relatively little interest in determining the best frequency for screening using discriminate analysis or in examining alternative and less expensive means of screening. Until further studies are conducted, I am afraid we are stuck with the current arbitrary recommendations.—D.M. Nathan, M.D.

Health Care Expenditures for People With Diabetes Mellitus, 1992
Rubin RJ, Altman WM, Mendelson DN (Lewin-VHI, Inc, Fairfax, Va)
J Clin Endocrinol Metab 78:809A–809F, 1994   112-95-11–9

Objective.—Diabetes mellitus represents an important public health and clinical problem. It also has an important economic impact, particularly when the costs of diabetes-related complications are included. The prevalence of diabetes and the annual health care costs for people with diabetes in 1992 were estimated.

Methods.—The analysis was based on data from the 1987 National Medical Expenditure Survey. Diabetics were identified by self-reports of a physician's diagnosis of diabetes and confirmed by a history of taking diabetic medications, a diabetes-specific health care episode, or the purchase of diabetic equipment. Estimates of total expenditures included such items as home health care, prescription drugs, and durable medical equipment.

Findings.—Per individual, annual health care expenditures in 1992 were nearly $9,500 for diabetics vs. $2,600 for nondiabetics. Expenditures were even higher for confirmed diabetics at nearly $11,200. Diabetics made up 4.5% of the United States population and accounted for nearly 15% of total United States health care spending. For confirmed diabetics, the figures were 3% and 12%, respectively.

Conclusion.—Health care for patients with diabetes accounted for about one seventh of health care expenditures in 1992. Any health care reform program should be structured to promote those forms of care that are likely to improve the health of people with diabetes as they decrease the cost of caring for them.

▶ For all who hunger to know how much various diseases cost, this study represents the most satisfying estimate that I have seen of the cost of diabetes in the United States. Most previous studies have tried to estimate the cost attributable to diabetes care, multiply that number by the number of diabetics in the population, and come up with an estimate of specific costs associated with diabetes. The difficulty is that they often include only the cost that is directly attributable to diabetes care and miss what may be as much as 50% of the cost of having diabetes, i.e., the cost of caring for its myriad complications.

This study looked at a national sample of patients, calculated the total cost of health care for those who were identified as having diabetes, and compared it with the total health care cost of patients without the diagnosis of diabetes. In so doing, they captured the entire health care expenditure associated with diabetes.

The results are sobering. First, the percent of patients with diagnosed diabetes estimated from their database was very close to the prevalence of diagnosed diabetes in the National Diabetes Data Group Studies (approximately 4%). Second, the total cost calculated for the diabetic population of the United States was $105 billion per year, accounting for almost 15% of United States health care expenditures. Finally, the calculations did not include patients with undiagnosed diabetes, which may provide a population as large as that of patients with diagnosed diabetes. Although the health care costs for such patients would not typically include diabetic medications and supplies, these patients are at risk of complications. The treatment of such complications will inevitably add to the horrendous human and financial cost of diabetes.—D.M. Nathan, M.D.

Long-Term Improvement of Glycemic Control by Insulin Treatment in NIDDM Patients With Secondary Failure

Lindström T, Olsson AG, Eriksson P, Arnqvist HJ (Univ Hosp, Linköping, Sweden)

Diabetes Care 17:719–721, 1994   112-95-11–10

Background.—In patients with NIDDM and secondary failure to oral hypoglycemic agents, insulin treatment markedly improves metabolic control and the lipid profile when they are measured after 2–3 months. However, the initial improvement subsequently disappears in patients who have been followed for 6–8 months. To investigate further, patients with NIDDM with secondary failure were studied after 2–3 years of insulin treatment.

Study Design.—Twenty-one NIDDM patients with secondary failure were studied while they were still receiving oral hypoglycemic agents and after a median 27 months (range, 24–35) of insulin treatment.

Outcome.—Long-term insulin treatment markedly improved glycemic control, reducing hemoglobin A (HbA_{1c}) from 8.2% during treatment with oral hypoglycemic agents to 6.9%. Likewise, the fasting and postprandial glucose concentration decreased significantly. Fasting and postprandial insulin concentrations increased, and C peptide concentrations decreased. Body weight increased during insulin treatment, but most of the weight gain occurred within 4–5 months of insulin treatment; no significant increase in body weight occurred between 12 and 36 months. Plasma triglyceride concentrations decreased significantly from 2.8 to 1.8 mM, mainly because of reductions in very-low-density lipoprotein fraction. None of the patients had severe hypoglycemia that required the help of another person.

Conclusion.—Significant improvements in glycemic control and lipoprotein concentrations persist after insulin treatment for 2–3 years in NIDDM patients with secondary failure. These improvements occur despite an increase in body weight and hyperinsulinemia.

▶ The authors of this article set up something of a straw man that they can then burn quite effectively. They argue that when insulin therapy is added to patients who have failed oral hypoglycemic agents, the insulin therapy initially works and then stops working.

In fact, there are almost no long-term (more than 1 year) studies that have examined this issue. Moreover, no long-term studies have taken an aggressive posture in treating NIDDM with insulin; however, short-term studies that have used insulin aggressively have uniformly demonstrated improvement in glycemia.

This study used twice-daily mixed insulin and even 3–4 times daily intensive therapy in a small number of patients. It demonstrated quite convincingly that such a treatment approach results in a persistent improvement in glycemia to the near-normal range. Although weight gain occurs, as previously demonstrated in short-term studies, it tends to level out after the first year without further weight gain.

The study also demonstrated the expected improvement in triglycerides and VLDL cholesterol, as demonstrated in other studies. Levels of HDL cholesterol increased, albeit not significantly. Finally, the mean total insulin dose in these patients was less than 60 units per day. When calculated by body weight, the mean daily dose of insulin was almost identical to that used by adult IDDM patients in the Diabetes Control and Complications Trial (approximately .7 units per kg per day).

One of the remaining questions is whether the same results would have been obtained with insulin alone. Short-term studies have suggested that the results would have been very similar, although at the expense of a slightly greater dose of insulin. Therefore, similar to the demonstration of lower glycemia in the variable-dose insulin treatment group in the University Group Diabetes Project, this study verifies the long-term efficacy of modestly intensive treatment regimens in maintaining glycemia in the near-normal range in NIDDM. The United Kingdom Prospective Diabetes Study is likely to show the same thing.—D.M. Nathan, M.D.

Coronary Artery Disease and Coronary Artery Bypass Grafting in Diabetic Patients Aged ≥ 65 Years (Report From the Coronary Artery Surgery Study [CASS] Registry)
Barzilay JI, Kronmal RA, Bittner V, Eaker E, Evans C, Foster ED (Emory Univ, Atlanta, Ga; Univ of Washington, Seattle; Univ of Alabama, Birmingham; et al)
Am J Cardiol 74:334–339, 1994   112-95-11–11

Introduction.—Adult-onset diabetes mellitus has its highest prevalence and greatest impact on individuals aged 65 years and older, particularly in terms of the disproportionately high prevalence of coronary artery disease (CAD). Based on the Coronary Artery Surgery Study, the anatomical extent of CAD in diabetic patients aged 65 years and older, the impact of diabetes relative to other cardiovascular risk factors, and the efficacy of coronary artery bypass graft (CABG) surgery in older diabetics were assessed.

Patients.—A cohort of 317 patients with diabetes who were age 65 years or older and 1,843 age-matched nondiabetic patients was followed for a mean of 12.8 years; all had angiographically proven CAD.

Findings.—Compared with nondiabetic patients, diabetic patients were more likely to be women, to have higher systolic blood pressures, to have never smoked or not be current smokers, and to have evidence of peripheral vascular disease. Furthermore, diabetic patients were more likely to have higher grades of angina, more unstable angina, a higher number of coronary occlusions, and more severe proximal and distal coronary disease than nondiabetic patients. Both groups were similar with respect to traditional risk factors, including total cholesterol levels, family history of CAD, previous myocardial infarction, and a history of hypertension or left ventricular hypertrophy. The mortality rate was higher in diabetic patients, and diabetes was an independent predictor of mortality, conferring a 57% increased risk of dying. Its effects on mortality were as powerful as that of smoking, age, and congestive heart failure, and even more powerful than those of hypertension and left ventricular hypertrophy. Despite the deleterious effect of diabetes on coronary vasculature, diabetic patients who underwent CABG had a significantly lower mortality rate than medically treated patients; CABG conferred a 44% reduction in the risk of dying. The degree of mortality reduction with surgery was similar in diabetic and nondiabetic patients.

Conclusion.—Elderly diabetic patients have a greater severity and diffuseness of CAD and a higher mortality rate than elderly nondiabetic patients, despite the presence of similar traditional risk factors and the reduced likelihood of diabetics being current smokers. Diabetes itself appears to be the main risk factor for advanced CAD, and efforts at modifying or preventing CAD in the elderly diabetic patient should be strongly directed at ameliorating the diabetic state itself. A coronary artery bypass graft is similarly effective as a therapeutic option for elderly diabetic patients with CAD, as it is for their nondiabetic counterparts.

▶ This report from the Coronary Artery Surgery Study (CASS) reminds us of the major impact that diabetes has on macrovascular disease, as previously documented by the Framingham Study and others.

There are several problems in the design of this study with regard to the accuracy of its assessment of the impact of diabetes on cardiovascular disease. It probably underestimates the real frequency of diabetes in the study population, because the diagnosis of diabetes was based on self-report and not on glucose tolerance testing. This can lead to misclassification of the "nondiabetic" control group. Nevertheless, I included the article because it makes several important points.

Despite the more advanced CAD noted in diabetic patients, the greater frequency of women, and the more frequent co-occurrence of peripheral vascular disease, CABG had beneficial effects in older diabetic patients similar to those in nondiabetic patients of a comparable age. Regardless of the beneficial impact of CABG on mortality, diabetic patients continue to have a worse survival rate than nondiabetic patients. The prevalence of NIDDM in the population older than age 65 years approaches 20%, and it may be considerably higher in certain minority populations.

Considering the epidemic proportion of diabetes and heart disease in the United States population, these diseases are likely to become increasingly dominant factors with regard to human, financial, and societal costs in the next century. Methods to prevent both diabetes and macrovascular disease within the diabetic population must be developed.—D.M. Nathan, M.D.

Diabetes and the Risk of Pancreatic Cancer

Gullo L, Pezzilli R, Morselli-Labate AM, and the Italian Pancreatic Cancer Study Group (Univ of Bologna, Italy; Istituto di Clinica Medica e Gastroenterologia, Bologna, Italy)
N Engl J Med 331:81–84, 1994   112-95-11-12

Background.—Although pancreatic cancer patients are known to have an increased frequency of diabetes, the nature of this relationship is not understood. Authorities disagree on whether diabetes is a risk factor for pancreatic cancer.

Methods.—Seven hundred twenty pancreatic cancer patients and 720 control patients from 14 centers in Italy were studied. All were interviewed in detail to elicit their clinical histories. The diagnosis of diabetes was based on American Diabetes Association criteria.

Findings.—Twenty-three percent of the pancreatic cancer patients and 8% of the control patients had diabetes. In 56% of the pancreatic cancer patients, diabetes was diagnosed concomitantly with the cancer or within 2 years before the diagnosis of cancer. However, when only patients with diabetes of 3 or more years' duration were included in the analysis, the relationship became nonsignificant. All the pancreatic cancer patients whose diabetes had been diagnosed before the cancer and all but 1 of the diabetic control patients had NIDDM.

Conclusion.—Diabetes is significantly associated with pancreatic cancer. However, no association was found between diabetes and pancreatic cancer in patients with long-standing diabetes. The increased prevalence of NIDDM in pancreatic cancer patients appears to result mainly from diabetes of recent onset, presumably caused by the tumor. There is no evidence to suggest that diabetes predisposes patients to pancreatic cancer.

▶ The usual clinical teaching was that pancreatic cancer could not cause diabetes, because the destruction of the pancreas associated with these usually small tumors was insufficient to cause a significant perturbation in insulin secretion. On the other hand, clinicians have often been struck by the frequent co-occurrence of adenocarcinoma of the pancreas and diabetes, uniformly of the NIDDM variety. This study helps clarify the issue.

Pancreatic cancer is associated with NIDDM. The most likely explanation, considering the positive family history of NIDDM in those patients with pancreatic cancer in whom diabetes develops, is that the increased stress or some humoral factor associated with pancreatic cancer precipitates NIDDM in patients who are susceptible.

Although new-onset NIDDM is too common to be an efficient way to screen for pancreatic cancer, the occurrence of new-onset glucose intolerance in the setting of a patient with back pain and weight loss should ring a diagnostic bell. (Of course, I hope that any patient with back pain and weight loss of otherwise unexplained etiology would be evaluated for occult neo-plasm.)—D.M. Nathan, M.D.

Human Islet Allograft Follow-Up: Long-Term Islet Function and Over 3 Years of Insulin Independence

Ricordi C, Rilo HLR, Carroll PB, Fontes P, Shapiro R, Tzakis AG, Alejandro R, Bebhoo R, Rastellini C, Fung JJ, Scantlebury VP, Starzl TE (Univ of Pittsburgh, Pa)

Transplant Proc 26:569, 1994   112-95-11–13

Background.—Human islet allotransplantation has been investigated as a therapeutic option for insulin-dependent patients. The goals of this treatment are stable long-term function of the islets and insulin independence. The success rate of islet allografts was reported.

Methods.—Three patient groups were studied: group I: liver-islet allo-graft after upper abdominal exenteration for tumors; group II: liver-islet allograft for end-stage liver disease associated with type I diabetes; and group III: kidney-islet allograft for end-stage renal disease secondary to type I diabetes. The study included 25 patients, with 11 in group 1, 3 in group II, and 11 in group III. An automated method was used to isolate islets from human cadaveric donor pancreata for transplantation.

Findings.—In group I, insulin independence lasting 9 months to more than 3 years was seen in 55% of patients. In 1 patient, insulin independence has lasted 41 months with a stimulated C peptide of more than 1.0 pmol/mL, normal glucose clearance, and near-normal hemoglobin A (HbA_{1c}) over time. In 73% of patients in group I, tumor recurrence was seen. Unfortunately, rejection episodes occurred in 64%. In group II, none of the patients became insulin independent, and 100% had rejection episodes. In group III, 100% of the patients experienced at least 1 episode of rejection, and none achieved insulin independence.

Conclusion.—Insulin independence and stable islet function can be achieved through islet allografting. However, despite improved methods of islet isolation and immunosuppression, rejection and primary non-function continue to be major problems.

▶ To dispel the overly optimistic and usually inaccurate reporting in the press of new developments in islet transplantation, which are often prompted by the need for start-up companies to raise venture capital, I have included this realistic update of the islet allograft transplant experience from a group that has done a large number of them. The report is sobering.

The only patients who currently achieve any significant duration of insulin independence are those without type I diabetes who receive an islet trans-plant, usually in the setting of total exenteration with liver, intestine, and islet transplantation. Such patients are fundamentally different than type I dia-betic patients, because they do not have an autoimmune disease and have imperfectly functioning livers and gastrointestinal tracts. Finally, they have had their entire pancreas removed (presumably), and therefore they have no glucagon to antagonize insulin activity. As a result, it is likely that the results seen in this setting may not be transferable to patients with IDDM; this appears to be the case in the experience reported. No patients with IDDM achieved more than partial islet function or insulin independence.

When judging the success of islet transplantation, we should continue to use stringent definitions, that is, normal glucose control without exogenous insulin. By this definition, islet transplantation remains highly experimental and at the moment not successful.

Whether the failure of islet transplantation resides in an inadequate volume of transplanted islets; inadequate viability; direct toxic effects of the immunosuppressants on the islets; the nonphysiologic placement of the islets, usually in the liver; recurrent autoimmune disease; or some combination of these factors and others remains unknown.

Islet volume does not appear to be the rate-limiting step, because earlier reports have suggested adequate C peptide secretion with transplanted islets in the range of 4,000–6,000 islet equivalents per kg.

Do not believe the headlines. The results continue to be disappointing.—D.M. Nathan, M.D.

Effect of Glycemic Control on Early Diabetic Renal Lesions
Barbosa J, Steffes MW, Sutherland DER, Connett JE, Rao KV, Mauer M (Univ of Minnesota, Minneapolis)
JAMA 272:600–606, 1994   112-95-11–14

Background.—Diabetic glomerulopathy ultimately results in overt renal disease in 25% to 40% of type I diabetic patients. Improved glycemic control in type I diabetic patients was hypothesized to prevent or minimize the development of diabetic lesions in the renal allograft.

Methods.—Forty-eight patients were enrolled in the prospective, controlled, randomized study. All were type I diabetics with terminal renal failure who were undergoing renal transplantation. The experimental group received maximized glycemic control, and the standard treatment group received the same care as other patients in the transplant clinic. Maximized glycemic control consisted of subcutaneous insulin that was given several times a day or continuously compared with once or twice per day in standard treatment.

Findings.—Compared with the maximized group, the standard treatment group had a more than twofold increase in the volume fraction of mesangial matrix per glomerulus. Patients who were given standard care had a threefold increase in arteriolar hyalinosis, a greater widening of the glomerular basement membrane, and an increase in volume fraction of the total mesangium that approached significance. Patients who were receiving maximized treatment had a higher incidence of severe hypoglycemic episodes.

Conclusion.—Hyperglycemia appears to be causally related to an important lesion of diabetic nephropathy, mesangial matrix expansion, in renal allografts that are transplanted into diabetic recipients. A similar trend among other important glomerular and vascular lesions that characterize the pathologic findings in diabetic nephropathy was also suggested.

▶ Any article that has 4 pages of methods and only 1 paragraph of results can be considered problematic, and this one is no exception. On the other hand, the authors performed a study that many have discussed but none have ever been able to complete.

Because of the huge volume of kidney transplants performed in patients with IDDM at the University of Minnesota, the authors were able to assign recent kidney transplant recipients randomly to either intensive or a standard treatment, similar to the method used in the Diabetes Control and Complications Trial. They then obtained renal biopsies to examine the impact of intensive therapy on the development of new kidney lesions that were characteristic of diabetic nephropathy.

Although the Diabetes Control and Complications Trial results may have made the authors' results somewhat anticlimactic, the renal biopsies demonstrated a beneficial impact of intensive therapy in preventing mesangial accumulation in these relatively new kidney transplants. Putting aside for a moment the 50% dropout rate, errors in study design with regard to randomization, and the almost certain lack of statistical significance of the results if they are corrected for multiple analyses, this study provides further support that intensive therapy plays a beneficial role in preventing the development of complications, even in the setting of kidney transplantation.

The authors demonstrated that intensive therapy achieves lower albeit not normal glycemia in this setting, which will be no surprise to care providers who try to manage patients who are treated with prednisone and other immunosuppressants. In addition, the risk of intensive therapy with regard to hypoglycemia was documented. Of particular note is that very few if any diabetic patients with a kidney transplant have ever lived long enough for documented diabetic nephropathy to return and cause kidney failure.

Balancing the risks and difficulties of implementing intensive therapy against the mortality from other causes in this population may mitigate against implementing intensive therapy as it is currently practiced in the renal transplant population.—D.M. Nathan, M.D.

Effects of Varying Carbohydrate Content of Diet in Patients With Non–Insulin-Dependent Diabetes Mellitus

Garg A, Bantle JP, Henry RR, Coulston AM, Griver KA, Raatz SK, Brinkley L, Chen Y-DI, Grundy SM, Huet BA, Reaven GM (Univ of Texas, Dallas; Stanford Univ, Calif; Univ of Minnesota, Minneapolis; et al)
JAMA 271:1421–1428, 1994   112-95-11–15

Introduction.—Diets that are high in carbohydrates and low in saturated fats and cholesterol are widely recommended for patients with NIDDM, but the validity of these recommendations has been questioned. Evidence suggests that high-monounsaturated-fat diets may provide a greater clinical benefit. The effects of variations in the carbohydrate content of a diet on glycemia and plasma lipoproteins in patients with NIDDM were studied.

Study Design.—Forty-two NIDDM patients who were receiving glipizide therapy were assigned to either a high-carbohydrate diet containing 55% of the total energy as carbohydrates and 30% as fats or to a high-monounsaturated-fat diet containing 40% carbohydrates and 45% fats. The amounts of saturated fats, polyunsaturated fats, cholesterol, sucrose, and protein were similar. The diets were prepared in metabolic kitchens, and they provided the sole nutrients for the research subjects for 6 weeks each. A subgroup of 21 patients continued the diet they received for an additional 8 weeks.

Results.—Compared with the high-monounsaturated-fat diet, the high-carbohydrate diet increased fasting plasma triglyceride levels by 24% and VLDL cholesterol by 23%. Furthermore, the high-carbohydrate diet increased the daylong levels of plasma triglycerides by 10%, increased plasma glucose by 12%, and increased plasma insulin by 9%. Plasma total cholesterol, LDL cholesterol, and HDL cholesterol levels remained similar on the 2 diets. The effects of both diets on plasma glucose, insulin, and triglyceride and VLDL cholesterol levels persisted during the extension studies.

Conclusion.—High-carbohydrate diets in NIDDM patients may cause persistent increases in plasma triglyceride and VLDL cholesterol levels, hyperinsulinemia, and deterioration in glycemic control. All these metabolic changes may be deleterious, with the potential for accelerating atherosclerosis and microangiopathy. Consumption of *cis*-monounsaturated fats provides a suitable alternative to replace carbohydrates in the diet of NIDDM patients. In planning a high-monounsaturated-fat diet, it is important not to exceed the required energy intake and to maintain a low intake of cholesterol-raising saturated fatty acids and *trans*-fatty acids.

▶ The controversy regarding the appropriate carbohydrate content in the diet of patients with diabetes originated in the failure of various "expert" bodies to make the distinction between insulin-dependent and noninsulin-dependent forms of diabetes mellitus.

In the preinsulin era, strict carbohydrate restriction (the Allen diet) was thought to be the only means of prolonging survival for patients with IDDM. Although the relative attributes of these diets were vigorously debated, the real answer to IDDM came about with the introduction of insulin therapy in 1922. In the insulin era, carbohydrates were recognized as being less pernicious for IDDM patients than the high fat that had been substituted for them.

Unfortunately, this same controversy has been expanded to include NIDDM, where dietary concerns are generally quite different than in IDDM. For example, in IDDM the major dietary issues include maintaining a relatively consistent and regular pattern of food and carbohydrate intake to facilitate matching insulin to carbohydrate. With intensive therapy, patients must be sophisticated with regard to their diets so that they can accurately select appropriate insulin doses. Heart-healthy, low-saturated-fat and low-cholesterol diets are of secondary importance.

On the other hand, in NIDDM, caloric control and weight loss are the major issues for the 80% to 90% of patients with NIDDM who are obese. Treatment of obesity should be the major focus for prevention and treatment of NIDDM. Unfortunately, because long-term caloric restriction and weight loss are rarely obtained, other dietary issues have come to the fore. Reduction in total fat content as a means of decreasing caloric intake and the most appropriate carbohydrate content of diabetic diets, as investigated in this article, have supervened.

Although the balance between carbohydrates and monounsaturated fats has been investigated in other articles, this comprehensive study was selected in part because of its careful provision of all food during the course of the study, which ensures that its observations are the result of the diets under study. Whereas the results of this study should not distract us from the major challenge, that is, to effect weight loss in obese individuals, it demonstrates that substitution of monounsaturated fats for carbohydrates appears to improve glycemia and lipid metabolism to a modest degree.

To the extent that elevated insulin levels cause mischief with regard to atherogenesis, this diet may also be beneficial. (I am more than a little bit tired of seeing a reduction of hyperinsulinemia used as a rationale for every possible treatment. We should keep in mind that elevated insulin levels are only theoretically associated with macrovascular disease in NIDDM; causality has certainly never been documented.)—D.M. Nathan, M.D.

Insulin in Ischaemic Heart Disease: Are Associations Explained by Triglyceride Concentrations? The Caerphilly Prospective Study
Yarnell JWG, Sweetnam PM, Marks V, Teale JD, Bolton CH (Llandough Hosp, Penarth, South Glamorgan, Wales; St Luke's Hosp, Guildford England; et al)
Br Heart J 71:293–296, 1994
112-95-11–16

Background.—Several risk factors have been established for ischemic heart disease (IHD). However, the factors identified account for only a portion of the actual cases. There have been several studies that have shown correlations between cardiovascular disease and hyperinsulinemia. The results of these studies have been controversial. The value of insulin as a predictive factor for the development of IHD in nondiabetic men was examined.

Methods.—A cohort of men from the town of Caerphilly, Wales, and surrounding areas were followed up for 5 years. Eligible men were 45–59 years of age. A total of 2,818 were enrolled. A standard medical and smoking history was obtained for each. The London School of Hygiene and Tropical Medicine chest pain questionnaire was given, and a 12-lead ECG was recorded. Fasting blood samples were obtained from 2,368 men. At follow-up 61 months later, the chest pain questionnaire was given again, and a second ECG was obtained. Any hospital admissions were coded using the International Classification of Diseases designation for definite acute myocardial infarction. Laboratory analysis included total immunoreactive insulin assay, total cholesterol, triglycerides, and glucose determinations. After eliminations were made, the remaining 2,287 men were included in the analysis, and insulin levels were measured in 2,022. Univariate and multivariate analyses were performed.

Findings.—During the follow-up (average, 5 years), 113 events indicating IHD occurred in 2,022 men. Of these, 50% were fatal and 39% were clinical but nonfatal events. In a univariate analysis of initial serum insulin concentration in men with and without IHD, the difference was not statistically significant. The relative odds increased with increasing insulin concentration in a statistically significant trend. Fasting serum insulin levels showed a positive association with several variables, the strongest of which were the triglycerides ($r = .48$) and body mass ($r = .39$). Multivariate analyses showed that adjustment for the confounding variables nearly eliminated the association between insulin concentration and IHD.

Conclusion.—Although men in whom IHD developed were found to have statistically significant higher serum insulin concentrations initially, the effect of insulin disappeared when it was adjusted for triglycerides and other variables. Further research on the role of plasma triglycerides in the development of IHD seems warranted.

▶ It has been more than a decade since the original publication of the 3 epidemiologic studies that documented an association between insulin levels and cardiovascular disease in nondiabetics. The Busselton Study in Australia and the Helsinki and Paris prospective studies examined men and women in the former and male civil servants in the latter 2 studies.

The large number of research subjects involved in each of the studies enabled the demonstration of an association between either fasting or postprandial insulin levels and incident cardiovascular disease. Notably, the only study that included women (Busselton) did not demonstrate an association. The results of the original studies were by no means consistent; some demonstrated relationships with postprandial and some with fasting insulin levels.

In this study, which includes a population-defined cohort of middle aged men in South Wales, after excluding patients with diabetes increasing levels of fasting insulin were associated with increasing risk of a cardiovascular disease event occurring during 5 years of follow-up. However, when it was adjusted for the level of obesity and baseline triglycerides, the effect disappeared.

Although it is difficult to impute causative relationships based on these epidemiologic studies, they suggest alternative explanations for the theory that hyperinsulinemia per se is atherogenic to explain the higher risk of cardiovascular disease associated with these patients.

A somewhat unusual finding in this study was the association of triglycerides as a univariate risk factor for cardiovascular disease, but there is no association between total cholesterol and outcome. Levels of HDL were not measured.—D.M. Nathan, M.D.

Evidence for Superantigen Involvement in Insulin-Dependent Diabetes Mellitus Aetiology

Conrad B, Weidmann E, Trucco G, Rudert WA, Behboo R, Ricordi C, Rodriquez-Rilo H, Finegold D, Trucco M (Rangos Research Ctr, Pittsburgh, Pa; Children's Hosp of Pittsburgh, Pa; Univ of Pittsburgh, Pa)
Nature 371:351–355, 1994   112-95-11–17

Background.—Insulin-dependent diabetes mellitus (IDDM) is considered to be a T-cell–mediated autoimmune disease that is triggered in a genetically predisposed individual by environmental factors that have not been identified.

Objective.—The possibility that a superantigen is a pathogenetic factor was explored by analyzing islet-infiltrating T (IIT) cells from 2 IDDM patients who had died at the onset of the disease from brain swelling secondary to ketoacidosis.

Findings.—Analysis of the T-cell receptor (TCR) Vβ repertoire of IIT cells from the first patient disclosed expression of Vβ7 in more than 30% of cells. The level of Vβ7 expression in the spleen, 11%, was similar to that noted in peripheral blood lymphocytes from nondiabetic individuals. Overexpression of about 25% was found in IIT cells from the second patient. The TCR Vβ7 chains exhibited extensive junctional diversity. When peripheral blood lymphocytes from nondiabetics were exposed to islet cell membrane preparations from diabetics, there was evidence that T-cell clones that were positive for Vβ7 were positively selected.

Interpretation.—A superantigen binding to pancreatic islet cell membranes is a pathogenetic factor in IDDM. Initial exposure to superantigen at a very early age may inactivate potentially autoreactive T-cell clones, but exposure years after birth may lead to the activation of many different T-cell clones that express the same TCR Vβ. In a genetically predisposed individual some of these cells may initiate the process that culminates in the destruction of β cells. Cytoplasmic antigens that become accessible to T and β lymphocytes because of initial islet cell damage may continue to stimulate self-antigen-selected T cell clones and β-cell responses, resulting in further β-cell destruction.

▶ The search continues for the elusive antigen that is involved in the autoimmune destruction of the β cell in IDDM. The past several years have focused on antibodies to glutamic acid decarboxylase (GAD), because relatively persistent antibody titers to GAD have been noted in most patients with phenotypic IDDM.

What is remarkable about this study is the careful examination of CD4 + T cells that were isolated from the pancreases of 2 youngsters who died shortly after being seen with phenotypic IDDM. Other studies have consistently documented the seminal role played by T-cell immunity in the destruction of the islet. The T-cell receptor of these islet-infiltrating T cells "overexpressed" the β-chain Vβ7 gene compared with splenic tissue from the patients or peripheral blood lymphocytes from nondiabetic individuals.

The Vβ region of the T-cell receptor has been demonstrated to be a site that binds to a class of molecules, including enterotoxin and other bacterial and viral products that stimulate a massive T-cell proliferation, perhaps by binding to Vβ and bringing the surfaces of the T-cell receptor and major histocompatability complex into close contact. These "superantigens" require the presence of and bind to major histocompatibility complex class II molecules.

Although the involvement of superantigens, which suggests a potential bacterial or viral role in the etiology of IDDM, is of some interest, these results are only suggestive and are by no means conclusive for superantigen involvement. This study opens a new door to the exploration of the etiopathogenesis of IDDM.—D.M. Nathan, M.D.

Glycemic Thresholds for Spontaneous Abortion and Congenital Malformations in Insulin-Dependent Diabetes Mellitus
Rosenn B, Miodovnik M, Combs CA, Khoury J, Siddiqi TA (Perinatal Research Inst, Cincinnati, Ohio; Univ of Cincinnati, Ohio)
Obstet Gynecol 84:515–520, 1994   112-95-11–18

Introduction.—For reasons that are not clear, women with IDDM (type I) are at risk of both spontaneous abortion and having an infant with major congenital anomalies. Whether and how these outcomes relate to measures of glycemic control were determined.

Objective and Methods.—Receiver-operating characteristic (ROC) curves were derived to relate the occurrence of spontaneous abortion and congenital malformations to the median preprandial blood glucose in the first trimester of pregnancy and the initial estimate of glycohemoglobin. The study group included 215 type I diabetic women who enrolled before 9 weeks' gestation.

Findings.—Fifty-two women (24%) in the study had spontaneous abortions. The areas under the glucose and glycohemoglobin curves were .69 and .66, respectively, both of which are statistically significant results. The risk of abortion increased markedly compared with the background risk for nondiabetic women when the glucose was higher than 130 mg/dL or the glycohemoglobin was greater than 12%. Fourteen of 229 infants born to women who enrolled before 14 weeks' gestation (6.1%) had major congenital malformations. Three of them were stillborn and 1 died neonatally. The areas under the glucose and glycohemoglobin curves were .73 and .66, respectively. The risk of malformations was increased when the median first trimester preprandial glucose was greater than 120 mg/dL or the initial glycohemoglobin exceeded 13%.

Conclusion.—Type I diabetic women whose initial pregnancy glycohemoglobin is greater than 12% or whose median first-trimester preprandial glucose exceeds 120 mg/dL are at an increased risk of aborting spontaneously and of having an infant with major congenital malformations.

▶ The risks for the offspring of pregnant women who are diabetic are well recognized. Historically, a higher incidence of congenital malformations and miscarriages has been noted in many studies. A clear benefit to achieving and maintaining near-normal glucose control was recognized well before the results of the Diabetes Control and Complications Trial (DCCT) became available. As a result, even before the DCCT, pregnant women with diabetes were encouraged to achieve tight control.

Much of the recent debate has focused on the need to implement intensive therapy before pregnancy. The impetus to control glycemia in the preconception period is based on the delay in the "diagnosis" of pregnancy until usually 4–6 weeks into the gestation and the recognition that most organogenesis has taken place by week 8 of gestation. Therefore, if glucose levels play a critical role in causing first-trimester miscarriages and/or congenital malformations, intensive therapy should be implemented before conception.

The importance of near-normal glucose control in the preconception period has been documented in some but not all studies. Moreover, insofar as the DCCT message is promulgated and adopted, it is hoped that most patients with IDDM will have a hemoglobin A_{1c} that is within the "safety range" suggested by the study, because they are adhering or attempting to adhere to intensive therapy independent of their plans for pregnancy.

Nevertheless, it would be reassuring for pregnant women with IDDM to know the relative risks for various levels of glycohemoglobin, or mean blood glucose, during the early part of pregnancy. This article provides a partial analysis of such data, and although it does not provide a risk function with regard to increasing levels of glycemia, it does suggest that a hemoglobin A_1 level of less than 7–8 SD above the mean during the first trimester represents a level that has a lower risk with regard to fetal outcome.—D.M. Nathan, M.D.

Differences in Peripheral and Autonomic Nerve Function Measurements in Painful and Painless Neuropathy

Veves A, Young MJ, Manes C, Boulton AJM (Manchester Royal Infirmary, England)
Diabetes Care 17:1200–1202, 1994   112-95-11-19

Background.—The cause, pathogenesis, and natural history of painful diabetic neuropathy have not been adequately described. The differences in peripheral and autonomic nerve function were examined in patients with painful and painless diabetic neuropathy.

Methods.—Thirty-eight patients without neuropathy, 32 with painless neuropathy, and 52 with painful neuropathy were investigated. The age ranges of the 3 groups were 29–71 years, 30–71 years, and 28–73 years, respectively. Neuropathic assessment was based on clinical symptoms, signs, and quantitative sensory testing.

Findings.—Patients with painful neuropathy had higher Neuropathy Symptom and Neuropathy Disability scores than those with painless neuropathy. There were no differences in quantitative sensory testing, including current perception threshold (CPT) measures, electrophysiologic measures, and autonomic nerve system function tests. When the neuropathy groups were compared with the group without neuropathy, significant differences were noted for all these measures. Current perception threshold measures correlated significantly with other peripheral nerve function assessments when all patients with diabetes were considered as 1 group. Peroneal nerve motor conduction velocity correlated with CPT at 2 kHz and the vibration perception threshold.

Conclusion.—Using conventional tests, no differences could be found in the function of small and large nerve fibers between painful and painless diabetic neuropathy. The CPT did not quantify painful symptoms, but it compared favorably with other quantitative sensory tests in determining peripheral neuropathy.

▶ Painful diabetic neuropathy remains a relatively rare but extremely difficult management problem, occurring in only a subset of patients with peripheral somatosensory neuropathy. Although the natural history of painful neuropathy includes waxing and waning of symptoms, it remains a persistent problem for most patients who experience it.

The list of therapies that are effective has increased modestly in the past decade, expanding from tricyclic antidepressants, with or without fluphenazine, carbamazepine, and diphenylhydantoin, to the inclusion of topical capsaicin, IV lidocaine, and mexiletene. Unfortunately, none of these treatments are uniformly effective, and many carry significant side effects.

The clinician and patient, frustrated by the sometimes unremitting course of the diabetic neuropathy, often surrender to the use of increasingly potent analgesics. The use of addictive narcotics in this setting is almost always a recipe for disaster because the risk of long-term addiction is high.

This study suggests that there is no clear difference in small and large nerve fiber function in patients with painful vs. painless diabetic neuropathy. Previous studies had suggested that small-fiber function, which mediates pain, was particularly abnormal in patients with painful neuropathy.

Although this article does not support that initial observation, it is not clear whether different types of painful neuropathy were included. For example, several studies have divided painful neuropathy on the basis of the type of dysesthetic symptoms, including lancinating pain vs. formication (burning). Whether these different clinical characteristics reflect a different underlying pathophysiology is not clear, although some investigators have noted differential responses to medications in patients with these different types of neuropathy.

In any case, this relatively careful look at painful neuropathy fails to demonstrate any unique sensory characteristics. Special sensory testing of these patients is not likely to provide useful information.—D.M. Nathan, M.D.

Abnormal Increases in Urinary Albumin Excretion During Pregnancy in IDDM Women With Pre-Existing Microalbuminuria
Biesenbach G, Zazgornik J, Stöger H, Grafinger P, Hubmann R, Kaiser W, Janko O, Stuby U (Gen Hosp, Linz, Austria)
Diabetologia 37:905–910, 1994   112-95-11–20

Background.—A subclinical rise in urinary albumin excretion, or so-called microalbuminuria, is characteristic of developing diabetic nephropathy. A slight increase in protein excretion may accompany the transient increase in glomerular filtration rate noted in healthy pregnant women.

Objective.—The effects of pregnancy on urinary albumin excretion were studied in a prospective series of 30 women with IDDM whose albumin excretion was normal before conception and 12 other women with IDDM who had preexisting microalbuminuria. None of the latter excreted more than .5 g of protein per 24 hours.

Observations.—The previously normoalbuminuric women had a mean increase of 385% in urinary albumin excretion at the end of the third trimester—from 9 to 44 µg/min. Mean fractional albumin excretion increased 352%. Baseline values were regained 3 months postpartum. The creatinine clearance increased 26% during pregnancy. In women with preexisting microalbuminuria, albumin excretion rose 678% from 63 to 492 µg/min, and the mean fractional albumin excretion increased 601%. As in the other women, albumin excretion was close to baseline 3 months after delivery. Glycated hemoglobin values were normal in the second and third trimesters. Four of the 12 initially microalbuminuric women had transient changes in the nephrotic syndrome in the last trimester. These women had increased systolic blood pressure develop at the same time, but their glycated hemoglobin levels remained normal.

Conclusion.—Women with IDDM who exhibit microalbuminuria are at increased risk of having transient nephrotic syndrome develop in late pregnancy.

▶ This article sheds light on the usual effect of pregnancy on albumin excretion in women with IDDM with and without abnormal albumin excretion at baseline. The common clinical observation has been that like their nondiabetic counterparts, women with IDDM have an increase in albumin excretion during pregnancy. The transience of the phenomenon is supported by the almost universal return to baseline values shortly after delivery. The mechanism of these changes is not clearly elucidated here. The renal plasma flow and glomerular filtration rate both increase; whether some additional change in the filtration constant, selectivity, or another factor also plays a role is not known.

The increase in albumin excretion in this population occurred even in the setting of significant improvement in hemoglobin A_{1c} during the pregnancy. Whether albumin excretion rates would have increased even more in the setting of poor glucose control also is not known.—D.M. Nathan, M.D.

A Subtype of Diabetes Mellitus Associated With a Mutation of Mitochondrial DNA

Kadowaki T, Kadowaki H, Mori Y, Tobe K, Sakuta R, Suzuki Y, Tanabe Y, Sakura H, Awata T, Goto Y-i, Hayakawa T, Matsuoka K, Kawamori R, Kamada T, Horai S, Nonaka I, Hagura R, Akanuma Y, Yazaki Y (Univ of Tokyo; Asahi Life Found, Tokyo; Natl Inst of Neuroscience, Kodaira, Japan; et al)
N Engl J Med 330:962–968, 1994   112-95-11–21

Background.—A mutation in mitochondrial DNA may cause diabetes and deafness. The mutation, which involves the substitution of guanine for adenine at position 3243 of leucine transfer RNA (tRNA), appears to interfere with RNA synthesis and binding of the transcription terminal factor, causing a defect in mitochondrial protein. To clarify the prevalence, clinical characteristics, and pathophysiology, 22 families with the mutation were identified and their clinical features were explored.

Methods.—The study sample included: group 1: 55 patients with IDDM and a history of diabetes in first-degree relatives; group 2: 85 patients with IDDM without family history; group 3: 100 patients with NIDDM and a history of diabetes in first-degree relatives; group 4: 5 patients with hearing loss and diabetes; and group 5: 39 unrelated patients with the mutation and multiple symptoms. In addition, 42 relatives of groups 1–4 and 127 relatives of group 5 were included. Questionnaires and direct examinations were used to confirm diagnoses. Molecular studies were done on the DNA using polymerase chain reaction, and insulin secretory capacity was evaluated. Statistical analysis was done using the Student's *t*-test and chi-square analysis.

Findings.—The mutation was seen in 52 patients with diabetes in 22 unrelated families who were identified as having the mutation. Diabetes appears to be transmitted maternally. The mutation can be associated with either IDDM or NIDDM. Sensory hearing loss can occur in patients with the mutation and diabetes. Hearing loss was often seen after the onset of diabetes in younger patients who had a lesser past history of obesity. More often, patients with the mutation seem to require insulin compared with those without it.

Conclusion.—This mutation of mitochondrial DNA may represent a cause of diabetes in Japan. The research also suggests an overlap between the cause of IDDM and NIDDM. Further research is needed to generalize this information to a broader population.

▶ Several distinct and heritable abnormalities have been identified as the cause of some cases of phenotypic NIDDM. These include the recent, newly heralded discovery of mutations in the glucokinase gene as a cause of maturity-onset diabetes in the young; familial abnormalities in the insulin gene that lead to abnormal processing and relatively ineffective secretion of mature insulin; and myriad abnormalities in the insulin receptor.

None of these accounts for more than a minor fraction of diabetes, although they may in combination with other defects contribute to a more substantial portion of NIDDM.

This article identifies a mutation in mitochondrial DNA that is associated with a distinct form of diabetes in Japan that includes deafness and other congenital abnormalities. Although it is clear that the mutation does not uniformly lead to diabetes and that it is almost certainly a relatively rare cause of diabetes, the patients with the mutation appear to have a form of diabetes that is phenotypically more similar to IDDM than it is to NIDDM.

Moreover, because these patients do not have obvious markers of autoimmunity, the mutation represents another path by which patients can become insulin deficient. Although it is tantalizing to wonder whether this mutation, which was identified in some persons without diabetes and in persons with phenotypic NIDDM, may contribute to NIDDM, it appears unlikely. Mitochondrial DNA is maternally transmitted and as would be expected, neither the mutation nor diabetes is passed from the father to the children.

However, there is no evidence of NIDDM being maternally transmitted in the large populations that have been studied. Although the mutation was identified in a small percent of patients with phenotypic NIDDM, it is by no means clear in the absence of specific genetic or phenotypic markers of NIDDM that the mutation played any role in their diabetes.

This study again informs us that the causes of all forms of diabetes are probably heterogeneous and perhaps multiple. The specific mechanism by which the mutation in mitochondrial DNA causes diabetes remains speculative.—D.M. Nathan, M.D.

Hyperinsulinemia Induces a Reversible Impairment in Insulin Receptor Function Leading to Diabetes in the Sand Rat Model of Non-Insulin-Dependent Diabetes Mellitus

Kanety H, Moshe S, Shafrir E, Lunenfeld B, Karasik A (Chaim Sheba Med Ctr, Tel Hashomer, Israel; Hebrew Univ-Hadassah Med School, Jerusalem)
Proc Natl Acad Sci U S A 91:1853–1857, 1994   112-95-11-22

Background.—Commonly, NIDDM is seen in patients who experience weight gain. In human beings, hyperinsulinemia and insulin resistance occur after overeating, followed by hyperglycemia. It is unclear whether hyperinsulinemia or insulin resistance is the primary event. Using the sand rat model, the events that lead from overeating to diabetes and the activity of insulin transmembrane changes and insulin receptor (IR) function were studied.

Methods.—Different stages of diabetes in the sand rat were evaluated. The rats were placed in 5 groups according to metabolic and disease status: group A: normoglycemia/normoinsulinemic; group B: hyperinsulinemic/normoglycemic; group C: hyperinsulinemic/hyperglycemic; recovered A: hyperglycemic/hyperinsulinemic converting to normoglycemic/normoinsulinemic on a modified diet, and recovered B: hyperglycemic/hyperinsulinemic converting to normoglycemic/hyperinsulinemic on a modified diet. Albino rats were used as controls. Insulin was injected by the portal vein. Controls received only phosphate-buffered saline. Tissues were removed, prepared, and their protein content assayed. Insulin-binding in the membranes was measured using ^{125}I-labeled insulin as a tracer. The ratios of bound to free insulin were used to measure the IR present. Data were analyzed using the Student's t-test. Assays for IR tyrosine kinase (TK) activity and dephosphorylation were conducted.

Findings.—Compared with controls, nondiabetic sand rats had a lower number of insulin receptors in the liver. Also of note was normal IR TK activity with a high adenosine triphosphate K_m for phosphorylation reaction. In the sand rats, overeating produced an overall drop in insulin-induced receptor tyrosine kinase activity. With overeating, examination of muscle showed a decrease in IR and an increase in TK activity. Imposing dietary restrictions on diabetic subjects corrected altered receptor kinase activation. When overeating occurred and liver receptors were scarce, hyperinsulinemia resulted, reducing receptor kinase activity and leading to insulin resistance.

Conclusion.—Hyperinsulinemia is suspected as being the cause of impaired insulin-stimulated insulin receptor TK activity, leading to insulin resistance and glucose intolerance. Further research is needed to investigate the cellular mechanism of this process and its implications in human beings.

▶ The primary role of insulin resistance in the genesis of impaired glucose tolerance and perhaps in NIDDM has been reasonably well established. A decreasing ability to secrete insulin and maintain normoglycemia in the face of increasing insulin resistance has also been noted as perhaps being the rate-limiting step in the development of NIDDM.

Although many small studies have demonstrated increased insulin resistance using insulin clamp methods before the appearance of any abnormal glucose metabolism, many other studies have inferred the presence of insulin resistance solely on the basis of elevated fasting or postprandial insulin levels. (Clearly, this is much easier to measure than performing insulin clamp studies.)

This study tries to elucidate whether hyperinsulinemia is a primary phenomenon or whether insulin levels rise because of a fundamental abnormality in the IR (or postreceptor) that leads to hyperinsulinemia as a compensatory mechanism. The authors used an animal model of NIDDM, the sand rat (gerbil). In captivity the sand rat, like other wild animals, has the tendency to overeat and relax. Obesity, hyperinsulinemia, and in some cases, hyperglycemia develop in these sand rats.

The authors manipulated the diet of the sand rat to create a model of obesity as a cause of NIDDM. (It is critical to note that although most patients with obesity have increased insulin resistance, less than 20% have NIDDM. As a result, the model of overeating as a cause of diabetes leaves much to be desired. Other factors must be involved.)

The results of this study suggest that hyperinsulinemia precedes abnormalities in IRs and IR kinase activity. Restoration of a high-fiber, low-calorie diet in animals who were both hyperglycemic and hyperinsulinemic restored normoglycemia, with a partial correction of insulin receptor TK. Full recovery of the TK was not seen until the hyperinsulinemia was also corrected.

To the extent that these sand rats are relevant models for human NIDDM, they suggest that hyperinsulinemia may be the primary factor in the development of insulin resistance. The unraveling of the temporal sequence in the development of NIDDM in human beings will be much more difficult.—D.M. Nathan, M.D.

Advanced Glycation End Products (AGEs) on the Surface of Diabetic Erythrocytes Bind to the Vessel Wall Via a Specific Receptor Inducing Oxidant Stress in the Vasculature: A Link Between Surface-Associated AGEs and Diabetic Complications

Wautier J-L, Wautier M-P, Schmidt A-M, Anderson GM, Hori O, Zoukourian C, Capron L, Chappey O, Yan S-D, Brett J, Guillausseau P-J, Stern D (Hopital Lariboisiere, Paris; Columbia Univ, New York; Hopital Broussais, Paris, et al)
Proc Natl Acad Sci U S A 91:7742–7746, 1994   112-95-11–23

Background.—Vascular complications are a significant source of morbidity and mortality in patients with diabetes. The extent of vascular complications has been associated with increased adherence of diabetic erythrocytes to endothelial cells (ECs) and to the accumulation of a class of glycated proteins, advanced glycation end products (AGEs). The formation of AGEs on the surface of diabetic erythrocytes may mediate their interaction with ECs, resulting in binding and induction of vascular dysfunction.

Methods and Findings.—Eighteen patients with diabetes and 18 healthy persons were studied. In addition, diabetic and normal rat erythrocytes were transfused into normal rats. In the first study, increased binding of diabetic erythrocytes to ECs was blocked by erythrocyte preincubation with anti–AGE immunoglobulin G (IgG) or EC preincubation with antibodies to the receptor for AGE (RAGE). The presence of RAGE in the vessel wall was confirmed by immunoblotting of cultured human ECs and immunostaining of normal and diabetic human tissue. Diabetic erythrocyte binding to endothelium produced an oxidant stress. The infusion of erythrocytes from diabetic rats into normal rats had an accelerated, early phase of clearance that was partly prevented by the RAGE antibody. Liver tissue from rats that were infused with diabetic erythrocytes demonstrated increased levels of thiobarbituric acid–reactive substances, which was prevented by pretreatment with anti-RAGE IgG or probucol.

Conclusion.—Erythrocyte surface AGEs can function as ligands that interact with endothelial RAGE. The extensive contact of diabetic erythrocytes bearing surface-related AGEs with vessel wall RAGE may play a significant role in vascular complications.

▶ The putative protean effects of AGEs continue to be advanced by several groups. Not only do AGEs mediate structural effects, such as changing the physical characteristics of collagen, but they apparently bind to a relatively specific receptor and cause changes in mesangial matrix, basement membrane, and immunoglobulins. In addition to binding to proteins, AGEs bind to fats and even to nucleic acids.

What is missing for many of these effects, which were demonstrated in animal models and in vitro, is a convincing link to the pathogenesis of diabetic complications in human beings. The most convincing data remain the effect of glycosylation on lens protein, which leads to cataract formation, and on tendon collagen, which leads to a variety of cheiropathies, including Dupuytren's contractures, the "prayer sign," and others.

This article provides yet another possible mechanism for the development of diabetic complications that may be mediated by AGEs. The authors demonstrate binding of erythrocytes with AGEs to endothelial receptors. They further demonstrate decreased erythrocyte survival, a presumed result of the altered clearance of these AGE-bound erythrocytes. Finally, they suggest that these erythrocytes may mediate oxidant stress.

Although this study is nicely done, the relevance of the findings, especially considering the absence of convincing data that erythrocyte turnover is altered significantly in human diabetes, must be questioned. I am virtually certain that glycation plays a role in the pathogenesis of diabetic complications.

How great a role and for which complications remain open questions.—D.M. Nathan, M.D.

The Linked Roles of Nitric Oxide, Aldose Reductase and, (Na+,K+) -ATPase in the Slowing of Nerve Conduction in the Streptozotocin Diabetic Rat
Stevens MJ, Dananberg J, Feldman EL, Lattimer SA, Kamijo M, Thomas TP, Shindo H, Sima AAF, Greene DA (Michigan Diabetes Research and Training Ctr, Ann Arbor; Univ of Michigan, Ann Arbor)
J Clin Invest 94:853–859, 1994   112-95-11–24

Background.—Metabolic and vascular defects have both been implicated in the pathogenesis of diabetic neuropathy. However, the interrelationships among them are not well understood. Evidence combined from several studies provides a framework for a potential novel metabolic-vascular pathogenetic matrix for diabetic neuropathy involving aldose reductase, nitric oxide (NO), and (Na+, K+)-adenosine triphosphatase (ATPase). The potential role of aldose reductase-related defects in NO synthesis or action in the pathogenesis of the reduced nerve conduction velocity (NCV) and/or nerve (Na+, K+)-ATPase activity in the streptozotocin-diabetic (STZ-D) rat model was studied.

Methods and Findings.—The ability of N-nitro-L-arginine methyl ester (L-NAME), a specific NO synthase inhibitor and arginine analogue that competes for the enzyme's substrate binding site, to block the salutary effect of aldose reductase inhibitor treatment on NCV in the STZ-D rat and to reproduce the slowed NCV of STZ-D in rats that were not diabetic was assessed. The increased NCV afforded by aldose reductase inhibitor treatment in rats that were acutely diabetic was reversed by L-NAME without affecting the attendant correction of nerve sorbitol and *myco*-inositol. Prolonged L-NAME administration fully reproduced the nerve conduction slowing and (NA+, K+)-ATPase impairment characteristic of diabetes.

Conclusion.—The aldose reductase-inhibitor-sensitive component of conduction slowing and the decreased (NA^+, K^+)-ATPase activity in the rat that was diabetic may partly reflect impaired NO activity. Therefore, the pathogenesis would be a dual metabolic-ischemic process.

▶ Here is another iteration of the aldose reductase theory of diabetic complications. When we last read about aldose reductase, it was implicated as the mediator of sugar alcohol (sorbitol) accumulation and trapping in the presence of hyperglycemia in a variety of tissues that were susceptible to diabetic complications. The accumulation of sorbitol was postulated to lead to diabetic complications by depleting myoinositol and perhaps other intracellular osmolytes such as taurine, which altered phosphoinositide metabolism and reduced (Na^+, K^+)-ATPase activity.

All these changes have been postulated at various times to cause axoglial dysfunction, affect nerve conduction, and promote the peripheral somatosensory polyneuropathy characteristic of diabetes mellitus.

A different clinical form of diabetic neuropathy, which includes the cranial and peripheral mononeuropathies and is usually focal, asymmetric, and self-limited, is thought to be a consequence of vascular obstruction of the vasa nervorum.

This article suggests that yet another type of vascular abnormality, decreased endoneurial blood flow, may also account for peripheral neuropathy by causing ischemia of the nerves. The authors note that aldose reductase-mediated events may also affect NO synthesis. They speculate that to the extent that microvascular disregulation is mediated by deficient NO-mediated vasodilatation, aldose reductase and NO may both be involved in diabetic neuropathy. By using a specific NO synthase inhibitor, they reverse improvements in nerve conduction velocity associated with aldose reductase inhibition in diabetic rats. This is all obviously quite speculative.

Although abnormalities in NO and excessive activity of aldose reductase may play joint roles in the pathogenesis of diabetic neuropathy, whether they are both dysfunctional in diabetes and whether either or both are the cause of diabetic neuropathy rather than just of nerve conduction velocity abnormalities remain to be firmly established.

After years of human experimentation with specific inhibitors of aldose reductase without a clear benefit, I wonder whether we are facing years of similarly fruitless experimentation with promoters of NO synthase.—D.M. Nathan, M.D.

Suggested Reading

The following articles are recommended to the reader:

EURODIAB IDDM Complications Study Group: Microvascular and acute complications in IDDM patients: The EURODIAB IDDM Complications Study. *Diabetologia* 37:278–285, 1994.

► A relatively new epidemiologic study of IDDM in 16 countries in Europe. Describes "modern-day" metabolic control and occurrence of the long-term complications in IDDM.

Frank RN: The aldose reductase controversy. *Diabetes* 43:169–172, 1994.
► Reviews the aldose reductase-sorbitol theory of diabetic complications and the evidence that supports or fails to support it.

Gale EAM, Bingley PJ: Can we prevent IDDM? *Diabetes Care* 17:339–344, 1994.
► Reviews potential means of preventing IDDM, once vulnerable individuals are identified.

Cryer PE, Fisher JN, Shamoon H: Hypoglycemia. *Diabetes Care* 17:734–751, 1994.
► A masterful review of hypoglycemia associated with blood glucose-lowering medications. Discusses causes, pathophysiology, risks, hypoglycemic unawareness, and treatment in both IDDM and NIDDM.

McCarthy MI, Froguel P, Hitman GA: The genetics of non-insulin-dependent diabetes mellitus: Tools and aims. *Diabetologia* 37:959–968, 1994.

Jarrett RJ: Why is insulin not a risk factor for coronary heart disease? *Diabetologia* 37:945–947, 1994.

Reaven GM, Laws A: Insulin resistance, compensatory hyperinsulinaemia, and coronary heart disease. *Diabetologia* 37:948–952, 1994.
► Reviews pro and con arguments regarding role of hyperinsulinemia in the genesis of the increased risk for coronary artery disease in diabetes mellitus.

Newgard CB: Cellular engineering and gene therapy strategies for insulin replacement in diabetes. *Diabetes* 43:341–350, 1994.

Updike J: *The Afterlife and Other Stories.* New York, Alfred A. Knopf, 1995.
► Relax and enjoy these 16 stories, each of which is masterful and touching in different ways.

12 Reproductive Endocrinology

Introduction

As in previous years, the section on reproductive endocrinology contains many basic science and clinical articles, so selecting a fair representation has been difficult.

We have largely confined our selection to articles that are of significant interest to clinical reproductive endocrinologists; unfortunately, this meant that we had to exclude many excellent studies of animal models of reproduction or of basic biochemical or molecular genetics, fields that in years to come may be highly relevant to clinical endocrinology.

The subsections include abstracts of 8 articles on male reproduction and 16 articles on female reproduction, which include studies of women during their reproductive life and after menopause.

William D. Odell, M.D., Ph.D., M.A.C.P.

Male Reproduction

Characterization of Mutant Androgen Receptors Causing Partial Androgen Insensitivity Syndrome

De Bellis A, Quigley CA, Marschke KB, El-Awady MK, Lane MV, Smith EP, Sar M, Wilson EM, French FS (Univ of North Carolina, Chapel Hill; Children's Hosp Med Ctr, Cincinnati, Ohio)

J Clin Endocrinol Metab 78:513–522, 1994

112-95-12-1

Background.—Mutations in the androgen receptor (AR) gene that cause androgen insensitivity syndrome (AIS) result in a spectrum of sex phenotypes that ranges from complete female (complete AIS) to nearly complete male (partial AIS). The AR gene mutations in 3 unrelated families with partial AIS were identified and characterized.

Methods.—The AR gene in three 46,XY individuals with partial AIS was studied using polymerase chain reaction and denaturing gradient gel electrophoresis.

Results.—One research subject had ambiguous genitalia, clitoromegaly, posterior labial fusion, and a urogenital sinus at birth. Sequence analysis of exon C detected a single base mutation that converted a leucine residue at position 616 to arginine. Androgen-binding studies in cultured genital skin fibroblasts revealed a binding affinity for the synthetic androgen methyltrienolone similar to that of control fibroblasts. The mutant AR exhibited greatly reduced binding to an androgen-response element DNA sequence, but it retained a low level of transcriptional activity at physiologic androgen concentrations that were consistent with the individual's phenotype of partial AIS. The second research subject also exhibited a distinctly ambiguous external genital phenotype. A single base mutation was identified in exon G, which converted arginine at position 840 to histidine. Genital skin fibroblasts in this research subject demonstrated a sevenfold lower androgen-binding affinity than control fibroblasts, and the mutant receptor had reduced transcriptional activity. The third research subject had the phenotype of complete androgen resistance at birth. Sequence analysis of exon H detected a mutation that converted the valine residue at position 889 to methionine. The mutant receptor had apparently normal androgen-binding capacity, but it had reduced androgen-binding capacity when it was examined by expression of the recreated mutant AR in COS 7 cells.

Summary.—The identification of single base mutations in 3 unrelated families with partial AIS was reported and the clinical, functional, and molecular heterogeneity in partial AIS were demonstrated.

Single Strand Conformation Polymorphism Analysis of Androgen Receptor Gene Mutations in Patients With Androgen Insensitivity Syndromes: Application for Diagnosis, Genetic Counseling, and Therapy

Hiort O, Huang Q, Sinnecker GHG, Sadeghi-Nejad A, Kruse K, Wolfe HJ, Yandell DW (Medizinische Universität, Lübeck, Germany; Tufts-New England Med Ctr, Boston; Massachusetts Eye and Ear Infirmary, Boston)
J Clin Endocrinol Metab 77:262–266, 1993   1 1 2-95-12–2

Background.—Androgen insensitivity syndrome (AIS) is a defect of the androgen receptor protein that manifests itself in defective sexual differentiation in karyotypic males. The familial form is an X-linked trait that is transmitted through female carriers, heterozygotes for the gene defect. Rapid mutational analysis of the androgen receptor gene in initial AIS diagnosis, genetic counseling, and molecular subclassification of affected patients and their families was investigated.

Methods.—The DNA from peripheral leukocytes of 6 patients with varying degrees of AIS and female family members was studied. Exons 2 to 8 of the androgen receptor gene were analyzed using single strand conformation polymorphism analysis and direct DNA sequencing.

Results.—Single-base DNA sequence variations within the hormone-binding domain were identified in all 6 patients. All mutations caused amino acid substitutions. One patient, who had incomplete androgen insensitivity, was a mosaic for the mutation. Four of the 5 mothers and 1 sister were carriers of the mutation that was present in the patient.

Discussion.—The androgen receptor gene is associated with diverse molecular defects that result in complex clinical manifestations. Screening whole blood DNA for germ-line androgen receptor gene mutations facilitates rapid diagnosis and carrier identification in most families. Because the screening techniques are inexpensive and require a small number of cells, they can be used routinely to diagnose all cases of genital abnormalities and provide genetic counseling to patients with AIS and their families. A detailed molecular classification of androgen receptor gene defects will facilitate future development of conservative therapies for many of these patients.

▶ These 2 articles (Abstracts 112-95-12–1 and 112-95-12–2) represent only a small part of a large number of mutations described in the androgen receptor gene of patients with partial or complete androgen resistance. The androgen, like all nuclear hormone receptors, possesses 3 general domains or portions: a hormone (androgen)-binding domain; a DNA-binding domain; and a third domain without a known function but which can be used to measure the receptor by immunoassays.

Many patients with complete androgen resistance have mutations resulting in stop codes for transcription that lead to production of no androgen receptor or to markedly truncated forms. The patients described in these 2 articles had partial AIS. These patients (with 1 exception) all had single base mutations leading to single amino acid substitution in the hormone-binding domain of the androgen receptor.

The exception was the patient in the study of DeBellis (Abstract 112-95-12–1) and associates, who had a single base mutation resulting in decreased DNA binding.

If the literature for all patients with clinically diagnosed androgen resistance syndrome is surveyed, increasing numbers of defined mutations will be described. However, no abnormality in the androgen receptor was identifiable in some patients, suggesting that abnormalities in genes whose expression is controlled by the androgen receptor may form the basis for some patients with androgen resistance syndrome.—W.D. Odell, M.D., Ph.D.

Effects on Behavior of Modulation of Gonadal Function in Men With Gonadotropin-Releasing Hormone Antagonists

Loosen PT, Purdon SE, Pavlou SN (Vanderbilt Univ, Nashville, Tenn; Dept of Veterans Affairs Med Ctr, Nashville, Tenn)
Am J Psychiatry 151:271–273, 1994   112-95-12–3

Purpose.—Administration of GnRH analogues reduces the endogenous secretion of testosterone, LH, and FSH. The effects of a new, potent GnRH antagonist Nal-Glu on spermatogenesis, sexual function, and behavior in normal men were studied.

Methods.—Eight normal men, ages 24–49 years, were given 10 mg of Nal-Glu daily by subcutaneous injection for 20 weeks. After 2 weeks, IM testosterone enanthate, 25 mg once per week, was added to the regimen to keep testosterone levels in the low-normal range. Behavior, libido, and sexual functioning were assessed at baseline, after 10 and 20 weeks of treatment, and at 10 weeks after Nal-Glu administration had ended. Libido and sexual functioning were assessed using a 5-item questionnaire.

Results.—Complete azoospermia was reached within 6–12 weeks after initiation of Nal-Glu administration, and mean serum testosterone, LH, and FSH concentrations fell to hypogonadal levels. Nal-Glu and low-dose testosterone administration reduced measures of outward-directed anger in all men, sexual desire in 3 men (38%), and mean anxiety scores in 5 men (63%). Measures of anger control, inward-directed anger, and affective state were unaffected. All measures of endocrine function rapidly normalized after Nal-Glu was discontinued.

Conclusion.—Measures of outward-directed anger are most sensitive to small reductions in circulating testosterone concentrations.

Effect of a Long-Lasting Gonadotrophin Hormone-Releasing Hormone Agonist in Six Cases of Severe Male Paraphilia
Thibaut F, Cordier B, Kuhn J-M (Psychiatric Hosp, Sotteville les Rouen, France; C Nicolle Hosp, Bois Guillaume, France)
Acta Psychiatr Scand 87:445–450, 1993   112-95-12–4

Objective.—Antiandrogenic drugs such as medroxyprogesterone acetate or cyproterone acetate can reduce sex drive and interest in sex in sex offenders. However, these drugs do not modify the direction of sexual interest and carry some theoretical risks. Gonadotropin luteinizing releasing hormone analogue (GnRHa) can lead to reversible castration, with the only side effects being those related to hypoandrogenism. Preliminary results of GnRHa treatment in 6 men with severe paraphilia were examined.

Patients.—The mean age of the patients was 25 years. Three were mildly to moderately mentally retarded, 2 had borderline personality disorder, and 1 had mixed bipolar disorder; 4 had been convicted of sexual offenses. All the men asked for treatment for their uncontrollable deviant sexual behavior. Treatment was with depot GnRHa, IM triptorelin, 3.75 mg/mo. All patients received concurrent psychotherapy.

Outcomes.—For 5 of the patients, triptorelin treatment stopped their deviant sexual behavior and decreased their sexual fantasies and activities. The only significant side effects were those related to hypoandrogenism. A gradual decrease in plasma testosterone to castration levels accompanied the clinical improvement within the first month. The benefits of treatment were maintained for as long as 3 years. In 1 patient, treatment interruption led to a relapse within 10 weeks.

Conclusion.—The reversible castration achieved with GnRHa may be a promising treatment for severe paraphilia. It reduces deviant sexual activity and produces fewer side effects than other antiandrogenic drugs. Treatment with GnRHa may also favor the use of concurrent psychotherapy.

▶ These 2 studies (Abstracts 112-95-12–3 and 112-95-12–4) of GnRH agonist or antagonist treatment of eugonadal men strikingly demonstrate the behavioral modification that results when normal androgen production is decreased.

Although as endocrinologists we are only occasionally asked to see or treat men with paraphilia, the use of GnRH agonists administered once monthly would seem to offer advantages over high-dose progestational compounds.—W.D. Odell, M.D., Ph.D.

Relatively Low Levels of Dimeric Inhibin Circulate in Men and Women With Polycystic Ovarian Syndrome Using a Specific Two-Site Enzyme-Linked Immunosorbent Assay

Lambert-Messerlian GM, Hall JE, Sluss PM, Taylor AE, Martin KA, Groome NP, Crowley WF Jr, Schneyer AL (Massachusetts Gen Hosp, Boston; Oxford Brookes Univ, Headington, England)
J Clin Endocrinol Metab 79:45–50, 1994   112-95-12–5

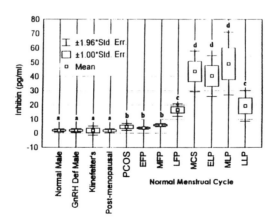

Fig 12–1.—Mean dimeric inhibin levels in serum from several fertile and infertile groups of men and women. Mean values and SEMs are shown for normal fertile men ($n = 13$), men with GnRH deficiency ($n = 11$)or Klinefelter's syndrome ($n = 3$), postmenopausal women ($n = 13$), women with polycystic ovarian syndrome (PCOS) ($n = 8$), and normal women across each phase of the menstrual cycle ($n = 3$). Groups with *different letter symbols* have significantly different means ($P < .05$). (Courtesy of Lambert-Messerlian GM, Hall JE, Sluss PM, et al: *J Clin Endocrinol Metab* 79:45–50, 1994.)

Introduction.—The endocrine feedback role of dimeric inhibin on FSH secretion from the pituitary has been well established in many species but not in man. It may be that the inhibin immunoassay used most widely in the human is a heterologous assay with an antiserum that exclusively recognizes the inhibin α-subunit in both its monomeric form and in inhibin dimers. A new ultrasensitive enzyme-linked immunosorbent assay (ELISA) that is specific for the dimeric form α/β only was used to quantify serum inhibin levels in a variety of fertile and infertile men and women.

Results.—The specificity of the new dimeric inhibin ELISA was confirmed by the absence of significant cross-reactivity with activin, transforming growth factor-β, mullerian inhibiting substance, LH, FSH, TSH, human chorionic gonadotropin (hCG), hCGα, or the inhibin α-subunit. The sensitivity limit of this assay was 1 pg/mL. Serial dilutions of human male and female serum samples paralleled the recombinant 32-kilodalton (kDa) dimeric inhibin standard curve. Complete recovery of exogenous 32-kDa recombinant inhibin was obtained in both follicular and luteal phase serum pools. Mean inhibin levels ranged from 5.7 pg/mL in the early follicular phase to 49 pg/mL in the midluteal phase of the normal menstrual cycle (Fig 12–1) and were elevated during ovulation induction (1,250 pg/mL) and pregnancy (500 pg/mL). Mean levels of dimeric inhibin in the normal follicular phase and in women with polycystic ovarian syndrome were comparable. Dimeric inhibin was virtually undetectable in normal men (< 2 pg/mL), and mean levels did not differ significantly from GnRH-deficient men and men with Klinefelter's syndrome. In addition, dimeric inhibin from all these men was indistinguishable from levels observed in postmenopausal women (1.7 pg/mL).

Discussion.—These results confirm the pattern of inhibin fluctuation in the normal menstrual cycle. The relatively high dimeric inhibin levels at midcycle and in the luteal phase of the normal menstrual cycle, after gonadotropin stimulation, and during pregnancy suggest that dimeric inhibin is predominantly produced by dominant follicles, corpora lutea, and placental tissues. The extremely low levels of inhibin in men suggest that (1) some forms of circulating and bioactive inhibin in the human are not detected by the new 2-site assay, either because of conformation or the presence of a unique binding protein for endogenous inhibin that does not bind to recombinant 32-kDa inhibin, or (2) dimeric inhibin may not be an important endocrine regulator of FSH in the human male.

▶ Previous immunoassays for inhibin have had a striking cross-reaction with the α-subunit of inhibin, and may react with the inhibin-related molecules, activin and transforming growth factor–β as well.

The assay used in this important clinical study was a 2-site, or sandwich-type, assay that was specific for intact inhibin and showed no reaction to the related molecules. In addition, the assay had much greater sensitivity than the previous assays.

Strikingly, inhibin was not detectable in the blood of normal men nor in GnRH-deficient men or men with Klinefelter's. These studies raise the question of whether inhibin is an important regulator of FSH secretion in men.—W.D. Odell, M.D., Ph.D.

Androgen Receptor Distribution in Rat Testis: New Implications for Androgen Regulation of Spermatogenesis
Vornberger W, Prins G, Musto NA, Suarez-Quian CA (Georgetown Univ, Washington, DC; Univ of Illinois, Chicago)
Endocrinology 134:2307–2316, 1994   112-95-12–6

Objective.—The cell site(s) of androgenic regulation of spermatogenesis within the testis is still not clear. Some studies demonstrate the presence of androgen receptor (AR) in somatic cells, whereas others show AR both at the level of somatic cells and germ cells. The distribution of AR in the adult rat testis was reexamined using a novel tissue-embedding protocol for immunocytochemistry.

Methods.—Tissues were processed using a technique that preserves antigenicity without compromising tissue preservation. The distribution of AR was ascertained by immunostaining with a rabbit polyclonal antibody.

Findings.—In the interstitium, intense AR immunostaining was detected within smooth muscle cells that form the walls of blood vessels, indicating that these cells were targets for androgens. Not all Leydig cells immunostained positive for AR, suggesting that these cells had a different functional activity within the population. In the seminiferous tubules, AR immunostaining occurred in all peritubular myoid cell nuclei but not in the distal layer of lymphatic endothelial cells. Specific AR immunostaining was also detected in Sertoli's cell nuclei and in elongated spermatid cytoplasm, and the intensity of staining varied as a function of the cycle of seminiferous epithelium. In elongated spermatids, AR immunostaining was seen solely in the nuclei of step 11–elongated spermatids, those in which nuclear elongation is apparent but chromatin condensation has not yet occurred. However, with the onset of condensation, nuclear AR immunostaining disappeared concomitant with the appearance of AR immunostaining of the cytoplasm of germ cells in step 12–elongated spermatids.

Conclusion.—In the adult rat testis, AR immunostaining is present in the nuclei of some Leydig cells, smooth muscle cells surrounding blood vessels, peritubular myoid cells, Sertoli's cells, and step 11–elongated spermatids. The presence of AR in Leydig cells supports the hypothesis that androgens modify Leydig cell activity in an autocrine fashion. The stage-specific AR immunoreactivity in Sertoli's cells seems to be indicative of a specific androgen response during these stages, whereas peritubular myoid cells may participate in the tonal maintenance of spermatogenesis. The specific presence of AR in step 11–elongated spermatids suggests that androgens can act directly on germ cells to regulate spermatogenesis, which is in contrast to earlier dogma.

▶ Many studies in rodents indicate that testosterone or dihydrotestosterone may be the major regulator of spermatogenesis. The roles of FSH and LH may be only to stimulate androgen production and to facilitate its delivery to Sertoli's cells and some stages of spermatids.

This study located the AR in rat testes, not by its androgen binding properties but by an antiserum produced against a region of the AR itself. Similar studies should be now performed on human testes, which could lead to development of additional ways to distinguish various causes of oligospermia or azoospermia in men.—W.D. Odell, M.D., Ph.D.

Preservation of Fertility Despite Subnormal Gonadotropin and Testosterone Levels After Cessation of Pulsatile Gonadotropin-Releasing Hormone Therapy in a Man With Kallmann's Syndrome
Bagatell CJ, Paulsen CA, Bremner WJ (Univ of Washington, Seattle)
Fertil Steril 61:392–394, 1994   112-95-12-7

Background.—Idiopathic hypogonadotropic hypogonadism (IHH) is characterized by low or low-normal gonadotropin levels, subnormal testosterone (T) levels, and failure to undergo puberty, presumably because of an isolated GnRH deficiency. In most men with IHH, pulsatile GnRH administration normalizes gonadotropin and T levels, and in many patients it initiates and maintains spermatogenesis. In almost all such men, discontinuance of treatment results in a return to pretreatment status. A patient was described in whom spermatogenesis persisted but who successfully fathered a child despite subnormal serum LH and T levels 1 year after pulsatile GnRH was discontinued.

Case Report.—The patient was initially seen in 1980 at age 23 years for failure to go through puberty. The initial workup showed normal thyroid function tests, PRL, and GH levels, very low serum T levels, and undetectable gonadotropins. There was no response to clomiphene citrate stimulation. Anosmia was confirmed by formal assessment. Serum gonadotropins were undetectable on repeat testing. Treatment with human chorionic gonadotropin (hCG), 2,000 IU IM 3 times per week was begun, and 18 months later the patient's wife became pregnant. For 8 years, the patient was intermittently treated with hCG, pulsatile GnRH, and T enanthate. Although his serum gonadotropin levels were very low or undetectable when hCG and GnRH were not given, 3 more children were conceived with hormonal therapy. After completing research protocols with pulsatile GnRH in 1990, T enanthate was prescribed. The patient had T shots irregularly in the first few months after discontinuing GnRH, then he received no shots for the 12 months preceding his next clinic visit. A month later, another pregnancy was confirmed in his wife.

Conclusion.—This patient with IHH and anosmia, or Kallmann's syndrome, was successfully treated with various hormonal regimens. Four children were conceived with hCG or pulsatile GnRH treatment. After GnRH was discontinued, the patient displayed continuing spermatogenesis despite low serum FSH and LH levels. This case adds to the recognized recovery range in IHH.

▶ This is an interesting case. Although paternity was not proven, this case report supports others that indicate IHH may partially recover with time or after treatment with exogenous gonadotropins or pulsatile GnRH.—W.D. Odell, M.D., Ph.D.

Finasteride (MK-906) in the Treatment of Benign Prostatic Hyperplasia
Stoner E, for the Finasteride Study Group (Merck Research Labs, Rahway, NJ)
Prostate 22:291–299, 1993   112-95-12–8

Introduction.—Finasteride is a potent inhibitor of 5α-reductase that has no androgenic, estrogenic, or progestational properties nor an affinity for the androgen receptor. The safety, tolerability, and efficacy of finasteride in the treatment of benign prostatic hyperplasia (BPH) were studied.

Study Design.—In a multicenter, randomized, double-blind, placebo-controlled study, 750 men with BPH were treated with finasteride, 1 or 5 mg, or placebo daily for 12 months. The patients' ages ranged from 46 to 83 years; all had maximum urinary flow rates of less than 15 mL/sec, prostate volume of 30 cm^3 or greater, and symptoms of urinary tract obstruction.

Outcome.—Compared with placebo, 5 mg of finasteride reduced serum dihydrotestosterone by 62%, serum prostate-specific antigen by 46%, prostate volume by 22%, and obstructive symptoms; increased maximum urinary flow rate by 1.7 mL/sec; and decreased total urinary symptom scores by 3.3 points (Fig 12-2). Finasteride, 1 mg/day, produced similar responses except for urinary symptoms, which did not differ significantly from placebo. Furthermore, men treated with 5 mg of finasteride had significantly greater improvements in urologic status and troublesome symptom score compared with those who were treated with placebo. Not all patients responded to finasteride therapy: At 12 months, about half the patients had a 20% decrease in prostate volume, and one third had an increase in maximum urinary flow rate of 3 mL/sec or more. Except for mild-to-moderate impotence, finansteride was gen-

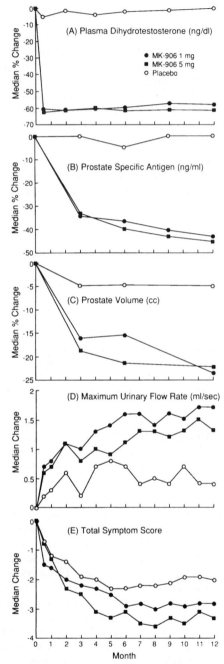

Fig 12–2.—Biochemical and clinical effects of finasteride (1 and 5 mg) therapy in patients with benign prostatic hyperplasia. (Courtesy of Stoner E, for the Finasteride Study Group: *Prostate* 22:291–299, 1993.)

erally well tolerated. Only 1 patient discontinued treatment because of impotence.

Conclusion.—Finasteride is an effective medical therapy for a significant proportion of patients with BPH. Its excellent safety and tolerability can be attributed to its specific mode of action and the limited role of 5α-reductase in male reproductive tissue.

▶ Inhibitors of 5α-reductase are playing increasing roles in clinical endocrinology. Their use in placebo-controlled studies of treatment of symptomatic BPH have led to better understanding of the long-term effects of transurethral prostatectomy and of which portion of symptoms that were previously ascribed to BPH was actually the result of changes in bladder control and tone.

Note the decreased urinary symptom score in the placebo-treated group of patients. Although dihydrotesterone concentrations in blood fell to the same degree in men who received both 1-mg and 5-mg doses, urinary symptoms decreased significantly more than placebo only in the group that received 5 mg.—W.D. Odell, M.D., Ph.D.

Female Reproduction

Effects of Finasteride, a 5α-Reductase Inhibitor, on Circulating Androgens and Gonadotropin Secretion in Hirsute Women
Fruzzetti F, De Lorenzo D, Parrini D, Ricci C (Univ of Pisa, Italy)
J Clin Endocrinol Metab 79:831–835, 1994   112-95-12-9

Introduction.—Finasteride is a 5α-reductase inhibitor that blocks the formation of dihydrotestosterone (DHT) without blocking testosterone (T) secretion. The effects of a short-term treatment with finasteride were assessed on gonadotropin and androgen secretion in hirsute women.

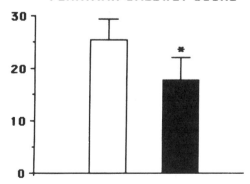

FERRIMAN GALLWEY SCORE

Fig 12–3.—Ferriman-Gallwey score (mean ± SD) before (*white bar*) and after (*black bar*) 3 months of finasteride therapy. *P < .001. (Courtesy of Fruzzetti F, De Lorenzo D, Parrini D, et al: *J Clin Endocrinol Metab* 79:831–835, 1994.)

Study Design.—Ten hirsute women, aged 16–28 years, were treated with daily oral 5-mg does of finasteride for 3 months. Gonadotropin secretion, basal and stimulated androgen secretion, and hair growth on the Ferriman-Gallwey grading scale were assessed after 1 and 3 months of treatment.

Results.—Finasteride significantly decreased DHT serum levels and serum 3α-diol G concentrations. The decrease in DHT levels paralleled the significant decrease in the Ferriman-Gallwey score by 27.8% (Fig 12–3), despite a significant increase in plasma T levels. Finasteride did not affect basal and GnRH-stimulated gonadotropin secretion nor modify the pulsatility of LH secretion. There were no significant changes in estradiol, PRL, free T, androstenedione (A), dehydroepiandrosterone sulfate (DHEAS), and sex hormone–binding globulin concentrations. Serum cortisol concentrations decreased significantly after 1 month of treatment, but they returned to pretreatment levels after 3 months. Finasteride did not modify the responses of T, A, and DHEAS to ACTH-(1–24) injection, but they blunted the cortisol response to corticotropin stimulation.

Conclusion.—These preliminary results indicate that finasteride improves hirsutism in affected women without any discernible effect on gonadotropin secretion.

▶ This study may result in a new and more effective treatment of hirsutism. Larger and longer clinical studies appear to be warranted.—W.D. Odell, M.D., Ph.D.

Urine hCG β-Subunit Core Fragment, a Sensitive Test for Ectopic Pregnancy

Cole LA, Kardana A, Seifer DB, Bohler HCL Jr (Yale Univ, New Haven, Conn)
J Clin Endocrinol Metab 78:497–499, 1994   112-95-12–10

Introduction.—The placenta produces human chorionic gonadotropin (hCG) as well as free α- and β-subunits. A portion of the hCG molecules is cleaved or nicked, and the resultant hCG is unstable, making more nicked free β-subunit and α-subunit. The nicked β-subunit may be the substrate for β-core fragment production, which appears in the urine of pregnant women, the main hCG/β-subunit in pregacy urine. To find more sensitive biological markers for ectopic pregnancy, the levels of hCG, free β-subunit, and β-core were compared in the urine of women with tubal and with intrauterine pregnancies.

Methods.—Urine was obtained in the emergency department from 12 women with tubal pregnancies and from 36 women with normal pregnancies. The levels of hCG, free β-subunit, and β-core were assayed.

Sandwich-type assays were used that were specific for each hCG-related molecule.

Results.—The hCG levels were measured with 2 assays; the levels in tubal pregnancies were $1/38$th and $1/48$th of the levels in normal pregnancies. The free β-subunit levels in tubal pregnancies were $1/28$th of the normal level. The β-core levels differed the most, with the levels in tubal pregnancies being $1/149$th of those seen in normal pregnancies. Another volunteer who provided urine samples during the 15 days before diagnosis of tubal pregnancy had hCG levels $1/97$th and $1/126$th, free β-subunit levels $1/8$th, and β-core levels $1/413$th that of median normal pregnancy levels.

Discussion.—Measuring the urine β-core levels yields a more sensitive indication of ectopic pregnancy than hCG measurement. Therefore, it may be a more useful test for rapid diagnosis of tubal pregnancy in the emergency department. It can also be used to screen for or detect a subclinical ectopic pregnancy.

▶ It is surprising that the major hCG-related molecule in pregnancy urine is not hCG but the isolated, cleaved, β-subunit metabolite "β-core." Specific measurement of this molecule seems to offer better sensitivity in detecting tubal pregnancies than measurement of hCG itself.—W.D. Odell, M.D., Ph.D.

No Adverse Effects of Medroxyprogesterone Treatment Without Estrogen in Postmenopausal Women: Double-Blind, Placebo-Controlled, Crossover Trial
Prior JC, Alojado N, McKay DW, Vigna YM (Univ of British Columbia, Vancouver, Canada; Mem Univ of Newfoundland, St John's, Canada)
Obstet Gynecol 83:24–28, 1994   112-95-12-11

Background.—Because of its beneficial effects, progestin has been recommended in addition to estrogen therapy for menopausal women. However, concerns about adverse effects may make physicians reluctant to prescribe this treatment and patients reluctant to comply. Whether cyclic medroxyprogesterone treatment without estrogen causes adverse symptoms in postmenopausal women was investigated.

Methods.—Fourteen women were initially enrolled in the placebo-controlled, double-blind, crossover trial. For 2 consecutive months; medroxyprogesterone and placebo were both given 10 days per month in random order. The participants recorded their physiologic and emotional experiences using a 0–4 scale on a daily diary form. Nonparametric tests were used to compare the sum of the scores for the 10 days of medroxyprogesterone with the sum of the scores for the 10 days of placebo.

Findings.—Eleven postmenopausal women aged 43 to 63 years completed the study. Scores did not differ significantly between the 10 days on which medroxyprogesterone was received and the 10 days on which placebo was received. The median composite score for premenstrual-like symptoms was 26 during medroxyprogesterone treatment and 25 during placebo administration.

Conclusion.—Given alone, medroxyprogesterone does not cause adverse symptoms in postmenopausal women. As a result, medroxyprogesterone therapy itself does not explain the adverse effects reported by women who receive combined hormones. Further research should focus on the multiple hormonal, pharmacologic, and social factors that may be associated with adverse symptoms during hormonal treatments.

▶ This is a most interesting controlled study of the effects of medroxyprogesterone or placebo on the emotional and physiologic symptoms in postmenopausal women. In clinical practice, many women think the progestational agent makes them feel depressed, anxious, and less energetic. This well-controlled study suggests that the progestational agent is not the culprit.—W.D. Odell, M.D., Ph.D.

Metabolic Effects of Once-A-Month Combined Injectable Contraceptives
Giwa-Osagie OF, and the World Health Organization Task Force on Long-Acting Systemic Agents for Fertility Regulation (Univ of Lagos, Nigeria)
Contraception 49:421–433, 1994   112-95-12–12

Introduction.—Once-a-month injectable contraceptives are highly effective and produce an improved menstrual pattern compared with progestogen-only contraceptives. A summary was provided of longitudinal and cross-sectional studies of healthy women regarding the metabolic effects of once-a-month combined injectable contraceptives. These included dihydroxyprogesterone acetophenide, 150 mg, and estradiol enanthate, 10 mg; depot-medroxyprogesterone acetate, 25 mg, and estradiol cypionate, 5 mg; norethisterone enanthate, 50 mg, and estradiol valerate, 5 mg; and 17 α-hydroxyprogesterone caproate, 250 mg, and estradiol valerate, 5 mg.

Findings.—Once-a-month combined injectable contraceptives do not produce the distinct changes in glucose tolerance and insulin levels that have been reported among users of combined oral and progestogen-only contraceptives. However, more long-term studies are needed of women who have used once-a-month injectables for at least 1 or 2 years. Similarly, treatment for as long as 12 months with once-a-month injectables produces either no significant or minor changes on lipids or changes that are mostly favorable. These observations have also been reported by the Special Programme of Research, Development and Research Training in Human Reproduction in its multicenter study on Cyclofem and Mesigyna, which includes the largest body of data on lipid levels in users of once-a-month injectables. This study also demonstrates that once-a-month injectables are associated with minor changes in coagulation parameters that usually remain within the normal range and may not be of clinical significance. There are no persistent changes in PRL, and serum cortisol, binding globulins, and liver function are not affected. The effect of these injectables on vitamin and protein metabolism remains to be defined.

Conclusion.—The safety of once-a-month combined injectable contraceptives was demonstrated. These contraceptives produce no significant changes in carbohydrate metabolism, and their effects on lipids and hemostasis are minor and more favorable than those caused by combined contraceptives.

▶ This is a well-written review that compares the metabolic effects of 4 once-a-month combined injected contraceptives, all of which appear to be well tolerated and effective. Given adequate medical or paramedical resources and disposable or carefully sterilized medical supplies, this could be an effective contraceptive in rural areas of developing countries. However, from my experience in many developing countries, problems in obtaining adequate supplies of safe syringes and needles are huge.—W.D. Odell, M.D., Ph.D.

Oral Contraception and Stroke: Evidence From the Royal College of General Practioners' Oral Contraception Study
Hannaford PC, Croft PR, Kay CR (Univ of Manchester, England)
Stroke 25:935–942, 1994   112-95-12–13

Introduction.—A nested case-control analysis of data collected by the Royal College of General Practitioners' (RCGP) Oral Contraception Study explored the association between oral contraceptive use and the risk of stroke.

Methods.—The RCGP Oral Contraception Study database consists of 23,000 women who used oral contraceptives and similar number who never used oral contraceptives. From these groups, 253 women who had a stroke or amaurosis fugax between 1968 and 1990 were identified, and 3 age-matched controls for each stroke patient were assigned. The records of all the women were examined to compare possible group differences in social class, parity, smoking, oral contraceptive use, and history of hypertension or toxemia in pregnancy.

Results.—Oral contraceptive use, smoking, lower social class, and a history of hypertension were the factors associated with an increased risk of stroke. Smoking doubled the risk compared with not smoking, and the risk increased with the severity of the smoking habit. A history of oral contraceptive use significantly increased the stroke risk, and current pill use increased the risk further, an effect that was not substantially altered by the presence of hypertension. The risk of fatal stroke (usually a subarachnoid hemorrhage) doubled with either past or present pill use, although this effect in former users was restricted to smokers. Oral contraceptives with a higher progestogen dose increased the risk of stroke more than low-dose pills, and of the progestogens, norethindrone acetate, lynestrenol, and ethynodiol diacetate increased the risk more than levonorgestrel or other agents.

Discussion.—These findings are difficult to interpret. Although hypertension and oral contraceptive use are clearly independent risk factors for stroke, women who continued to use the pill after a diagnosis of hypertension had the same relative risk as hypertensive women who had never used the pill. Whereas certain progestogens most significantly increased the risk of stroke, the risk may actually have been associated with the high doses of estrogen with which they were combined. However, low-dose formulas of combined contraceptives appear to be associated with less risk than higher-dose preparations.

▶ Once again we are reminded that smoking increases the risk of stroke in oral contraceptive users. Clinicians, educate your patients!—W.D. Odell, M.D., Ph.D.

A Syndrome of Female Pseudohermaphrodism, Hypergonadotropic Hypogonadism, and Multicystic Ovaries Associated With Missense Mutations in the Gene Encoding Aromatase (P450arom)
Conte FA, Grumbach MM, Ito Y, Fisher CR, Simpson ER (Univ of California, San Francisco; Univ of Texas, Dallas)
J Clin Endocrinol Metab 78:1287–1292, 1994   112-95-12–14

Introduction.—Features of a new syndrome of aromatase deficiency resulting from molecular defects in the CYP19 (P450arom) gene were reported in a 46,XX girl. Only 1 well-documented case of aromatase deficiency in a female infant has been recorded.

Case Report.—Girl, 14 years, had been followed up from infancy to 8 years of age and was then lost to follow-up for 6 years. She was born after a normal full-term pregnancy during which no medications had been taken. The child had ambiguous genitalia at birth, including a 2-cm phallic-like structure bound down in chordee; a nonadrenal form of female pseudohermaphrodism was diagnosed. A laparotomy at 17 months revealed normal female internal genital structures and ovaries with a normal histologic appearance. Both basal and LHRH-induced FSH levels were strikingly elevated at this time. The patient developed normally during infancy and childhood and had plasma LH and FSH levels in the normal range at 8 years of age. When seen again at age 14 years, she had not experienced breast development, a pubertal growth spurt, or menarche; her bone age was 10 years.

Results.—Examination of the patient at age 14 years revealed plasma concentrations of testosterone (3,294 pmol/L) and androstenedione (9,951 pmol/L) to be elevated; a nonadrenal source was indicated by ACTH and dexamethasone tests. Plasma estradiol levels were less than 37 pmol/L, and plasma gonadotropin levels were in the castrate range. Multiple 4- to 6-cm ovarian cysts were observed bilaterally through pelvic sonography and MRI. Estrogen replacement therapy was begun that resulted in suppression of gonadotropins, androstenedione, and testosterone and in breast development, a pubertal growth spurt, and regression of ovarian cysts. Analysis of genomic DNA from ovarian fibroblasts, which were obtained previously at laparotomy, demonstrated 2 single base changes in the coding region of the P450arom gene, 1 at 1,303 basepairs (C-T), R435C, and the other at 1,310 basepairs (G-A), C437Y, in exon 10. Molecular genetic studies indicated that the patient was a compound heterozygote for these mutations.

Conclusion.—This syndrome of female pseudohermaphrodism, hypergonadotropic hypogonadism, and multicystic ovaries resulted from P450arom deficiency. Although they are rare in this form, partial defects in P450arom may be responsible for some underestrogenized women with hirsutism, multicystic ovaries, and abnormal menstrual periods. This suggests that survival of the conceptus can occur in the complete or near-complete absence of estrogen synthesis by the implanting blastocyte, fetus, and placenta.

▶ I have always enjoyed reading a description of a new clinical syndrome. This patient with 2 basepair changes in the P450 aromatase gene represents the second reported case of a patient with aromatase deficiency.—W.D. Odell, M.D., Ph.D.

A Double-Blind Cross-Over Controlled Study to Evaluate the Effect of Human Biosynthetic Growth Hormone on Ovarian Stimulation in Previous Poor Responders to In-Vitro Fertilization
Hughes SM, Huang ZH, Morris ID, Matson PL, Buck P, Lieberman BA (St. Mary's Hosp, Manchester, England; Univ of Manchester, England)
Hum Reprod 9:13–18, 1994   112-95-12-15

Introduction.—Despite more successful ovulation induction regimens, a significant group of patients fail to show adequate follicular development. The effect of exogenous human biosynthetic growth hormone (HGH) on the response to ovarian stimulation using a buserelin/human menopausal gonadotropin (hMG) regimen in previous poor responders was evaluated.

Study Design.—In a prospective, double-blind, placebo-controlled, crossover study, 40 patients who had previously shown a "poor response" to ovarian stimulation despite receiving doses of hMG of 300 IU or more per day were treated. Only women with serum FSH or LH of 10 IU per liter between days 2 and 5 of a menstrual cycle were considered. The urinary 24-hour GH secretion was normal in all patients.

Treatment Protocol.—All patients received a course of combined buserelin acetate, 500 mg/day, and hMG. When pituitary desensitization was confirmed, the exogenous gonadotropins were started, along with a second daily injection of either placebo or 12 IU of HGH for up to 12 days or until human chorionic gonadotropin (hCG) was administered.

Outcome.—Thirty-three patients completed the study. Of these, 21 achieved hCG criteria in both arms of the study, thereby providing complete placebo-controlled comparative data. Although these women had gonadotropins within the normal range on a single sample before the study, a repeat sampling taken before the second arm of the study at least 3 months later revealed supranormal values.

After 8 days of co-treatment with HGH, the number of cohort follicles that measured 14–16.9 mm in diameter increased significantly, but this increase did not persist to the day of hCG administration. Serum estradiol on the 8th day of hMG or on the day of hCG, length of the follicular phase, and the total dose of hMG used did not differ significantly between the placebo and HGH cycles. The expected yield of oocytes was low, and it did not improve with HGH administration. Serum fasting insulin concentrations were signficantly increased on days 8 and 13 of hMG in those cycles that received HGH.

Conclusion.—The administration of HGH does not improve the ovarian response to ovulation induction in previously poor responders. The reliability of solitary perimenstrual gonadotropin assays in assessing the pituitary-ovarian axis is questionable. Several consecutive readings should be taken in women who have had suboptimal responses to hMG therapy.

▶ This study was performed to vertify or refute results of a "pilot" study by Ibrahim and associates (*Fertil Steril* 55:202, 1991) suggesting that cotreatment with GH and gonadotropins might increase likelihood of fertility in women undergoing in vitro fertilization who were selected to be resistant to ovarian stimulation by gonadotropins alone.

Growth hormone treatment is expensive, and without definitive proof, many other groups have added it to gonadotropins in the belief that it is helpful.

The authors are to be complimented for performing this double-blind, crossover study that evaluated the efficacy of GH. Their carefully controlled study shows that GH does not improve the ovarian response in such patients.—W.D. Odell, M.D., Ph.D.

The Antiprogestin RU486 Delays the Midcycle Gonadotropin Surge and Ovulation in Gonadotropin-Releasing Hormone-Induced Cycles
Batista MC, Nieman LK, Cartledge TP, Loriaux DL, Zellmer AW, Merriam GR

(Natl Inst of Child Health and Human Development, Bethesda, Md; Natl Insts of Health, Bethesda, Md)
Fertil Steril 62:28–34, 1994   112-95-12–16

Objective.—In a previous study, the antiprogestin RU486 was found to delay the timing of the gonadotropin surge and ovulation without suppressing folliculogenesis or E_2 secretion. To assess the site(s) of progesterone (P) action in the control of ovulation, RU486 was studied to determine whether it can delay the midcycle gonadotropin surge independent of hypothalamic inhibition.

Study Design.—Six women with hypothalamic amenorrhea who were undergoing ovulation induction with GnRH pulses of unvarying frequency and dose participated in a prospective, crossover, single-blinded clinical study. All women were treated with RU486 or placebo at a low dose of 1 mg per day for 5 days, starting when the dominant follicle reached 14-16 mm. Blood samples and ovarian ultrasound examinations were performed daily in the later follicular phase and every 3-4 days during the remainder of the cycle.

Results.—RU486 consistently delayed the timing of the midcycle gonadotropin surge by a mean of 3.3 days compared with placebo (Fig 12-4). Luteinizing hormone and FSH levels remained unchanged or decreased during RU486 treatment, which also inhibited ovarian steroidogenesis and delayed the timing of peak E_2 concentrations and preovulatory P rises. However, it did not suppress follicular growth in most patients. Despite similar hormonal changes, 2 women exhibited more prolonged follicular maturation in both RU486 and placebo cycles, and

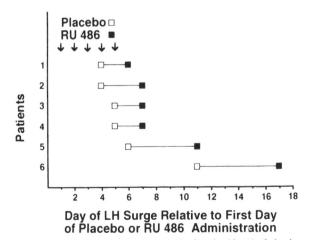

**Day of LH Surge Relative to First Day
of Placebo or RU 486 Administration**

Fig 12–4.—Day of the midcycle LH peak relative to the first day (day 1) of placebo or RU486 administration in 6 women with hypothalamic amenorrhea treated with pulsatile GnRH. Placebo or RU486 (1 mg/day) was given orally for 5 days (*arrows*), starting when the dominant follicle reached 14-16 mm. Symbols connected with a line represent the same patient. (Courtesy of Batista MC, Nieman LK, Cartledge TP, et al: *Fertil Steril* 62:28-34, 1994.)

ovulation occurred only after treatment was discontinued. It is possible that GnRH replacement was insufficient to induce a completely normal follicular phase, and this coupled with a pituitary suppressive effect of RU486 resulted in more severe disruption of follicular maturation than in the other patients who exhibited normal GnRH-induced folliculogenesis.

Conclusion.—The antiprogestin RU486 delays the midcycle gonadotropin surge and ovulation despite the external administration of constant pulsatile GnRH signals, suggesting that RU486 does not act primarily on the hypothalamus to delay ovulation. Instead, RU486 appears to antagonize P at the pituitary level to suppress gonadotropin and steroid hormone secretion. As a result, P acts on the pituitary independent of any hypothalamic effects to regulate the timing of the midcycle gonadotropin surge and ovulation.

▶ Many years ago, studies from our laboratory (Odell and Swerdloff: *Proc Natl Acad Sci U S A* 61:529, 1968; Swerdloff et al: *Endocrinology* 90:1529, 1972) suggested that an ovarian signal received by the hypothalamic/pituitary system initiated the LH/FSH ovulatory surge and that this signal was composed of estradiol and small amounts of progesterone produced by the maturing follicle.

This study, which used the antiprogestin RU486, supports this hypothesis and adds evidence that the pituitary gland is the site of progesterone effects.—W.D. Odell, M.D., Ph.D.

The Effects of 2-Year Treatment With the Aminobisphosphonate Alendronate on Bone Metabolism, Bone Histomorphometry, and Bone Strength in Ovariectomized Nonhuman Primates
Balena R, Toolan BC, Shea M, Markatos A, Myers ER, Lee SC, Opas EE, Seedor JG, Klein H, Frankenfield D, Quartuccio H, Fioravanti C, Clair J, Brown E, Hayes WC, Rodan GA (Merck Research Labs, West Point, Pa; Beth Israel Hosp, Boston)
J Clin Invest 92:2577–2586, 1993   112-95-12–17

Introduction.—The greatest contributor to the bone loss seen in patients with menopausal osteoporosis is the increase in bone turnover with bone resorption exceeding bone formation that occurs with the loss of ovarian function. Alendronate sodium (ALN), an aminobisphosphonate, inhibits bone resorption in women with postmenopausal osteoporosis. The efficacy of ALN in preventing estrogen deficiency and bone loss and in increasing bone strength in baboons was assessed. The effects of ALN at the tissue level also were studied.

Methods.—Twenty-eight adult female baboons were assigned to 1 of 4 groups, with each group consisting of 7 baboons. Three groups underwent surgical removal of the ovaries and uterus (OVX groups). Two

OVX groups were treated with IV ALN, .05 or .25 mg/kg, every 2 weeks for 2 years; the third OVX group received saline solution only. Serum and urine chemistries were analyzed every 3 months. All the baboons were killed after 2 years, and the spine and femora were removed for analysis.

Results.—The ovariectomized animals had significantly higher serum levels of alkaline phosphatase, osteocalcin, and tartrate-resistant acid phosphatase compared with the animals with intact ovaries. These levels remained high in the OVX animals that were treated with saline solution only, but they were reduced to non-OVX levels with low-dose ALN and to even lower levels with high-dose ALN treatment. Similarly, the saline-treated OVX animals maintained elevated urinary excretion of the bone collagen crosslink lysylpyridinoline/creatinine, which was reduced to non-OVX levels with either low- or high-dose ALN. Bone volume was significantly greater in the group that was treated with high-dose ALN; the other 3 groups did not differ significantly. Measures of tissue level bone turnover and bone remodeling were improved by ALN in a dose-dependent manner, although bone formation parameters did not differ significantly with the dose. Bone mineral density also showed dose-dependent increases. Bone strength in the high-dose group was twice as great as in the saline group and was also greater than the non-OVX group.

Discussion.—Ovariectomized baboons had an increase in bone turnover and bone loss similar to that of women. Treating the baboons with ALN for 2 years inhibited bone turnover and bone loss and increased bone strength to levels comparable to those of nonovariectomized baboons.

▶ Etidronate has not been approved for prevention or treatment of osteoporosis in the United States, and long-term data on its effectiveness in preventing fractures are controversial. Alendronate sodium is an aminobisphosphonate, which is a potent group for inhibition of bone resorption.

This carefully designed prospective study in baboons, which is seemingly a suitable model for human menopausal osteoporosis, demonstrates the effectiveness of alendronate in preventing bone loss. It is unfortunate that an estrogen-treated control group was not included so that the results of the bisphosphonate could be compared with estrogen.—W.D. Odell, M.D., Ph.D.

The Effect of the Hypoestrogenic State, Induced by Gonadotropin-Releasing Hormone Agonist, on Doppler-Derived Parameters of Aortic Flow

Eckstein N, Pines A, Fisman EZ, Fisch B, Limor R, Vagman I, Barnan R, Ayalon D (Ichilov Hosp, Tel Aviv, Israel; Sheba Med Ctr, Tel Hashomer, Israel; Beilinson Med Ctr, Petach Tikva, Israel)
J Clin Endocrinol Metab 77:910–912, 1993   112-95-12–18

Background.—Gonadotropin-releasing hormone agonists (GnRH-a) induce a pseudomenopausal state through a downregulation mechanism. An acute reduction in estrogen levels in women with functional ovaries during GnRH-a treatment may induce changes in Doppler-derived parameters of aortic flow.

Methods.—Fifteen healthy women, aged 25–42 years, were studied. All had symptomatic fibroids or endometriosis or were candidates for GnRH-a therapy before in vitro fertilization (IVF).

Findings.—In all women, serum E_2 levels dropped to castration levels 3 weeks after treatment was begun. There were no significant changes in blood pressure, but peak flow velocity and cardiac index were reduced significantly. The flow velocity integral was also decreased, but it was nonsignificant. Mean acceleration was significantly lowered. There were no significant changes in acceleration time or ejection time.

Conclusion.—Acute estrogen deprivation significantly reduced peak aortic flow velocity, cardiac index, and mean acceleration. The changes observed in left ventricular hemodynamic parameters probably did not affect the regular daily performance of the patients treated.

▶ It has often been said that the lower cardiovascular mortality in postmenopausal women who receive estrogen replacement compared with those who do not receive estrogens results from the estrogen-induced effects on plasma lipids. However, several studies indicate that estrogens may directly affect cardiovascular function. This study is a recent example of these data.

Previously, Pines and colleagues (*Am J Obstet Gynecol* 164:806, 1991) demonstrated beneficial increases in Doppler-derived parameters of aortic blood flow after 10 weeks of estrogen replacement in postmenopausal women.—W.D. Odell, M.D., Ph.D.

Antioxidant Potential of Specific Estrogens on Lipid Peroxidation

Subbiah MTR, Kessel B, Agrawal M, Rajan R, Abplanalp W, Rymaszewski Z (Univ of Cincinnati, Ohio)
J Clin Endocrinol Metab 77:1095–1097, 1993   112-95-12–19

Background.—Coronary heart disease (CHD) is the leading cause of death in postmenopausal women. Estrogen administration in these women reduces the risk of CHD by 50%, but an increase in HDL ac-

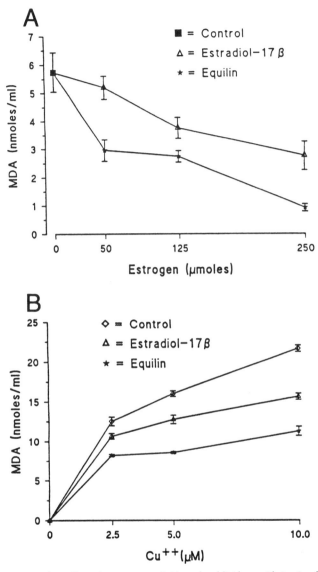

Fig 12–5.—Antioxidant effect of estrogens on Cu^{++}-catalyzed lipid peroxidation in whole plasma. **A,** dose response to estrogens at constant Cu^{++} concentration (2.5 μM); **B,** Cu^{++}-dependent lipid peroxidation at constant estrogens concentration (125 μmol/mL). (Courtesy of Subbiah MTR, Kessel B, Agrawal M, et al: *J Clin Endocrinol Metab* 77:1095–1097, 1993.)

counts for only 25% to 50% of the cardioprotective effect of estrogen. Peroxidation of lipoproteins plays a key role in atherogenesis as a result of excess uptake of oxidized LDL by macrophages. Estrogen may display antioxidant potential, but structural differences in the estrogen molecule may influence that potential.

Method.—In in vitro studies, the effects of 2 human (estrone and estradiol-17β) and equine (equilenin and equilin) estrogens on copper-mediated oxidation of LDL were measured by the formation of malonaldehyde (MDA). The effects of these estrogens on the oxidation of cholesterol moiety in LDL and fatty acid oxidation in whole plasma were also measured.

Results.—All estrogens exhibited some antioxidant activity on peroxidation of LDL, but equine estrogens, particularly equilin, appeared to be more potent than estrone and estradiol-17β. Similarly, equilin was significantly more effective than estradiol-17β in inhibiting the formation of oxysterols and preventing the formation of MDA in whole plasma consistently at different estrogen and copper concentrations (Fig 12-5). Only equilin and equilenin suppressed fatty acid oxidation in human macrophages, whereas estradiol-17β and estrone had no effect.

Conclusion.—A variety of estrogen preparations that are currently used in postmenopausal hormone replacement therapy and conjugated equine estrogens, particularly equilin, are effective in inhibiting both fatty acid and cholesterol oxidation. The clinical significance of the lipoprotein peroxidation potential of estrogens should be studied in women before and after administration of various estrogens.

▶ This is yet another potential mechanism for an estrogen-associated reduction in cardiovascular mortality in postmenopausal women.—W.D. Odell, M.D., Ph.D.

Induction of Amenorrhea During Hormone Replacement Therapy: Optimal Micronized Progesterone Dose. A Multicenter Study

Gillet JY, Andre G, Faguer B, Erny R, Buvat-Herbaut M, Domin MA, Kuhn JM, Hedon B, Drapier-Faure E, Barrat J, Lopes P, Magnin G, Leng JJ, Bruhat MA, Philippe E (Saint Roch Hosp, Nice, France)
Maturitas 19:103–115, 1994   112-95-12–20

Introduction.—Uterine bleeding is a common reason for discontinuing hormone replacement therapy (HRT). A schedule of estrogen-progestin combination lowers the frequency of irregular or regular bleeding as it effectively prevents endometrial hyperplasia. The effects of oral micronized progesterone on the endometrium and bleeding pattern were assessed in a multicenter study.

Methods.—Study participants were 101 healthy, nonhysterectomized postmenopausal women who had a mean age of 53.9 years. All had amenorrhea for at least 12 months, and none had reported any spotting or breakthrough bleeding when they were previously taking HRT. Women who wanted to have regular monthly bleeding received percutaneous 17β-estradiol, 3 mg/day, given from day 1 to day 25 of each calendar month and associated with micronized progesterone, 300 mg/day, from day 16 to day 25. No treatment was administered during days 26–30 to 31 in this high-dose treatment regimen (high E-P group). Those who did not want to reinduce regular bleeding (the low E-P group, which consisted of all but 3 of the 101 women) received lower doses of 17β-estradiol, 1.5 mg/day, and oral micronized progesterone, 100 mg/day, which were given on 2 different schedules. The women were assessed at entry and between days 17 and 25 of the third and the sixth month of therapy.

Results.—The 3 women who chose the high E-P regimen were younger than the other women and had a shorter duration of menopause. None had been previously treated with an HRT. Two independent pathologists examined endometrial biopsy specimens that were obtained at least 6 months after the start of HRT. Findings in the low E-P group were quiescent without mitosis (61%), mildly active with very rare mitoses (23%), partial secretory endometrium (8%), a subatrophy (4%), or inadequate tissue (4%). Neither pathologist found evidence of hyperplasia. From a total of 525 cycles, cyclic withdrawal bleeding was reported in 6.6% of cases at 3 months and 9.4% at 6 months. Spotting was noted by 20% of women in the third month, but it had decreased to 8.2% by the sixth month. Amenorrhea was recorded by 93.3% of women in the low E-P group at 3 months and by 91.6% at 6 months.

Conclusion.—Unopposed estrogen therapy increases abnormal vaginal bleeding and the risk of endometrial cancer. A low dose of oral progesterone, 100 mg/day, which was given over 25 days, was found to induce amenorrhea and protect the endometrium by fully inhibiting mitoses in the majority of postmenopausal women. Such a regimen should increase compliance and avoid the need for repeated intrauterine investigations.

▶ A number of studies now demonstrate that combined estrogen/progestogen replacement therapy in postmenopausal women is effective against osteoporosis and that it leads to amenorrhea *without* endometrial hyperplasia.

This study demonstrated that oral progesterone, 100 mg/day, which is given for 25 days each month combined with low doses of estradiol, 1.5 mg/day, was effective in terms of bleeding patterns and resulted in absent menses in 80% of women.

This combined oral replacement resulted in a quiescent endometrium. The effects on lipids were not included in this report. Bone mineral density also was not evaluated, but presumably this combination would assist in preventing osteoporosis.—W.D. Odell, M.D., Ph.D.

Effect of Continuous Combined Estrogen and Desogestrel Hormone Replacement Therapy on Serum Lipids and Lipoproteins

Marsh MS, Crook D, Whitcroft SIJ, Worthington M, Whitehead MI, Stevenson JC (Wynn Inst for Metabolic Research, London; King's College School of Medicine and Dentistry, London)
Obstet Gynecol 83:19–23, 1994   112-95-12–21

Background.—No reports have been published on the effects of desogestrel on serum lipid and lipoprotein levels when it is used in continuous combined hormone replacement therapy. The effects of this therapy with desogestrel and 17β-estradiol (E2) on serum lipid and lipoprotein levels were investigated.

Methods.—Fifty-seven healthy postmenopausal women younger than age 60 received continuous oral desogestrel, .15 mg/day, and continuous micronized 17β-E2, 1 mg/day. Fasting venous blood samples were obtained before and after 6 and 12 months of treatment for determination of serum lipid and lipoprotein levels.

Findings.—Thirty-two women completed the treatment. By the 6-month assessment, all serum lipid and lipoprotein levels had decreased significantly, and they remained low at 12 months. After 1 year, HDL cholesterol levels decreased a mean of 12.8%. This was primarily caused by a decrease in HDL$_2$ subfraction, which decreased by 25.7%. Both LDL cholesterol and triglyceride levels decreased by 7.7%, and lipoprotein (a) levels decreased 17.6%.

Conclusion.—The combination of hormone replacement treatment in this study profoundly affected serum lipid and lipoprotein levels. The decrease in HDL cholesterol levels was unexpected, considering these levels increase when desogesterol is combined with ethinyl estradiol in contraceptive pills. The reduction of HDL cholesterol levels may be harmful. When desogesterol, .15 mg/day, is combined with continuous micronized 17β-E2 at 1 mg/day *continuously*, the predominate effects of the progestogen are to reduce both HDL cholesterol levels and the HDL$_2$ subfraction.

▶ This combination of oral desogestrel, .15 mg/day, with micronized 17β-estradiol, 1 mg/day, resulted in a surprising drop in HDL. The dose of the progestogen may be important in producing these undesirable effects on lipids.—W.D. Odell, M.D., Ph.D.

Long-Term Effects of Oral and Transdermal Hormone Replacement Therapies on Serum Lipid and Lipoprotein Concentrations

Whitcroft SI, Crook D, Marsh MS, Ellerington MC, Whitehead MI, Stevenson JC (King's College, London; Wynn Inst, London)
Obstet Gynecol 84:222–226, 1994   112-95-12–22

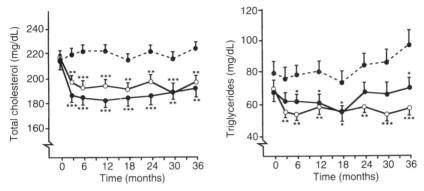

Fig 12–6.—Serum total cholesterol and triglyceride concentrations in women treated with hormone replacement therapy. Data are derived from the combined (estrogen/progestin) phase of therapy. *Vertical bars* represent means and standard errors; *dashed lines and solid circles*, reference group (*n* = 29); *solid lines and solid circles*, oral therapy (*n* = 30); *solid lines and open circles*, transdermal therapy (*n* = 31). *P < .05; **P < .01; ***P < .001: differences between treatment group and reference group by analysis of variance. (Courtesy of Whitcroft SI, Crook D, Marsh MS, et al: *Obstet Gynecol* 84:222-226, 1994.)

Objective.—A previous study has described the short-term changes in serum lipid and lipoprotein concentrations induced by postmenopausal estrogen-progestin therapy. Whether these changes are maintained in the long term was evaluated.

Study Design.—Fasting serum lipid and lipoprotein concentrations were monitored for 3 years in 61 healthy postmenopausal women who were randomly assigned to either oral or transdermal hormone replace-

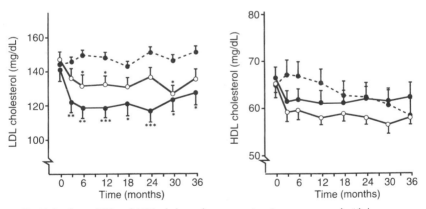

Fig 12–7.—Serum LDL and HDL cholesterol concentrations in women treated with hormone replacement therapy. Data are derived from the combined (estrogen/progestin) phase of therapy. *Vertical bars* represent means and standard errors; *dashed lines and solid circles*, reference group (*n* = 29); *solid lines and solid circles*, oral therapy (*n* = 30); *solid lines and open circles*, transdermal therapy (*n* = 31). *P < .05; **P < .01; ***P < .001: differences between treatment group and reference group by analysis of variance. (Courtesy of Whitcroft SI, Crook D, Marsh MS, et al: *Obstet Gynecol* 84:222-226, 1994.)

ment therapy. Oral therapy consisted of continuous conjugated equine estrogen, .625 mg/day, with sequential dl-norgesterel, .15 mg/day, for 12 days each cycle. Transdermal therapy consisted of patches that delivered continuous 17β-estradiol (E2), .05 mg/day, with sequential norethindrone acetate, .25 mg/day, for 14 days each cycle. The reference group included 29 healthy postmenopausal women who did not request treatment. Blood samples were obtained during the estrogen-progestin phase in hormone users.

Outcome.—Serum total cholesterol concentrations fell signficantly by 12.1% with oral therapy and by 8.4% with transdermal therapy (Fig 12-6). Decreases in LDL cholesterol concentrations largely accounted for the reduction in total cholesterol concentrations, although transdermal therapy appeared to have less effect on LDL than oral therapy (6.6% vs. 14.2%) (Fig 12-7). These changes were apparent at 3 months and were maintained for 3 years. Serum triglyceride concentrations fell by 2.5% with oral therapy and 16.4% with transdermal therapy. These changes were evident at 6 months in both groups, but they were maintained during the 3 years only by transdermal therapy. Both therapies reduced HDL cholesterol concentrations, which fell by 7.8% with oral therapy and 10.7% with transdermal therapy. These changes occurred within 3 months of therapy, and they were maintained over 3 years; likewise, HDL cholesterol fell significantly in untreated postmenopausal women in a manner similar to that seen in treated women.

Summary.—Hormone replacement therapy induces potentially beneficial changes in LDL cholesterol, total cholesterol, and triglyceride concentrations that are maintained in the long term. Both therapies also reduce HDL concentrations, contrary to common perceptions that estrogens raise HDL concentrations. It appears that changes in HDL cholesterol that are seen with current low-dose regimens are more subtle and that progestins such as levonorgestrel may increase HDL catabolism and overcome an estrogen-induced increase in HDL protein synthesis. Further studies are needed to confirm the long-term effects of hormone replacement therapy on HDL.

▶ This study used a lower dose and a shorter exposure to the progestogen, and the combination of estrogen/progestin lowered both total cholesterol and LDL cholesterol. There was also a decrease in HDL cholesterol. As with previous studies, transdermal estrogens had less of an effect on LDL cholesterol than did oral estrogens.—W.D. Odell, M.D., Ph.D.

The Effect of 25-mg Percutaneous Estradiol Implants on the Bone Mass of Postmenopausal Women
Holland EFN, Leather AT, Studd JWW (Chelsea and Westminster Hosp, Lon-

don)
Obstet Gynecol 83:43–46, 1994   112-95-12-23

Background.—All drugs should be given in the lowest dose needed to provide adequate response. The lowest available dose of percutaneous implant—25 mg of estradiol—controls the symptoms of menopause and provides a physiologic profile of circulating estrogens. The effect of this dose on bone mineral density in postmenopausal women was studied.

Methods.—Eighteen healthy postmenopausal women received implant treatment for 1 year. Before and after the year of treatment, dual energy x-ray absorptiometry was done at the lumbar spine and proximal hip, using a quantitative digital radiography densitometer. Measures of estradiol and FSH levels before and after treatment were also obtained. Changes in bone mineral density were compared with those of 18 women who did not receive this treatment.

Findings.—After 1 year, bone mineral density in the treated women increased a median of 5.7% at the lumbar spine, 3.4% at the femoral neck, and 3.4% at the hip. Bone mineral density significantly increased from baseline at all sites except the Ward triangle. The median post-treatment estradiol level was 320 pmol/L, and the median FSH level was 28 IU/L.

Conclusion.—Percutaneous 25-mg estradiol implants signficantly increased bone mineral density at the spine and hip in postmenopausal women. Postmenopausal bone loss was effectively prevented at this dose. Serial bone densitometry is needed to ensure that patients are responding appropriately to low-dose treatment.

▶ This is an effective, low-dose implant method of delivering long-term estrogen treatment to menopausal women. In women who had a uterus, cyclic oral medroxyprogesterone was added. The effects on plasma lipids were not reported.—W.D. Odell, M.D., Ph.D.

Oral Contraceptives and Risk of Breast Cancer in Women Aged 20–54 Years

Rookus MA, van Leeuwen FE, for the Netherlands Oral Contraceptives and Breast Cancer Study Group (The Netherlands Cancer Inst, Amsterdam)
Lancet 344:844–851, 1994   112-95-12-24

Background.—Many studies have investigated the relationship between oral contraceptive (OC) use and breast cancer risk. However, findings have been inconsistent. A case-control study of OC use and breast cancer risk was conducted in The Netherlands, where the percentage of women taking OCs is among the highest in the world.

Methods.—Nine hundred eighteen women with breast cancer, aged 20–54 years at diagnosis, were pair-matched by age with women who were selected randomly from municipal registries. Data on OC use were obtained from women and their prescribers and combined using standard decision rules.

Findings.—Oral contraceptive use for 12 years or more was associated with a relative risk (RR) of 1.3. This positive trend was noted in women younger than 36 years of age and in women 46–54 years of age but not in those aged 36–45 years. Compared with shorter-term use, women who used OCs for 4 years or more had a 2.1 RR of having breast cancer before 36 years of age. The risk increased in women younger than 36 years who used OCs in the longer term, beginning before they were 20 years of age. Recent use correlated with an increased risk of breast cancer in 46- to 54-year-old women.

Conclusion.—Four or more years of OC use, especially if it began before 20 years of age, is associated with a greater risk of development of breast cancer at a younger age. Limited evidence suggests that the excess risk disappears as the cohort of young OC users ages, but further research is needed to confirm this.

▶ It is important to emphasize that overall the risk of breast cancer was not increased by the use of oral contraceptives. The suggestion that the use of oral contraceptives before age 20 years and for a total of 4 or more years may be associated with a small increased risk of breast cancer at a young age is of concern.

Breast cancer is not a common disease in women younger than age 34, and in this study only 4 cases and 4 controls were identified. However, previous meta-analyses and the United Kingdom national case-control study reanalyses of 2 previous studies (Wingo et al: *Obstet Gynecol* 78:161, 1991; Paul et al: *Int J Cancer* 46:366, 1990) also indicate that use of oral contraceptives before age 20 years may increase the risk of breast cancer at an early age.—W.D. Odell, M.D., Ph.D.

Oral Contraceptive Use and Mortality During 12 Years of Follow-Up: The Nurses' Health Study
Colditz GA, for the Nurses' Health Study Research Group (Harvard Med School, Boston)
Ann Intern Med 120:821–826, 1994   112-95-12-25

Objective.—Data from a prospective cohort investigation, the Nurses' Health Study, were analyzed to determine the mortality risk in women who had used oral contraceptives at any time. The study population included 166,755 women who were 30–55 years of age when the study began in 1976 and who were followed through 1988 for a total of 1.3 million person-years.

Findings.—Deaths during the entire follow-up period totaled 2,879. Initially, 55% of the participants reported having used oral contraceptives at some time, and 5% were current users. The total mortality in women who had used oral contraceptives at any time did not differ from that of women who had never used them. Those who had ever used them had a lower risk of death from coronary heart disease, although the effect was not a significant one. There was no significant association between OC use and cancer death, including liver cancer. Women who were using oral contraceptives in 1976 had a significantly increased risk of subsequently dying of breast cancer. Total cardiovascular mortality did not differ from that in women who had never used oral contraception. There was no evident trend in risk for an increasing duration of past contraceptive use.

Conclusion.—There were no indications in this study that even long-term use of oral contraception adversely affects survival.

▶ This large study of nurses indicates that long-term oral contraceptive use is not associated with increased mortality, including death from breast cancer. Compare these findings with those of the preceding study (Abstract 112-95-12-24) by Rookus from The Netherlands.—W.D. Odell, M.D., Ph.D.

Suggested Reading

The following articles are recommended to the reader:

Groome NP, Illingworth PJ, O'Brien M, et al: Detection of dimeric inhibin throughout the human menstrual cycle by two-site enzyme immunoassay. *Clin Endocrinol* 40:717–723, 1994.

Saez JM: Leydig Cells: Endocrine, paracrine, and autocrine regulation. *Endocr Rev* 15(5):574–626, 1994.

Randall VA: Androgens and human hair growth (Review). *Clin Endocrinol* 40:439–457, 1994.

Hsueh AJW, Billig H, Tsafriri A: Ovarian follicle atresia: A hormonally controlled apoptotic process. *Endocr Rev* 15(6): 707–724, 1994.

Kyei-Mensah A, Jacobs HS: Ovarian stromal hypertrophy (Commentary). *Clin Endocrinol* 41:555–556, 1994.

Dewailly D, Robert Y, Helin I, et al: Ovarian stromal hypertrophy in hyperandrogenic women. *Clin Endocrinol* 41:557–562, 1994.

Bhasin S, Berman N, Swerdloff RS: Follicle-stimulating hormone (FSH) escape during chronic gonadotropin-releasing hormone (GnRH) agonist and testosterone treatment. *J Androl* 15(5):386–391, 1994.

Sohn MHH: Current status of penile revascularization for the treatment of male erectile dysfunction. *J Androl* 15(3):183–186, 1994.

Subject Index*

A

Abdominal
  adipocytes, adrenergic regulation of
    lipolysis during exercise in, 93: 269
  adipose tissue
    accumulation, waist circumference
      and abdominal sagittal diameter in
      estimate of, 95: 219
    morphology and metabolism of, in
      men, 94: 260
  adiposity, hormonal relationships to, in
    non–insulin-dependent diabetes, in
    elderly, 95: 73
  sagittal diameter in estimate of
    abdominal visceral adipose tissue
    accumulation, 95: 219
  surgery, GH therapy in, 94: 8
Abortion
  spontaneous
    in diabetes mellitus,
      insulin-dependent, glycemic
      thresholds for, 95: 322
    thyroid antibodies and, 94: 278
Abscess
  adrenal, as complication of adrenal
    fine-needle biopsy, 94: 157
Absorptiometry
  dual-energy x-ray
    for bone loss, age-associated, 95: 86
    for bone mass and bone density
      development in spine and femoral
      neck, in children and adolescents,
      95: 57
    for bone mineral density at lumbar
      spine and proximal femur in
      osteoporosis, 93: 157
    precision in determining bone mineral
      density and content at various sites,
      93: 156
  dual-photon, for bone mass and body
    composition in normal women,
    93: 160
  single-photon, of bone metabolism and
    bone density after partial
    gastrectomy, 93: 159
Acetazolamide
  /danazol in hormonal migraine, 93: 364
Acipimox
  in hypertriglyceridemia, 93: 340
Acquired immunodeficiency syndrome (see
    AIDS)
Acromegaly
  bromocriptine in

comparison of octreotide,
  bromocriptine, or combination of
  both, 95: 12
outcome of, 94: 12
Cushing's disease coexisting with,
  94: 24
ectopic GH-RH secretion by bronchial
  carcinoid causing, 93: 243
GH therapy and gastrointestinal
  malignancies, 95: 6
growth hormone receptor antibodies
  with GH-like activity in,
  spontaneous occurrence of, 93: 6
lanreotide in, 95: 13; 94: 14
octreotide in (see Octreotide, in
  acromegaly)
treatment
  medical, benefits vs. risks of, 95: 33
  outcome, audit of, 94: 12
tumor suppressor gene mutations and,
  94: 12
ACTH, 95: 19-21; 94: 22-26; 93: 15-23
  (See also Corticotropin)
  in blood
    hypothalamic hypophysial, 94: 2
    portal (in rat), 94: 3
  plasma, in Addison's disease diagnosis,
    94: 148
  precursor secretion in small cell lung
    cancer cell lines, effect of
    bromocriptine on, 94: 193
  receptor gene abnormalities causing
    glucocorticoid deficiency, 95: 134
  responses to CRH vs. metyrapone in
    hypopituitarism, in children, 95: 20
  -secreting bronchial carcinoids (see
    Carcinoids, ACTH-secreting)
  -secreting islet cell tumors, 95: 186
  -secreting tumors causing Cushing's
    disease, localization with
    somatostatin analogue scintigraphy,
    95: 12
  secretion
    ectopic, 95: 184–187; 94: 191–194
    pituitary, regulation during chronic
      stress, 95: 33
  stimulation, elevated plasma
    19-hydroxyandrostenedione levels
    in Cushing's disease after, 94: 140
  syndrome, ectopic
    adrenalectomy in, bilateral, 95: 132
    mineralocorticoid excess and
      inhibition of 11β-hydroxysteroid
      dehydrogenase in, 94: 129
    non–small cell, surgical management
      of, 94: 191

---

* All entries refer to the year and page number(s) for data appearing in this and previous
editions of the YEAR BOOK.

virilizing, superimposed on congenital
adrenocortical hyperplasia, 93: 187
Adrenocorticotropic
hormone (*see* ACTH)
Adrenocorticotropin (*see* Corticotropin)
Adrenomedullin
15-52, short-lived vasodilator activity in
hindlimb vascular bed (in cat),
95: 156
vasodilator activity in hindlimb vascular
bed, short-lived (in cat), 95: 156
Adrenoreceptor(s), 94: 164–165
α, venular *vs.* arteriolar smooth muscle,
sensitivity preservation during
reduced blood flow (in rat),
93: 214
α$_1$-, role in catecholamine-mediated
lymphatic constriction (in dog),
93: 216
α$_2$-
high-affinity platelet, density decrease
in elderly, 94: 74
role in catecholamine-mediated
lymphatic constriction (in dog),
93: 216
β-
blockade, effect on post-exercise
oxygen consumption, 95: 207
insulin effect on adipose tissue
metabolism in situ and, 93: 208
β$_1$-, β$_2$-, and β$_3$-, coexistence in fat cells
and differential activation by
catecholamines (in dog), 94: 167
β$_2$-, decreased expression in fat cells,
lipolytic catecholamine resistance
due to, 94: 169
cytoplasmic domains of, antagonism of
catecholamine receptor signaling by
expression of, 94: 164
Adriamycin
in adrenocortical carcinoma, advanced,
93: 194
intrahepatic, in hepatoma associated
with hypoglycemia and
overproduction of insulin-like
growth factor-II, 95: 189
in thyroid cancer, anaplastic, 95: 285
Aerobic
training, effect on 24-hour energy
expenditure, in women, 94: 212
Affective disorder
seasonal, pituitary-adrenal responses to
CRH in, 93: 167
African Americans (*see* Blacks)
Age
appendicular bone mass in older women
and, 94: 110

-associated bone loss, and weight,
95: 86
bone, initial, effect on growth hormone
therapy in Turner's syndrome,
93: 53
effect on catecholamine responses to
standing and exercise, plasma,
95: 208
growth hormone secretion and
clearance rates in boys and, 93: 44
-related changes
in cortico-releasing factor,
somatostatin, neuropeptide Y,
methionine enkephalin and
β-endorphin in specific brain areas
(in rat), 93: 66
in thyroid hormone action, 95: 93
-related decline in resting metabolic
rate, and sodium-potassium pump
activity, 94: 99
-related differences in pituitary gland
morphology on MRI, 93: 67
skin collagen changes and, 94: 79
vertebral density and, postmenopausal,
93: 81
Aging, 95: 63–93; 94: 71–101; 93: 61–93
adrenal, 95: 90–91
bone, 95: 86–90
effect of dehydroepiandrosterone on,
95: 117–118
effect of 5α-dihydrotestosterone,
testosterone, estradiol, and estrone
levels in prostatic tissue, 94: 88
effect on hormones (in rodents),
93: 62, 63
of endocrine system, biopathology of,
95: 93
growth hormone and, 94: 100
interleukin-6 production changes and
(in mice), 94: 73
mechanisms, 94: 73–75; 93: 65–67
pituitary, 95: 65–67; 94: 75–78;
93: 67–70
process, effect of vitamin E therapy on,
94: 67
thyroid, 95: 84–86; 93: 70–73
trophic factors in, 95: 93
Agitation
extreme, after crack cocaine ingestion,
95: 150
Agranulocytosis
methimazole-induced, granulocyte
colony-stimulating factor in,
95: 258
AIDS
cortisol resistance in, 93: 167
GH therapy in, 94: 8

Author Index